Professor von Zerssen
mit herzlichen Grüßen!

Andreas Marneros
Ming T. Tsuang

Bonn   30.6.1990

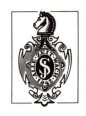

A. Marneros · M.T. Tsuang (Eds.)

Affective and Schizoaffective Disorders

Similarities and Differences

Contributors
J. Angst, P. Berner, D. Bunk, B.J. Carroll, W. Coryell,
A. Deister, C. Eggers, H.M. Emrich, H. Häfner,
K. Heinrich, H. Helmchen, K.R.R. Krishnan, W. Maier,
M. Maj, A. Marneros, T.F. McNeil, H.-J. Möller,
B. Müller-Oerlinghausen, E.S. Paykel, C. Perris, B. Pitt,
P. Propping, A. Rohde, R.-D. Stieglitz, M.T. Tsuang,
D. von Zerssen, G. Winokur, and others

Springer-Verlag Berlin Heidelberg New York
London Paris Tokyo Hong Kong

Professor Dr. med. ANDREAS MARNEROS
Psychiatrische Universitätsklinik
Sigmund-Freud-Strasse 25, 5300 Bonn 1, FRG

MING T. TSUANG, M.D., Ph.D., D.Sc.
Professor and Director of Psychiatric Epidemiology
Harvard Schools of Medicine and Public Health
Brockton/West Roxbury VA Medical Center
940 Belmont Street, Brockton, MA 02401, USA

With 34 Figures and 93 Tables

ISBN 3-540-52071-6 Springer-Verlag Berlin Heidelberg New York
ISBN 0-387-52071-6 Springer-Verlag New York Berlin Heidelberg

Library of Congress Cataloging-in-Publication Data. Affective and schizoaffective disorders:
similarities and differences / [edited by] A. Marneros, M.T. Tsuang; contributors, J. Angst . . .
[et al.]. p. cm. ISBN 0-387-52071-6 (U.S.: alk. paper) 1. Affective disorders. 2.
Schizoaffective disorders. I. Marneros, A. (Andreas). II. Tsuang, Ming T. III. Angst, Jules.
[DNLM: 1. Affective Disorders, Psychotic. 2. Psychotic Disorders. WM 207 A2562]
RC537.A29   1990 616.89'5—dc20 DNLM/DLC for Library of Congress.

© Springer-Verlag Berlin Heidelberg 1990
Printed in Germany

Typesetting: Best-set Typesetter Ltd., Hong Kong
2125/3130(3011)-543210 – Printed on acid-free paper

Preface

Several contributions in our first book about schizoaffective disorders (Marneros and Tsuang, *Schizoaffective* Psychoses, Springer-Verlag, 1986) supported the assumption that schizoaffective disorders differ in relevant ways from schizophrenic disorders. The classification of schizoaffective disorders as a subgroup of schizophrenia has also been criticized, and empirical research in clinical, genetic, therapeutic, and prognostic areas supports the idea that there are some strong similarities between schizoaffective and affective disorders. Of course, there are not only similarities between these two groups, but also differences just as there are between schizoaffective and schizophrenic disorders.

It is precisely the existence of similarities and differences between schizoaffective disorders and the other two so-called typical mental disorders, i.e., schizophrenia and affective disorders, which makes them a challenge in psychiatric research, a challenge to the traditional dichotomy in the classification of disorders which originated with Kraepelin. This challenge is certainly proving fruitful in psychiatric research. These "cases in between" may well demonstrate that separating, dividing, and limiting is not always meaningful. Sometimes it can be more meaningful to unify; to unify in the sense of building bridges between typical groups.

It is here that the assumption of a "psychotic continuum" can become relevant, and the investigation of schizoaffective disorders is of prime importance in research on a possible continuum of psychosis.

Schizoaffective disorders should not be bounced like a ping-pong ball between other groups of psychotic disorders. In this volume we have tried to describe and define what separates and what unites affective and schizoaffective disorders. The present volume also shows clearly that operational research on schizoaffective disorders has made great progress in recent years, but what we wrote in our first book remains valid: more research on this field yielding unambiguous, nondogmatic answers is still necessary.

Summer 1990

A. Marneros, Bonn, FRG
M.T. Tsuang, Boston, USA

Acknowledgements

This volume and the conference on which it is based were made possible through the generous support of Janssen GmbH, Neuss, Ciba-Geigy GmbH, Wehr/Baden, Hoffmann-La Roche AG, Grenzach-Wyhlen, Kanoldt Arzneimittel GmbH, Höchstädt/Donau, Organon GmbH, Oberschleißheim, and Boehringer Ingelheim KG, Ingelheim am Rhein. We would like to express our thanks and appreciation.

We acknowledge with gratitude the great help of Drs. A. Rohde and A. Deister in the organization of the conference and the publication of this volume.

Finally, we would like to thank Dr. Thiekötter and the staff at Springer-Verlag for their patience and expertise.

The Editors

Contents

Contents

List of Contributors

You will find the address at the beginning of the respective contribution

Angst, J. 168
Berner, P. 4
Black, D.W. 23
Bunk, D. 89
Carroll, B.J. 208
Cording, C. 33
Coryell, W. 186
Deister, A. 130, 146, 157
Eggers, C. 89
Emrich, H.M. 262
Gross, G. 168
Häfner, H. 277
Hallmayer, J. 201
Heinrich, K. 218
Helmchen, H. 53
Huber, G. 168
Jünemann, H. 146, 157
Kieffer, W. 4
Krishnan, K.R.R. 208
Lichtermann, D. 201
Maier, W. 201
Maj, M. 8
Marneros, A. 1, 130, 146, 157

McNeil, T.F. 72
Minges, J. 201
Möller, H.-J. 33, 231
Müller-Oerlinghausen, B. 251
Nasrallah, A. 23
Paykel, E.S. 107
Perris, C. 8
Pitt, B. 102
Propping, P. 195
Rayasam, K. 208
Rohde, A. 130, 146, 157
Staab, B. 146, 157
Stassen, H.H. 168
Stieglitz, R.-D. 53
Stone, M.H. 168
Tegeler, J. 218
Thies, K. 251
Tsuang, M.T. 1, 123, 274
Volk, J. 251
von Zerssen, D. 33
Winokur, G. 23
Wittchen, H.-U. 33
Zaudig, M. 33

Are the Schizoaffective Disorders a Ping-Pong Ball Between Schizophrenia and the Affective Disorders?

A. MARNEROS[1] and M.T. TSUANG[2]

In our first book on this topic (Marneros and Tsuang 1986a), we investigated the differences and similarities between the schizoaffective disorders and other atypical disorders (Marneros and Tsuang 1986b; Perris 1986; Pichot 1986; Strömgren 1986; Tsuang and Marneros 1986). Taking a historical point of view, Angst (1986) pointed out that the concept of schizoaffective disorders is not new, having clearly emerged in the work of Kahlbaum (1863), who described the "vesania typica circularis." Angst showed that the idea of schizoaffective disorder has always been present in European psychiatry but that it never achieved the prominence of Kraepelin's (1920) concept of a dichotomy. Although Kraepelin himself recognized the existence of a group between schizophrenia and the affective disorders, he considered this intermediate area to be a great weakness of his *Zweiteilungsprinzip* -- the principle of the dichotomy of psychoses.

One of the conclusions of our first workshop was that the definitions of schizoaffective disorder given by Kasanin in 1933 and subsequently by others no longer correspond to the modern operational definitions of schizoaffective disorder. Perris reported findings supporting the distinction between cycloid psychoses and the schizoaffective disorders. Pichot noted that the concept in French psychiatry of "bouffee delirante" is not identical to the modern concept of schizoaffective disorder, nor are the so-called reactive or psychogenic psychoses of Scandinavian psychiatry, described by Strömgren.

Having concluded that, despite some overlap, the schizoaffective disorders are not identical to other groups of so-called atypical disorders, we asked ourselves whether the WHO classification of the schizoaffective disorders as a subgroup of schizophrenia was completely warranted. The findings of Angst, Berner, Huber, Marneros, Meltzer, Taylor, Tsuang and Winokur (all contributions in Marneros and Tsuang 1986) raise serious questions about how certain we can be about this categorization. The authors cite differences between the schizoaffective and schizophrenic groups in terms of social and premorbid characteristics, genetic and biological data (although the latter are still extremely rare and unreliable), and most importantly, differences in course and psychopathological, psychological, and social outcome.

[1] Psychiatrische Universitätsklinik, Sigmund-Freud-Straße 25, 5300 Bonn 1, FRG
[2] Harvard Schools of Medicine and Public Health, Brockton/West Roxbury VA Medical Center, 940 Belmont Street, Brockton, MA 02401, USA

Affective and Schizoaffective Disorders
Edited by A. Marneros and M.T. Tsuang
© Springer-Verlag Berlin Heidelberg 1990

Schizoaffective Disorders: Cases-In-Between?

The differences between schizoaffective disorder and the classical group of psychotic disorders – schizophrenia and affective psychoses – support the hypothesis that schizoaffective disorder is composed of "cases-in-between" schizophrenia and affective psychoses, similar to Kurt Schneider's definition. The boundaries, however, between schizoaffective disorder and schizophrenia on the one hand and affective disorder on the other hand are fuzzy rather than clear-cut.

The concept of schizoaffective disorder as the "cases-in-between" and, more importantly, its mobile and fluid boundaries with schizophrenia and the affective disorders pose certain problems. Not only are there difficulties regarding the classification and the definition of homogeneous schizoaffective subtypes for fundamental research in genetics, biology, pharmacology, etc., but there are also difficulties for clinical practice concerning treatment and prophylaxis. In terms of nosology, considering schizoaffective disorder as the "cases-in-between" is not only a challenge to Kraepelin's *Zweiteilungsprinzip*, but also to Jaspers' hierarchical principles. If genetic, premorbid, and social features, course, and outcome can be used as criteria of diagnostic validity, then we have to reject these hierarchical principles or, perhaps, reverse them in favor of affectivity.

A point of discussion at our first workshop was whether schizoaffective disorder should be considered a variant of the affective disorders. The simplest solution is to recategorize schizoaffective disorder under "affective disorders." But is the simplest solution also the best solution? What makes us so certain about our categorical model of classification? Is it really always possible to arrange the pathological alterations of mental life (the psychopathological constellations) into clearly separate patterns? Or is it better to accept the suggestion, made repeatedly, that schizoaffective disorder could best be thought about and researched if we adopt a model of "a psychotic continuum." Whatever the range of answers to this question, we believe that Strauss' (1983) statement, characterizing the schizoaffective disorders as the "key to understanding the psychoses," is still valid.

References

Angst J (1986) the Course of Schizoaffective Disorders. In: Marneros A, Tsuang MT (eds) Schizoaffective Psychoses. Springer: Berlin Heidelberg New York London Paris Tokyo
Berner P, Lenz G (1986) Definitions of Schizoaffective Psychosis: Mutual Concordance and Relationship to Schizophrenia and Affective Disorder. In: Marneros A, Tsuang MT (eds) Schizoaffective Psychoses. Springer: Berlin Heidelberg New York London Paris Tokyo
Gross G, Huber G, Armbruster B (1986) Schizoaffective Psychoses – Long-Term Prognosis and Symptomatology. In: Marneros A, Tsuang MT (eds) Schizoaffective Psychoses. Springer: Berlin Heidelberg New York London Paris Tokyo
Kahlbaum J (1963) Die Gruppierung der psychischen Krankheiten und die Einteilung der Seelenstörungen. Kafemann, Danzig
Kasanin J (1933) The acute schizo-affective psychoses. Am J Psychiatry 13:97–126

Kraepelin E (1920) Die Erscheinungsformen des Irreseins. Z Ges Neurol Psychiatrie 62:1–29
Marneros A, Tsuang MT (eds) (1986a) Schizoaffective Psychoses. Springer: Berlin Heidelberg
    New York London Paris Tokyo
Marneros A, Tsuang MT (1986b) Schizoaffective Disorders: present Level and Future Per-
    spectives. In: Marneros A, Tsuang MT (eds) Schizoaffective Psychoses. Springer: Berlin
    Heidelberg New York London Paris Tokyo
Marneros A, Rohde A, Deister A, Risse A (1986) Schizoaffective Disorders: The Prognostic
    Value of the Affective Component. In: Marneros A, Tsuang MT (eds) Schizoaffective
    Psychoses. Springer: Berlin Heidelberg New York London Paris Tokyo
Meltzer HY (1986) Biological Studies of the Nosology of the Major Psychoses: A Status
    Report on the Schizoaffective Disorders. In: Marneros A, Tsuang MT (eds) Schizoaffec-
    tive Psychoses. Springer: Berlin Heidelberg New York London Paris Tokyo
Perris C (1986) The Case for the Independence of Cycloid Psychotic Disorder from the
    Schizoaffective Disorders. In: Marneros A, Tsuang MT (eds) Schizoaffective Psychoses.
    Springer: Berlin Heidelberg New York London Paris Tokyo
Pichot P (1986) A Comparison of Different National Concepts of Schizoaffective Psychosis.
    In: Marneros A, Tsuang MT (eds) Schizoaffective Psychoses. Springer: Berlin Heidelberg
    New York London Paris Tokyo
Strauss JS (1983) Schizo-affective disorders: "Just another illness" or key to understanding the
    psychoses? Pychiatr Clin 16:286–296
Strömgren E (1986) Reactive (Psychogenic) Psychoses and Their Relations to Schizoaffective
    Psychoses. In: Marneros A, Tsuang MT (eds) Schizoaffective Psychoses. Springer: Berlin
    Heidelberg New York London Paris Tokyo
Taylor MA (1986) The Validity of Schizoaffective Disorders: Treatment and Prevention
    Studies. In: Marneros A, Tsuang MT (eds) Schizoaffective Psychoses. Springer: Berlin
    Heidelberg New York London Paris Tokyo
Tsuang MT, Marneros A (1986) Schizoaffective Psychosis: Questions and Directions. In:
    Marneros A, Tsuang MT (eds) Schizoaffective Psychoses. Springer: Berlin Heidelberg
    New York London Paris Tokyo

What Are the Schizophrenic and the Affective Aspects of Schizoaffective Disorders?

P. Berner and W. Kieffer[1]

Concepts of schizoaffective psychoses differ extensively relative to the criteria used to define their schizophrenic and affective components (Berner and Lenz 1986). These definitions originate not only from pragmatic or empirical considerations, but to a high degrees also from theoretical reflections which must be taken into account if the conceptualization of schizoaffective disorders as a separate entity is to increase scientific insight. The hypotheses about the nature of "psychoses of uncertain origin" have, during the past decades, gradually evolved from the assumption of distinct disease entities towards vulnerability models. The question of whether different types of vulnerability give rise to schizophrenia and mood disorders, or whether the existence of schizoaffective psychoses points to a common basis for both diseases remains open however. All theoretical reflections on this subject must take into account the relationship between changes of mood and activation on the one hand and cognitive disturbances on the other. Braden (1984) reviews this problem with special reference to schizoaffective psychosis and proposes a "two-factor vulnerability model" for it: the first factor is a vulnerability to an episode of psychotic illness characterized by psychomotor and vegetative activation; the second is a vulnerability to disorganization and cognitive disturbance in response to increased activation. Braden demonstrates that this concept is more consistent with clinical observations than other assumptions (such as the separate-process or the single-process model). It postulates that "cognitive symptoms depend on the level of activation and also on preexisting central nervous system . . . deficits." The question arises, however, whether all cognitive disturbances observable in excited episodes must be attributed to the presence of the second factor, because it seems conceivable that a primary activation entails secondary modifications of certain cognitive functions. In this perspective it might be appropriate to envisage different kinds of cognitive symptoms – some may be the direct consequence of the activation, whereas others may appear because the "dynamic" dysregulation raises latent cognitive deficiencies to the level of clinical relevance. Furthermore, activation need not be the only energetic source of cognitive disturbances; the "dynamic restriction" (Janzarik 1959) occurring in depressive states may, for instance, also be accompanied by perceptual and conceptual modifications. Finally, it must be taken in to consideration that primary cognitive disturbances may provoke or facilitate secondary changes of

---

[1] Vienna University Clinic, Währinger Gürtel 18–20, 1090 Vienna, Austria

Affective and Schizoaffective Disorders
Edited by A. Marneros and M.T. Tsuang
© Springer-Verlag Berlin Heidelberg 1990

mood and energy which also may give rise to clinical features suggesting the presence of a "schizoaffective psychosis."

Broad definitions of schizoaffective psychoses have their roots in the traditional German dichotomy of endogenous psychoses, which assumes that schizophrenia is a disease that disrupts cognitive function while manic-depressive illness is a disorder of mood – or, in the terminology of more modern approaches, of the "dynamic" (Janzarik 1959). The reflections detailed above suggest that schizoaffective psychoses conceived as a combination of cognitive and dynamic disturbances may include disorders of heterogenic origin: Only some of them may fit into the "two-factor vulnerability model," whereas for others a "linked-process model" (Braden 1984) seems to be more appropriate. The latter can be applied to two different conditions: In some patients belonging to the group with mood disorders a basic process may produce activation dysregulations which trigger a second pathological process producing certain cognitive symptoms. In some schizophrenic patients, on the other hand, the basic cognitive disturbances may release dynamic changes manifesting themselves as affective symptomatology.

In order to test such hypotheses one may assume that the cognitive disturbances directly related to schizophrenic vulnerability are, at least in part, different from those related to activation dysregulations. Opinions as to which symptoms correspond to these "specific" hard-core schizophrenic cognitive disturbances diverge: Many studies suggest that formal thought disorders lie at the center of this core (Mundt and Lang 1987). Discrepencies arise, however, with respect to the question of which "reported" subjective psychotic experiences may be attributed to a supposed basic cognitive disturbance. It is frequently assumed that Schneiderian first-rank symptoms have their roots exclusively therein and must therefore be regarded as belonging to the hard-core cognitive symptomatology, whereas second-rank symptoms may result either from cognitive impairments or from perceptual disturbances brought about by "dynamic derailments." In support of the assumed causal relationship between first-rank symptoms and self-experienced basic cognitive disturbances, Klosterkötter (1988) has recently demonstrated how the former may gradually emerge from the latter: The morbid schizophrenic process disturbs the processing of information, leads to overinclusion and response interference, distorts external and internal perception, and thus provokes auto- and heteropsychic depersonalization and cenesthopathies. These "irritating" experiences are progressively "externalized," resented as alien, interpreted in reference to common and personal beliefs or "attribution styles," and finally crystallize as characteristic first-rank symptoms. Formal thought disorders are, in this perspective, supposed to originate from the same basic cognitive dysfunction as first-rank symptoms, but they are considered of less interest for the establishment of diagnosis because of the above-mentioned difficulties in recognizing them reliably. Dynamic derailments, whose frequent occurrence during the course of illness has already been mentioned in all classical descriptions of this disorder, are, in contrast, thought to be a secondary consequence of the "irritation" caused by the cognitive impairments. The affective blunting appears partially as a real deficiency resulting from severe forms of the morbid process, and partially as a protective withdrawal.

The observation that first-rank symptoms may result from cognitive primary disturbances has, however, not really devalued Janzarik's psychopathological studies. These illustrate how first-rank symptoms may be generated by dynamic derailments, because they effect an actualization of specific values: in states of expansion the positive elements of the structure are actualized, while in states of restriction the negative ones prevail, since positive values find no actualization. In states of dynamic instability, rapid changes in actualization of differently invested parts of the structure occur, whereby "ambivalently" invested elements of the value structure also rise to consciousness. Higher levels of instability lead to "delusional impressions" (feeling that one's surroundings are changed in a striking and puzzling way), delusional perceptions, illusions, and hallucinations. The rapid swings in drive, emotional resonance, and affectivity are overpowering, making one feel at their mercy; this may explain how feelings of will deprivation, alien influence, depersonalization, derealization, and ambivalence arise. Thus, dynamic instability appears to be the source of Schneider's first-rank symptoms and a part of Bleuler's basic symptoms. Janzarik's assumption that the dynamic instability may arise in abnormal mental conditions stemming from various origins creates doubts as to the specifity of these phenomena. These suspicions were also strengthened by a series of investigations (those reported by Mellor in 1982, for example). In particular, experiences with rapidly alternating "unstable" manic-depressive mixed states (Carlson and Goodwin 1973; Nunn 1979), which the school of Hamburg calls *Mischbilder* (or "mixed pictures," Mentzos 1967), and with *bouffées délirantes* (Magnan 1893) support the point of view that instability, giving rise to the aforementioned symptoms, occurs often in affective psychoses.

Janzarik, inclined to accept the concept of a unitarian psychosis, supposes that the real endogenous psychotic factor is, in fact, the propensity to dynamic instability. The manifestation of schizophrenic formal thought disorders and dynamic deficiency is, in his view, only the expression of a certain premorbid personality type which is independent of the predisposition to psychosis: These individuals are supposedly characterized by a constitutional dynamic weakness which Janet already had in mind when he coined (1889) his concept of "psychasthenia." Since the elements of the value structure are linked together by dynamic investments, persons characterized by this "forerunning deficiency" (Janzarik 1983) also have a weaker structure than others. They are therefore more prone to develop formal thought disorders which lead to structural disorganizations and these, in turn, aggravate the forerunning deficiency.

A review of the literature and the results of our own experiences suggest that the models of the Bonn school (Huber 1983, Klosterkötter 1988) and the Heidelberg school (Janzarik 1959, 1983) are valid for different groups of patients: First-rank symptoms may well arise from impaired information processing as well as from primary dynamic derailments. Thus, in our opinion, they are not suitable for distinguishing between schizophrenic and endogenous affective disorders. The Vienna school consequently relies primarily on formal thought disorders, even if their clinical recognition is often difficult, for diagnostic attribution to schizophrenia. Our model implies that different vulnerabilities lie at the root of schizophrenic and endogenous affective psychoses. If we assume what vulnerability for schizophrenia may be grasped only through the manifestation of formal thought disorders, how may we recognize vulnerability for manic-depressive illness? This question is especially difficult because changes in mood and drive also occur in schizophrenia, as mentioned above. According to our present state of knowledge, a given mood disorder may be attributed only cross-sectionally to an endogenous affective vulnerability through the presence of "biological symptoms" such as variations in biorhythms (which we do not consider simply as an expression of severity). From this point of view, true schizoaffective psychoses may be diagnosed only if the characteristic indicators of both vulnerability models are present. This, of course, applies only to research in view of the clinical difficulty in establishing formal thought disorders, and because biorhythmic variations may not manifest themselves in all phases thoughout the course of endogenous affective disorders. Seeing that specificity is far more important than sensitivity for research diagnostic purposes, we recommend that further investigations into schizoaffective psychoses take the proposed strict definitions for the schizophrenic and affective components into account.

References

Berner P (1977) Psychiatrische Systematik. Huber, Berlin

Berner P, Lenz G (1986) Definitions of schizoaffective psychosis: mutual concordance and relationship to schizophrenia and affective disorder. In: Marneros A, Tsuang MT (eds) Springer, Berlin Heidelberg New York Tokyo

Braden W (1984) Vulnerability and schizoaffective psychosis: a two-factor model. Schizophr Bull 10 (1):71–86

Carlson GA, Goodwin FK (1973) The stages of mania. A longitudinal analysis of the manic episode. Arch Gen Psychiatry 28:221–228

Huber G (1983) Das Konzept substratnaher Basissymptome und seine Bedeutung für Theorie und Therapie schizophrener Erkrankungen. Nervenarzt 54:23–32

Janet P (1889) L'automatisme psychologique. Essai de psychologie experimentelle sur les formes inférieures de l'activité humaine. Alcan, Paris

Janzarik W (1959) Dynamische Grundkonstellationen in endogenen Psychosen. Springer, Berlin Göttingen Heidelberg

Janzarik W (1983) Basisstörungen. Eine Revision mit struktur-dynamischen Mitteln. Nervenarzt 54:122–130

Kosterkötter J (1988) Basissymptome une Endphänomene der Schizophrenie. Springer, Berlin Heidelberg New York Tokyo

Magnan V (1893) Leçons cliniques, 2nd edn. Bataille, Paris

Mellor CS (1982) The present status of first-rank symptoms. Br J Psychiatry 140:423

Mentzos S (1967) Mischzustände und mischbildhafte phasische Psychosen. Enke, Stuttgart

Mundt CH, Lang H (1987) Die Psychopathologie der Schizophrenien. In: Kisker KP et al. (eds) Psychiatrie der Gegenwart, vol 4. Springer, Berlin Heidelberg New York Tokyo

Nunn CMH (1979) Mixed affective states and natural history of manic depressive psychosis. Br J Psychiatry 134:153–160

Definition and Classification of Schizoaffective Disorders Based on Long-Term Course

M. Maj[1] and C. Perris[2]

Introduction

The current conceptualization of schizoaffective disorders is fairly well synthesized by the definition proposed in the latest draft of the ICD-10 (World Health Organization 1989): "These are episodic disorders in which affective and schizophrenic symptoms are both prominent and present simultaneously."

Indeed, several sets of diagnostic criteria for these conditions have been provided during the past 15 years (Welner et al. 1974; Spitzer et al. 1975; Kendell 1986; American Psychiatric Association 1987). These criteria differ with respect to the number and nature of the affective and "schizophrenic" symptoms whose presence is required, or to the temporal relationship which is demanded between the occurrence of the affective and the "schizophrenic" symptoms. It must be recognized, however, that all of them consistently reflect an approach to the definition of schizoaffective disorders which is essentially cross-sectional.

Defined as above, schizoaffective disorders have been the subject of a considerable controversy during the past few decades. At least five different hypotheses about their nature have been put forward: (a) that they are always variants of schizophrenia; (b) that they are always variants of major affective disorders; (c) that they represent a "third psychosis", different from both schizophrenia and major affective disorders; (d) that they find their place in the intermediate position of a "continuum" whose poles are represented by the typical forms of schizophrenia and manic-depressive illness; (e) that they result from the simultaneous occurrence of a "true" schizophrenia and a "true" major affective disorder in the same patient, as a fortuitous event.

The last of these hypotheses is clearly not acceptable, since it would predict an annual incidence of schizoaffective disorders of about 2 per 10^8, compared with the observed incidence of 2 per 10^5 (Brockington and Meltzer 1983). It remains possible, however, that the association of a "true" schizophrenia and a "true" major affective disorder, rather than occurring by chance, is produced by an etiological factor which simultaneously activates the biological and/or psychological mechanisms responsible for the two syndromes.

---

[1] Department of Psychiatry, First Medical School, University of Naples, Piazza Miraglia 2, 80138 Napoli, Italy
[2] Department of Psychiatry, University of Umeå, 90185 Umeå, Sweden

Affective and Schizoaffective Disorders
Edited by A. Marneros and M.T. Tsuang
© Springer-Verlag Berlin Heidelberg 1990

Of the remaining four hypotheses, the first two are consistent with the Kraepelinian "binary" or "dichotomous" paradigm (according to which there are only two functional psychoses, and "mixed" psychotic syndromes can be only variants of either of them), whereas the third and the fourth contradict this paradigm (the former because it acknowledges the existence of a "third" psychosis, the latter because it questions the existence of a "discontinuity" between the two major psychoses and therefore revives, in practice, the concept of a "unitary" psychosis, repeatedly put forward during the nineteenth century).

The hypothesis that schizoaffective disorders are always variants of schizophrenia is disproved by currently available family studies, most of which show that the prevalence of schizophrenia in first-degree relatives of schizoaffective patients is clearly lower than in the relatives of schizophrenics (for a review, see Maj and Kemali 1987). On the other hand, outcome studies document that at least schizodepressive disorders cannot be interpreted in every case as variants of major affective disorders (Brockington et al. 1980a; Maj 1985). Furthermore, even the idea that schizoaffective disorders are variants sometimes of schizophrenia and sometimes of major affective disorders is not supported by the results of a recent family study (Maj 1989), suggesting that some schizoaffective forms escape the Kraepelinian binary paradigm.

The "continuum" hypothesis is not directly disproved by empirical studies, but it appears inconsistent with the finding of a low morbid risk for each of the major psychoses in the first-degree relatives of patients suffering from the other. Moreover, as pointed out by Shenton et al. (1987), if the "continuum" model were valid, the prevalence of schizoaffective disorders (that lie midway in the continuum) should be higher than that of both schizophrenia and major affective disorders, and not largely lower, as it is in fact.

The idea that schizoaffective disorders represent a "third psychosis" is inconsistent with the results of family studies, which show that a homotypical heredity taint is very rare in schizoaffective patients. It is important to stress, in this connection, that several empirical data have recently supported the independence from schizoaffective disorders, as currently defined, of the condition known as cycloid psychosis (Brockington et al. 1982; Perris 1986; Maj 1988). This last disorder has been regarded as an at least provisionally distinct diagnostic entity, on the basis of the reported familial consistency of its pattern and of the relative consistency among patients concerning course and outcome (Perris 1988). Research findings regarding cycloid psychotic disorder, however, should be considered not relevant to the issue of the nosological nature of schizoaffective disorders.

Thus, none of the above-mentioned hypotheses on the nature of schizoaffective disorders is supported by the available empirical evidence. What empirical studies seem to show, instead, is that such disorders represent a heterogeneous group of syndromes. In order to deal with this heterogeneity, a multiaxial approach, taking into account not only the cross-sectional symptomatology but also the long-term course, has been repeatedly invoked (Maj and Perris 1985; Levinson and Levitt 1987; Samson et al. 1988). A careful assessment of long-term course, in fact, is likely to provide a clue to the identification of more homogeneous subtypes of schizoaffective disorders and to a better understanding of their nature and their relationship to the major psychoses.

Surprisingly enough, however, only little attention has been paid in all these years to the long-term course of the disorders defined cross-sectionally as schizoaffective. As pointed out by Angst (1986), longitudinal studies have usually focused on the onset and the outcome of these conditions, disregarding what happens in between, that is, "the whole gestalt of the course over lifetime."

The present paper deals just with the definition and classification of schizoaffective disorders on the basis of long-term course. It includes a brief review of the relevant literature and presents the results of a study carried out in Naples.

Review of the Literature

Looking at schizoaffective disorders from a longitudinal viewpoint, a preliminary distinction should be drawn between the usually described "concurrent" forms, in which affective and "schizophrenic" symptoms appear in the same episode, and the less frequently recognized "sequential" forms, in which an affective and a schizophrenic syndrome occur in different episodes (Angst 1966; Maj and Perris 1985).

The possibility of a transition from a manic-depressive to a schizophrenic syndrome or vice versa, not accounted for by diagnostic error or by change in psychiatrists' diagnostic habits, has been repeatedly reported (see Maj and Perris 1985 and Angst 1986 for reviews), although the frequency of this shift has been variously estimated, mainly due to differences in the observation time and in the adopted diagnostic criteria (Angst 1986). For instance, Lewis and Piotrowski (1954) reported that 54% of a sample of patients defined as manic-depressive developed a clear-cut schizophrenic syndrome after 3–20 years, and the 2-year follow-up study by the World Health Organization (1979) found that 16% of patients diagnosed as schizophrenic who relapsed during the follow-up period experienced affective episodes, whereas Clark and Mallett (1963), in their 3-year follow-up study, found that progression from depression to schizophrenia occurred in 6% of cases and the reverse in no case.

The relationship between "sequential" and "concurrent" schizoaffective disorders has also been differently interpreted. Marneros et al. (1988) maintained that "the diagnostic value of the sequential schizoaffective symptomatology is equal to that of the concurrent symptomatology," and included patients suffering from either condition in a same sample. On the contrary, the latest draft of the ICD-10 (World Health Organization 1989) states that the term schizoaffective disorder "should not be applied to patients who exhibit schizophrenic symptoms and affective symptoms only in different episodes of illness." It is useful, in this connection, to emphasize that, according to Strauss (1983), "some patients with schizophrenia and major affective disorders go through a 'schizoaffective period' on the way to developing the clinical picture of the other disorder," which means that "concurrent" schizoaffective disorders may sometimes represent an intermediate stage within the course of the "sequential" ones.

As regards "concurrent" schizoaffective disorders, an assessment of long-term course can be found in the papers by Angst et al. (1980), Brockington et al. (1980a,b), Rzewuska and Angst (1982a,b), Maj (1985), and Marneros et al. (1986, 1988). All these studies consistently report that the course of these conditions is marked by an extreme variability of the clinical picture from one episode to another, which represents an important difference with respect to "pure" major affective disorders, in which interepisodic variability is much lower. For instance, in their follow-up investigation covering 14–17 years (at least five of them prospectively), Rzewuska and Angst (1982b) found that in patients with a diagnosis of bipolar affective disorder, 98.5% of the episodes were either manic or depressive, whereas in patients defined as schizoaffective, 54.6% of the episodes were schizoaffective, 34% affective, and 4.6% schizophrenic. The predominance of mixed episodes within the course of schizoaffective disorders has been confirmed by all the authors, who also agreed on the fact that "pure" schizophrenic episodes are the least common.

Bipolarity of course in schizoaffective disorders has been reported to be frequent (58% of cases according to Angst et al. 1980; 49.3% according to Marneros et al. 1988). An independent assessment of the course in patients defined cross-sectionally as either schizomanic or schizodepressive was performed by Brockington et al. (1980a,b) and Maj (1985): they both found that the most frequent pattern of course in schizomanics is bipolar (occurrence of schizomanic and pure depressive episodes), whereas in schizodepressives it is not bipolar (recurrent schizodepressive episodes), although the possibility of a unipolar recurrent schizomanic disorder was recognized. A bipolar course seems to be a predictor of a favorable outcome, both in schizomanics (Maj 1985) and in schizodepressives (Maj et al. 1987), and the same appears to be true for the occurrence of "pure" melancholic episodes in addition to the schizoaffective ones (Marneros et al. 1986). The favorable prognostic significance of the appearance of "pure" affective episodes was also reported by Clayton (1982), who, referring to data collected by Shopsin (1979), stated that schizoaffective patients frequently report an episode of pure affective illness without schizophrenic features in the past, and that this occurrence "should predict a more treatable condition and a better prognosis."

The characteristics of interepisodic intervals in schizoaffective disorders have rarely been explored. Rzewuska and Angst (1982b) reported that the presence of a residual symptomatology during the intervals is equally frequent among schizoaffectives (43.6%) and bipolars (42.5%), but that while in bipolars the most frequent symptom is dysphoria, followed by affective symptoms and hypochondriasis, in schizoaffectives the most prominent symptom is "disturbed contact" (48% of cases). Maj (1985), on the other hand, found that the mean scores on the items "lack of appropriate emotion" and "withdrawal" of the Comprehensive Psychopathological Rating Scale (CPRS) during interepisodic periods were significantly higher in schizodepressives than in "pure" depressives, whereas the mean scores on the items "hypochondriasis" and "lassitude" were significantly higher in the latter group. Finally, both Brockington et al. (1980a) and Maj et al. (1987) observed that the onset of the index episode against a background of previous schizophrenic symptoms is a predictor of a poor outcome in schizodepressive patients.

On the whole, the above-mentioned studies clearly show that patients defined cross-sectionally as being schizoaffective turn out to represent a very heterogeneous group when they are followed up longitudinally. Bipolarity of course and previous occurrence of "pure" affective episodes (two features which frequently coexist) seem to characterize schizoaffective forms with a long-term outcome similar to "pure" affective disorders, whereas the onset of schizoaffective episodes against the background of a residual schizophrenic symptomatology appears to be associated with a poor outcome. These two extreme patterns of course, already recognized by Schneider (1973), correspond to the affective subtype (recurrent) and the schizophrenic subtype (continuous with exacerbations) identified by Maj and Perris (1985) on the axis 2 (course) of their multiaxial classification of schizoaffective disorders. Whether further subtypes of these disorders can be singled out on the basis of long-term course remains an open research topic, which has been approached in the Naples study, presented in the following section.

The Naples Study

Subjects and Methods

The study was carried out in two samples of patients: "schizoaffectives" and "affectives". The schizoaffective sample consisted of 72 patients who were referred to the Center for the Prevention and Treatment of Affective Disorders at the First Psychiatric Department of Naples University during the period from January 1, 1979, to December 31, 1985; who fulfilled, on the occasion of their first visit at the Center, cross-sectional Research Diagnostic Criteria (RDC, Spitzer et al. 1975) for schizoaffective disorder; and who could be examined prospectively for at least 3 years and on the whole (that is, considering retrospective and prospective assessment) for at least 10 years. The sample included 33 men and 39 women with an age ranging, at the time of the first visit at the Center, from 20 to 51 years (mean ± SD 35.7 ± 7.0). Cross-sectional RDC diagnosis was schizoaffective disorder, manic type, in 29 of them and schizoaffective disorder, depressed type, in 43. The affective sample consisted of the first 29 patients with a cross-sectional RDC diagnosis of manic disorder and the first 43 patients with an RDC diagnosis of major depressive disorder referred to the Center since January 1, 1979, who could be examined prospectively for at least 3 years and on the whole for at least 10 years. They were 30 men and 42 women with an age ranging from 26 to 55 years (mean ± SD 41.0 ± 7.1). The duration of the observation period ranged from 10 to 28 years (mean ± SD 14.5

± 12.0) in the schizoaffective group, and from 10 to 30 years (mean ± SD 16.1 ± 13.6) in the affective one.

For each patient, retrospective assessment was made on the occasion of the first visit at the Center. The patient was interviewed by means of the Schedule for Affective Disorders and Schizophrenia (SADS, Endicott and Spitzer 1978). The interview was supplemented by the collection of all available information from relatives and medical records. Previous morbid episodes were classified, when possible, according to the RDC. Prospective evaluation was performed by interviewing the patient monthly or bimonthly and assessing his or her psycho-pathological state by CPRS (Åsberg et al. 1978). New morbid episodes were recorded and classified according to the RDC. Interepisodic symptoms were also recorded: they were defined as the symptoms occurring during the periods in which the patient did not fulfill the RDC for any psychiatric disorder (excluding the last visit before and the first visit after an episode). At the end of the follow-up period, the psychopathological and psychosocial outcome were evaluated in each patient by means of the Strauss-Carpenter Outcome Scale (Strauss and Carpenter 1972) and the Disability Assessment Schedule (Jablensky et al. 1980). On the basis of the score in section 5 ("global evaluation of social adjustment") of the DAS, the psychosocial outcome was rated as good (score of 1 or 2), intermediate (score of 3), or poor (score of 4, 5, or 6).

Results

The morbid episodes recorded during the observation period in patients defined cross-sectionally as being either schizoaffective or affective are summarized in Table 1. In patients diagnosed as schizoaffective, 48.5% of the episodes were schizoaffective, 30.9% affective, and 12.7% schizophrenic. Three percent of the episodes could not be classified according to the RDC (mostly because the number of affective symptoms was not sufficient to fulfill criterion B for a schizoaffective disorder), whereas for 4.8% of the episodes information was not

Table 1. Episodes recorded during the observation period in patients defined cross-sectionally as being either schizoaffective or affective

Type of episode (according to RDC)	Schizoaffectives		Affectives	
	No. of episodes	%	No. of episodes	%
Manic	34	10.3	130	34.9
Major depressive	68	20.6	201	54.0
Schizomanic	58	17.6	9	2.4
Schizodepressive	102	30.9	15	4.0
Schizophrenic	42	12.7	4	1.1
Other	10	3.0	7	1.9
Not classifiable	16	4.8	6	1.6

Table 2. Some characteristics of the course in patients defined cross-sectionally as being either schizoaffective or affective

Variable	No. of schizoaffectives (%)	No. of affectives (%)
Occurrence of pure affective episodes	26 (36.1)**	72 (100)
Occurrence of pure schizophrenic episodes	15 (20.8)**	2 (2.8)
Occurrence of schizo-affective episodes	72 (100)**	10 (13.9)
Occurrence of both pure affective and pure schizophrenic episodes	2 (2.8)	2 (2.8)
Bipolarity of course	22 (30.5)*	42 (58.3)
Polymorphism of course	43 (59.7)**	12 (16.7)
Occurrence of a single episode	6 (8.3)	5 (6.9)

Significant differences between patients defined as being schizoaffective or affective: $*P <$ 0.01, $**P < 0.001$.

sufficient to allow classification. In patients diagnosed as affective, 54% of the episodes were depressive, 34.9% were manic, 6.4% were schizoaffective, and 1.1% were schizophrenic; 1.9% did not fulfill criteria for any RDC category and 1.6% could not be classified due to the lack of sufficient information.

Table 2 shows that a course definable as "polymorphous" (that is, charact-erized by the occurrence of at least two types of episodes among the following: schizoaffective, affective, schizophrenic, and other) was observed in 59.7% of the patients defined cross-sectionally as being schizoaffective and in 16.7% of those defined cross-sectionally as being affective. This difference is statistically significant ($\chi^2 = 26.475$, df $= 1$, $P < 0.001$). Another significant difference concerned the frequency of a bipolar course (that is, a course marked by the appearance of both manic or schizomanic and depressive or schizodepressive episodes), which was observed in 58.3% of patients defined as affective and 30.5% of those defined as schizoaffective ($\chi^2 = 10.153$, df $= 1$, $P < 0.01$). Of course, the occurrence of pure affective episodes was significantly more frequent in patients diagnosed as affective, and that of schizoaffective and pure schizo-phrenic episodes in those diagnosed as schizoaffective. The occurrence, in independent episodes, of a pure affective and a pure schizophrenic syndrome (sequential schizoaffective disorder) was detected in two patients defined cross-sectionally as being schizoaffective and in two of those defined as being affective. In all these cases, the affective syndrome preceded the schizophrenic one. In six patients diagnosed as schizoaffective and in five of those diagnosed as affective the index episode was the only one which occurred during the observation period.

The patterns of course which could be identified in patients defined cross-sectionally as being schizoaffective are summarized in Table 3. The most fre-

Table 3. Patterns of course in patients defined cross-sectionally as being schizoaffective

Pattern of course	No. of patients (%)
A – Occurrence of schizomanic and depressive or of schizomanic, manic, and depressive episodes	20 (27.8)
B – Occurrence of schizodepressive episodes only	15 (20.8)
C – Occurrence of schizodepressive and schizophrenic episodes	11 (15.3)
D – Occurrence of schizomanic episodes only	6 (8.3)
E – Single schizoaffective episode	6 (8.3)
F – Occurrence of schizodepressive and depressive episodes	4 (5.5)
G – Occurrence of schizoaffective episodes and of 'mixed' episodes not fulfilling the RDC for schizoaffective disorder	4 (5.5)
H – Occurrence of schizomanic and schizophrenic episodes	2 (2.8)
I – Occurrence of schizomanic and schizodepressive episodes	2 (2.8)
J – Occurrence of affective, schizoaffective, and schizophrenic episodes	2 (2.8)

quent pattern was that characterized by a bipolar course with the appearance of schizomanic and pure depressive or of schizomanic, pure manic, and pure depressive episodes (27.8% of cases), followed by that marked by the occurrence of schizodepressive episodes only (20.8%) and by that characterized by the occurrence of schizodepressive and pure schizophrenic episodes (15.3%). In two cases, one or more schizoaffective episodes characterized the intermediate stage of the development of a sequential schizoaffective disorder (occurrence of pure affective episodes, followed by schizoaffective and pure schizophrenic ones).

Table 4 shows the depressive, manic, and "schizophrenic" CPRS items (from the list proposed by Maj and Perris 1985) which were the most frequently rated during the interepisodic periods in patients defined cross-sectionally as being schizoaffective. Four items were rated in at least six visits in more than one quarter of the patients: "reduced sleep," "reduced appetite," "lassitude," and "concentration difficulties." Only two "schizophrenic" items, that is "withdrawal" and "lack of appropriate emotion," were rated in at least ten patients. Six of the 11 patients presenting "withdrawal" and five of the ten patients presenting "lack of appropriate emotion" showed the pattern of course indicated as C in Table 3 (occurrence of schizodepressive and pure schizophrenic episodes).

At the end of the follow-up period, the mean global score on the Strauss-Carpenter Outcome Scale was found to be significantly lower in patients defined cross-sectionally as being schizoaffective than in those defined as being affective (12.1 $\pm$ 3.0 vs. 13.5 $\pm$ 2.5, $t = 3.05$, $P < 0.01$). As shown in Table 5, among the patients defined cross-sectionally as being schizoaffective, those with a unipolar schizoaffective course (patterns B and D of Table 3) and those with a course characterized by schizoaffective and pure schizophrenic episodes (patterns C

Table 4. Most frequent interepisodic symptoms in patients defined cross-sectionally as being schizoaffective

CPRS item	No. of patients in whom the item was rated in at least six visits (%)
Reduced sleep	30 (41.7)
Reduced appetite	26 (36.1)
Lassitude	25 (34.7)
Concentration difficulties	21 (29.2)
Inability to feel	16 (22.2)
Failing memory	13 (18.0)
Withdrawal	11 (15.3)
Pessimistic thoughts	11 (15.3)
Lack of appropriate emotion	10 (13.9)
Agitation	10 (13.9)

Table 5. Mean global score on Strauss-Carpenter Outcome Scale at the end of follow-up in patients defined cross-sectionally as being either schizoaffective (subdivided on the basis of pattern of course, see Table 3) or affective

Patients	No.	Global score on Strauss-Carpenter Outcome Scale (mean ± SD)
Schizoaffectives	72	$12.1 \pm 3.0^{**}$
Pattern of course A	20	13.0 ± 3.0
Patterns of course B+D	21	$12.0 \pm 2.5^*$
Patterns of course C+H	13	$11.4 \pm 3.5^*$
Pattern of course E	6	12.9 ± 2.1
Affectives	72	13.5 ± 2.5

Significant differences with respect to patients defined as being affective: $^*P < 0.02$, $^{**}P < 0.01$.

and H) also had a significantly poorer psychopathological outcome than patients defined cross-sectionally as being affective, whereas patients with a bipolar course marked by the presence of pure affective episodes (pattern A) and those with a single schizoaffective episode (pattern E) had a psychopathological outcome not different from affective patients.

The psychosocial outcome of patients defined cross-sectionally as being schizoaffective was good in 38 cases (52.7%), intermediate in 25 (34.7%), and poor in nine (12.5%). The corresponding figures in patients defined cross-sectionally as being affective were 57 (79.2%), 11 (15.3%), and four (5.5%), the difference being statistically significant ($\chi^2 = 11.165$, df $= 2$, $P < 0.01$). The psychosocial outcome in the different schizoaffective subtypes identified on the basis of the pattern of course is shown in Table 6. In patients whose course was

Table 6. Psychosocial outcome at the end of follow-up in subgroups of patients defined cross-sectionally as being schizoaffective, identified on the basis of pattern of course (see Table 3)

Pattern of course	No. of patients	Psychosocial outcome		
		Good	Intermediate	Poor
A	20	15	4	1
B	15	7	6	2
C	11	3	4	4
D	6	3	3	0
E	6	4	2	0
F	4	2	2	0
G	4	3	1	0
H	2	1	0	1
I	2	0	2	0
J	2	0	1	1

bipolar with pure affective episodes (pattern A) the psychosocial outcome was not different from affective patients, whereas in those with a unipolar schizoaffective course (patterns B and D) or with schizoaffective and pure schizophrenic episodes (patterns C and H) it was significantly poorer than in affectives ($\chi^2 = 8.392$, df = 2, $P < 0.02$ and $\chi^2 = 11.631$, df = 2, $P < 0.01$, respectively).

Discussion

The Naples study supports some of the findings obtained in the few previous longitudinal investigations of schizoaffective disorders and provides some new evidence in favor of the usefulness of the assessment of long-term course as a basis for a meaningful classification of patients defined cross-sectionally as being schizoaffective. In line with previous studies (Angst et al. 1980; Brockington et al. 1980a,b; Rzewuska and Angst 1982a,b; Marneros et al. 1986, 1988), it shows that the conditions defined as schizoaffective according to cross-sectional criteria turn out to be very heterogeneous when studied longitudinally, and that a polymorphous course (that it, a course marked by the occurrence of at least two different types of episodes among the following: schizoaffective, affective, schizophrenic, and other) is significantly more frequent in these conditions than in major affective disorders. In the course of the disorders diagnosed cross-sectionally as schizoaffective, schizoaffective episodes are confirmed to be the most frequent, followed by pure affective and pure schizophrenic ones. Bipolarity is confirmed to be common, although the percentage of bipolar cases observed in the Naples study is lower than that reported in some previous investigations (such as those by Angst et al. 1980 and Marneros et al. 1988): this is probably due in part to a definition of bipolarity requiring the occurrence of

both manic or schizomanic and depressive or schizodepressive episodes, whereas
(contrary to some previous studies) a course characterized by schizomanic
episodes only is not defined as bipolar. Finally, it is confirmed that the transition
from a pure affective to a pure schizophrenic syndrome is possible, although
rare, so that sequential schizoaffective disorder should be regarded as a meaningful diagnostic construct.

The Naples study supports the observation (Brockington et al. 1980b; Clayton 1982) that a frequent pattern of course in patients defined cross-sectionally as
being schizomanic is the bipolar one with the occurrence of schizomanic and
pure depressive or of schizomanic, pure manic, and pure depressive episodes. In
these forms, intervals between the episodes are usually free from a residual
schizophrenic symptomatology (although residual affective symptoms may be
present), and the outcome is not different from that of pure major affective
disorders. In some patients of this group, schizomanic episodes are only a
sporadic occurrence within a course dominated by pure affective episodes: in
these cases, schizomanic attacks tend to be more frequent in the earlier years of
the illness, which is in line with the view expressed by several authors (Carlson
and Strober 1978; Dunner and Rosenthal 1979; Ballenger et al. 1982; Rosen
et al. 1983; Joyce 1984) that manic episodes of the young frequently show mood-
incongruent psychotic features. Analogous to this first pattern of course may be
that characterized by the occurrence of schizodepressive and pure depressive
episodes: in the Naples study, this type of course was observed in only four
patients, who did not show any residual schizophrenic symptomatology between
the episodes and had a good or intermediate psychosocial outcome. The two patterns of course mentioned above correspond to the affective subtype (recurrent)
identified by Maj and Perris (1985) on the axis 2 (course) of their multiaxial
classification of schizoaffective disorders.

The other extreme pattern of course whose existence is also confirmed by
the Naples study is that marked by the appearance of schizodepressive and pure
schizophrenic episodes. In this subtype of schizoaffective disorder, already
recognized by Brockington et al. (1980a) and Maj et al. (1987), the frequency of
interepisodic residual schizophrenic symptoms is high (54.5% of patients presented the symptom "withdrawal" and 45.4% the symptom "lack of appropriate
emotion" in at least six visits), and the outcome is significantly poorer than that
of major affective disorders, from both the psychopathological and the psychosocial viewpoint. The literature on "depression in schizophrenia" and its
multiple determinants (Knights and Hirsch 1981; Galdi 1983) may be relevant
in this context. On the other hand, it should be stressed that the distinction
between depressive symptoms and the "negative" symptomatology of schizophrenia may sometimes be difficult (Kulhara et al. 1989), so that a proportion of
patients of this subgroup may be schizophrenics with prominent negative
symptoms, either primary or secondary to psychotic experiences or neuroleptic
treatment (Carpenter et al. 1985). In any case, this pattern of course corresponds to the schizophrenic subtype (continuous with exacerbations) identified
by Maj and Perris (1985) on the axis 2 of their classification. Whether the rare
cases (two in the Naples study) in which the course is characterized by schizo-

manic and pure schizophrenic episodes should be interpreted in the same way remains to be established.

The Naples study confirms that schizoaffective disorders with a "monomorphous" course (that is, those characterized by schizoaffective episodes only) are not uncommon. The most frequent pattern is that marked by the occurrence of multiple schizodepressive episodes, whereas the occurrence of multiple schizomanic episodes is much less common, and the bipolar course with schizodepressive and schizomanic episodes is very rare. The interpretation of these patterns remains problematic. Nevertheless, the outcome of these forms is clearly poorer in comparison not only with pure major affective disorders but also with the conditions in which schizoaffective episodes alternate with pure affective ones. Recurrent schizodepressive disorders may partially overlap with "delusional depressions" repeatedly described in the literature (Kantor and Glassman 1977; Charney and Nelson 1981; Price et al. 1984), although it should be specified that delusions may not be the only psychotic symptoms in schizodepressive patients. Some cases of this subgroup may also be the result of the superimposition of a manic or depressive syndrome on the substrate of a schizotypal personality, characterized by peculiarities and oddities of ideation, perception, and behavior, whose presence during the acute episodes may prompt a diagnosis of schizoaffective disorder, and whose persistence after recovery may be interpreted as a residual schizophrenic symptomatology. On the other hand, as pointed out by Akiskal and Puzantian (1979), a diagnosis of schizoaffective disorder may sometimes be made even if a major affective disorder occurs in a subject with an introverted personality, marked by a restricted range of affect, a tendency to social withdrawal, and a deficit of social skills. Also in this case, the patient, upon recovery, reintegrates into his introverted and socially restricted adjustment, which may be mistaken for a psychopathological residuum.

A relatively infrequent pattern of course identified in the Naples study is that characterized by the occurrence of schizoaffective episodes and of "mixed" episodes not fulfilling the RDC for schizoaffective disorder (mostly because the number of affective symptoms is not suffucent to meet criterion B). This pattern may pertain to the borderline between schizoaffective and cycloid disorders. According to the diagnostic criteria provided by Perris and Brockington (1981), cycloid episodes are marked by "mood swings not so pronounced as to justify a diagnosis of affective disorder," in addition to mood-incongruent delusions and/ or hallucinations and perplexity or puzzlement. Although these episodes tend to recur with the same characteristics in a given patient, it has been documented (Maj 1988) that cycloid episodes may occur in patients defined cross-sectionally as being schizoaffective, and that schizoaffective episodes may be recorded in patients diagnosed cross-sectionally as cycloid.

Finally, a very rare pattern of course is that marked by the appearance of pure affective, schizoaffective, and pure schizophrenic episodes. In these cases, one or more schizoaffective episodes may represent the intermediate stage of the evolution of a sequential schizoaffective disorder (or, in other terms, a concurrent schizoaffective disorder may be part of the development of a sequential one). The possible occurrence of this pattern was already recognized by Strauss

(1983) but has never, to our knowledge, been demonstrated in a longitudinal study.

Of course, it cannot be excluded that the results of the Naples study have been conditioned by the short duration of the observation period and by the relatively small size of the patient sample. In particular, the former factor may have biased the patterns of course identified in the study, while the latter may have produced an over- or underestimation of the frequency of the various patterns. Moreover, as always in research concerning schizoaffective disorders, hidden selection factors may have been at work in patients' recruitment (for instance, the fact that the unit in which patients were recruited is designed for prevention and treatment of affective disorders may have produced a bias in favor of the subtypes of schizoaffective syndromes with a predominant affective component).

In any case, the results of the study confirm that a careful assessment of long-term course in patients defined cross-sectionally as being schizoaffective can provide a clue to the identification of more homogeneous subtypes of schizoaffective disorders. They suggest that the currently predominant cross-sectional approach to the diagnosis and classification of these conditions may be inadequate, and that future diagnostic criteria should pay more attention to the variable represented by the course of the illness.

References

Akiskal HS, Puzantian VR (1979) Psychotic forms of depression and mania. Psychiatr Clin North Am 2:419–439

American Psychiatric Association (1987) Diagnostic and statistical manual of mental disorders, 3rd edn/revised. American Psychiatric Association, Washington DC

Angst J (1966) Zur Aetiologie und Nosologie endogener depressiver Psychosen. Eine genetische, soziologische und klinische Studie. Springer, Berlin Heidelberg New York

Angst J (1986) The course of schizoaffective disorders. In: Marneros A, Tsuang MT (eds) Schizoaffective psychoses. Springer, Berlin Heidelberg New York Tokyo, pp 63–93

Angst J, Felder W, Lohmeyer B (1980) Course of schizo-affective psychoses: results of a follow-up study. Schizophr Bull 6:579–585

Åsberg M, Perris C, Schalling O, Sedvall G (1978) The CPRS – applications of a psychiatric rating scale. Acta Psychiatr Scand [Suppl] 271:1–69

Ballenger JC, Reus VI, Post RM (1982) The 'atypical' clinical picture of adolescent mania. Am J Psychiatry 139:602–606

Brockington IF, Meltzer HY (1983) The nosology of schizoaffective psychosis. Psychiatr Dev 4:317–338

Brockington IF, Kendell RE, Wainwright S (1980a) Depressed patients with schizophrenic or paranoid symptoms. Psychol Med 10:665–675

Brockington IF, Wainwright S, Kendell RE (1980b) Manic patients with schizophrenic or paranoid symptoms. Psychol Med 10:73–83

Brockington IF, Perris C, Kendell RE, Hillier VE, Wainwright S (1982) The course and outcome of cycloid psychosis. Psychol Med 12:97–105

Carlson GA, Strober M (1978) Manic-depressive illness in early adolescence. J Am Acad Child Adolesc Psychiatry 17:138–153

Carpenter WT, Heinrichs DW, Alphs LD (1985) Treatment of negative symptoms. Schizophr Bull 11:440–452

Charney DS, Nelson JC (1981) Delusional and nondelusional unipolar depression. Further evidence for distinct subtypes. Am J Psychiatry 39:1181–1184

Clark JA, Mallett BL (1963) A follow-up study of schizophrenia and depression in young adults. Br J Psychiatry 109:491–499

Clayton PJ (1982) Schizoaffective disorders. J Nerv Ment Dis 170:646–650

Dunner DL, Rosenthal NE (1979) Schizoaffective states. Psychiatr Clin North Am 2:441–448

Endicott J, Spitzer RL (1978) A diagnostic interview: the Schedule for Affective Disorders and Schizophrenia. Arch Gen Psychiatry 35:837–862

Galdi J (1983) The causality of depression in schizophrenia. Br J Psychiatry 142:621–625

Jablensky A, Schwarz R, Tomov T (1980) WHO collaborative study on impairments and disabilities associated with schizophrenic disorders. Acta Psychiatr Scand [Suppl] 268: 152–163

Joyce PR (1984) Age of onset in bipolar affective disorder and misdiagnosis as schizophrenia. Psychol Bull 14:145–149

Kantor SJ, Glassman AH (1977) Delusional depression: natural history and response to treatment. Br J Psychiatry 131:351–360

Kendell RE (1986) The relationship of schizoaffective illnesses to schizophrenic and affective disorders. In: Marneros A, Tsuang MT (eds) Schizoaffective psychoses. Springer, Berlin Heidelberg New York Tokyo pp 18–30

Knights A, Hirsch SR (1981) "Revealed" depression and drug treatment for schizophrenia. Arch Gen Psychiatry 38:806–811

Kulhara P, Avasthi A, Chadda R, Chandiramani K, Mattoo SK, Kota SK, Joseph S (1989) Negative and depressive symptoms in schizophrenia. Br J Psychiatry 154:207–211

Levinson DF, Levitt MEM (1987) Schizoaffective mania reconsidered. Am J Psychiatry 144:415–425

Lewis N, Piotrowski Z (1954) Clinical diagnosis of manic-depressive psychosis. In: Hoch PM, Zubin J (eds) Depression. Grune and Stratton, New York, pp 25–38

Maj M (1985) Clinical course and outcome of schizoaffective disorders. A three-year follow-up study. Acta Psychiatr Scand 72:542–550

Maj M (1988) Clinical course and outcome of cycloid psychotic disorder: a prospective study. J Affective Disorders 14:129–135

Maj M (1989) A family study of two subgroups of schizoaffective patients. Br J Psychiatry 154:640–643

Maj M, Kemali D (1987) Nosological status of schizoaffective disorders: theoretical models and empirical evidence. Psychiat Psychobiol 2:163–172

Maj M, Perris C (1985) An approach to the diagnosis and classification of schizoaffective disorders for research purposes. Acta Psychiatr Scand 72:405–417

Maj M, Starace F, Kemali D (1987) Prediction of outcome by historical, clinical and biological variables in schizoaffective disorder, depressed type. J Psychiatr Res 21:289–295

Marneros A, Rhode A, Deister A, Risse A (1986) Schizoaffective disorders: the prognostic value of the affective component. In: Marneros A, Tsuang MT (eds) Schizoaffective psychoses. Springer, Berlin Heidelberg New York Tokyo, pp 155–163

Marneros A, Deister A, Rhode A, Jünemann H, Fimmers R (1988) Long-term course of schizoaffective disorders. I. Definitions, methods, frequency of episodes and cycles. Eur Arch Psychiatry Neurol Sci 237:264–257

Perris C (1986) The case for the independence of cycloid psychotic disorder from the schizoaffective disorders. In: Marneros A, Tsuang MT (eds) Schizoaffective psychoses. Springer, Berlin Heidelberg New York Tokyo, pp 272–308

Perris C (1988) The concept of cycloid psychotic disorder. Psychiatr Dev 6:37–56

Perris C, Brockington IF (1981) Cycloid psychoses and their relation to the major psychoses. In: Perris C, Struwe G, Jansson B (eds) Biological psychiatry 1981. Elsevier, Amsterdam, pp 447–450

Price LH, Nelson JC, Charney DS, Quinlan DM (1984) Family history in delusional depression. J Affective Disorders 6:109–114

Rosen LN, Rosenthal NE, Van Dusen PH, Dunner DL, Fieve RR (1983) Age at onset and number of psychotic symptoms in bipolar I and schizoaffective disorder. Am J Psychiatry 140:1523–1524

Rzewuska M, Angst J (1982a) Prognosis of periodic bipolar manic-depressive and schizoaffective psychoses. Arch Psychiatr Nervenkr 231:471–486

Rzewuska, M, Angst J (1982b) Aspects of the course of manic-depressive, schizo-affective and paranoid schizophrenic psychoses. Arch Psychiatr Nervenkr 231:487–501

Samson J, Simpson JC, Tsuang MT (1988) Outcome studies of schizoaffective disorders. Schizophr Bull 14:543–554

Schneider K (1973) Klinische Psychopathologie, 10th edn. Thieme, Stuttgart

Shenton ME, Solovay MR, Holzman P (1987) Comparative studies of thought disorders. II. Schizoaffective disorder. Arch Gen Psychiatry 44:21–30

Shopsin B (1979) Manic illness. Raven, New York

Spitzer RL, Endicott J, Robins E (1975) Research diagnostic criteria (RDC) for a selected group of functional disorders, 2nd edn. Biometrics Research, New York

Strauss JS (1983) Schizo-affective disorders: "just another illness" or a key to understanding the psychoses? Psychiatr Clin 16:286–296

Strauss JS, Carpenter WT (1972) The prediction of outcome in schizophrenia. I. Characteristics of outcome. Arch Gen Psychiatry 27:739–746

Welner A, Croughan JL, Robins E (1974) The group of schizoaffective and related psychoses. Critique, record, follow-up, and family studies. A persistent enigma. Arch Gen Psychiatry 31:628–631

World Health Organization (1979) Schizophrenia: an international follow-up study. Wiley, Chichester

World Health Organization (1989) ICD-10. 1989 draft of chapter V. WHO, Geneva

The Schizoaffective Continuum:
Non-Psychotic, Mood Congruent, and Mood Incongruent

G. WINOKUR, D.W. BLACK, and A. NASRALLAH[1]

Introduction

The evolutionary line in the development of the schizoaffective diagnosis is not easily traced. This is because we can estimate 24 or 25 different definitions of schizoaffective disorder. Several definitions are operational and well described (Marneros and Tsuang 1986; Levinston and Levitt 1987), while some encompass illnesses that share a lot in common with operational definitions of schizoaffective disorder such as benign stupors, reactive psychoses, good premorbid schizophrenia, cycloid psychoses, schizophreniform illnesses, remitting schizophrenia, and acute schizophrenia (Winokur 1984). Certainly, 24 or 25 definitions are a rough estimate; we made no systematic effort to obtain all of the possible definitions and related diagnoses. Assuming 24 possible definitions and criteria sets, it would be possible to study any patient group and come up with 48 to 50 different studies (assuming a separation of schizoaffective mania and schizoaffective depression).

The number of possible studies in which an investigator might compare one definition with another is, of course, astronomical. Assuming all 48 definitions are independent, 1128 comparative studies are possible. There would be 276 possible comparisons for the schizoaffective depressive and an equal number for the schizoaffective manic groups alone. Is it any wonder that we have considerable problems with the concept of schizoaffective disorder? This fact is simply a monument to the fecundity of psychiatry's ability to come up with new definitions.

In the United States, essential elements of schizoaffective disorder are captured in the *Research Diagnostic Criteria* (RDC, Spitzer et al. 1978). Patients with this diagnosis have an episode of mania or depression with a specified number of affective symptoms concomitant with specific psychotic features, such as mood-incongruent delusions or hallucinations. Patients could meet the RDC criteria if they had a period of time when there was an absence of affective symptoms, but showed above-type schizophrenic symptoms; this criterion is harder to document. The diagnosis of schizoaffective disorder in the American standard nomenclature (DSM-III-R, 1987) contains no rigorous criteria such as the RDC. The diagnoses of the affective disorders are broader in the DSM-III-R

[1] Department of Psychiatry, University of Iowa College of Medicine, Psychiatric Hospital, 500 Newton Road, Iowa City, IA 52242, USA

Affective and Schizoaffective Disorders
Edited by A. Marneros and M.T. Tsuang
© Springer-Verlag Berlin Heidelberg 1990

than they are in the RDC, and consequently some of the patients who received the diagnosis of schizoaffective disorder in the RDC would receive the diagnosis of affective disorder in DSM-III-R.

We had earlier used the RDC to evaluate a group of schizoaffective manics. We compared the schizoaffective manics with manics who had no schizophrenic-type symptoms and found no difference in course or family history. These findings suggest that the schizoaffective manics are simply manics with a some-what different clinical background. An additional finding was the possibe asso-ciation of a schizoaffective clinical picture in manic patients with endocrine abnormalities or in a postpartum state (Winokur et al. 1986).

In a new and large data set, we have chosen to evaluate patients on a continuum. We will compare nonpsychotic patients with depression and mania with manic or depressive psychotic patients with mood-congruent psychotic symptoms and with manics or depressives with mood-incongruent psychotic symptoms. We will compare these groups of depressives or manics, divided separately into the three groups, with the idea of determining how they may be similar in clinical picture, course of illness, and response to treatment.

Methodology

Two thousand fifty-four patients with an affective disorder were admitted to the University of Iowa Psychiatric Hospital between (January 1, 1970, and December 31, 1981. These patients had chart diagnoses of unipolar depression, manic disorder, involutional melancholia, manic-depressive psychosis, atypical depression, atypical manic disorder, atypical psychosis, schizoaffective disorder, secondary depression, neurotic depression, cyclothymia, or dysthymia. All patients were systematically evaluated for sex, marital status, age at index admission, previous hospitalization, age at index hospitalization, duration of illness at admission, precipitating events, organic features at admission, suicidal thoughts at admission, melancholia symptoms at admission, delusions and hallucinations, treatment and response for index hospitalization, previous treatments and response, previous suicide attempts, outcome at discharge, and death, including cause of death. Index admission was the last admission if there were more than one. Relapse after discharge was recorded and the patient was considered to have relapsed if on a subsequent clinic visit he or she reported three or more depressive symptoms from a symptom checklist or a manic syndrome was diagnosed by a psychiatrist. Suicide attempts were recorded if either serious or nonserious suicide attempts were recorded in the progress notes.

We recorded the presence of a nonaffective psychiatric illness that might have predated the depression for which a patient was diagnosed and admitted (secondary depression). In this study, depression was considered secondary if a severe or life-threatening medical illness or a nonaffective psychiatric condition was noted in the chart that predated or paralleled the depression. No secondary depressives are included in this study.

The methodology has been described previously (Black et al. 1987a,b; Winokur et al. 1988). For this study, we looked at patients with a DSM-III diagnosis of major depressive disorder or a DSM-III diagnosis of mania. Included are 604 unipolar depressives without psychotic symptoms, 76 unipolar depressives with mood-congruent psychotic symptoms, and 60 unipolar depressives with mood-incongruent psychotic symptoms. The other large category included 188 nonpsychotic manics, 113 mood-congruent psychotic manics, and 88 mood-incongruent psychotic manics. The depressives and the manics were evaluated separately using a $2 \times K$ chi-square analysis.

Our method looked at severity in a continuous and systematic way. The unipolar depressives and the manics with mood-incongruent symptoms were considered to be the ones who most clearly represented schizoaffective disorder according to the RDC. They were then compared with two groups with separate levels of severity; those with unipolar depression and congruent psychotic symptoms were presumed to be more severely affected than those without psychotic symptoms. We considered this true for the manics as well. Psychotic symptoms in this study included delusions and hallucinations, and the definitions of mood congruent and mood incongruent are defined in the DSM-III-R (American Psychiatric Association 1987).

Finally, the method offered a new possibility for analysis. We compared the unipolar depressives who had incongruent psychotic symptoms with the paralleled previously reported differences in patterns between nonpsychotic unipolars and manics.

Results

Comparisons among unipolar depressive are shown in Tables 1 and 2. Acute onset (duration of illness at admission) does not differentiate three groups, but the mood-incongruent psychotics were less likely to have had a chronic course prior to hospitalization (Table 1). Only 22% of the mood-incongruent group had been ill for 6 months before entering the hospital, as opposed to 32% of the mood-congruent group and 40% of the group of patients who had no psychotic symptoms. A simple explanation for this difference might be that the mood-incongruent psychotics have aberrant behavior that is not tolerated by families and are therefore brought for medical attention earlier.

Precipitating events occur more frequently in unipolar depressive without psychotic symptoms. It is entirely likely that this large group contains many patients who meet the diagnosis of "neurotic depression," which in general is associated with a lack of psychotic symptoms and a positive report on the part of the patient for precipitating factors (Winokur 1985; Winokur et al. 1987).

Table 2 shows that hallucinations are more frequent in the unipolar depressives with mood-incongruent psychotic symptoms. As both of the unipolar depressive psychotic groups have delusions, this is a striking finding. If one accepts the possibility that hallucinations are a sign of increased severity, this supports the idea that unipolar depressives with mood-incongruent psychotic symptoms

G. Winokur et al.

Table 1. Nonpsychotic unipolar depressives vs depressives with congruent and incongruent psychotic symptoms

	Unipolar depressives without Psychotic sx	Unipolar depressives with congruent psychotic sx	Unipolar depressives with incongruent psychotic sx	P
N	604	76	60	
Median age at admission	44	56	34	0.02
% female	64	68	73	N.S.
Duration of hospitalization <4 weeks	50%	38%	35%	0.001
7 or more hospitalizations previously	4%	4%	14%	0.004
Age first ill, mean	37	32	31	0.02
Duration of illness at admission ≤4 weeks	9%	9%	12%	N.S.
Previous suicide attempts	33%	26%	35%	N.S.

Table 2. Nonpsychotic unipolar depressives vs depressives with congruent and incongruent psychotic symptoms

	Unipolar depressives without psychotic sx	Unipolar depressives with congruent psychotic sx	Unipolar depressives with incongruent psychotic sx	P
Organic factors	14%	28%	19%	0.02
Hallucinations	0%	17%	50%	0.001
Marked improvement at discharge	61%	68%	57%	N.S.
ECT given	44%	67%	50%	0.01
Marked improvement with ECT	59%	56%	70%	N.S.
DST nonsuppression at 4 PM (≥5 mg/dl)	42%	81%	47%	0.01
Marked improvement or improvement on antidepressants	19%	14%	19%	N.S.
Antipsychotic maintenance	21%	35%	57%	0.001
Melancholia diagnosis positive	12%	41%	13%	0.001
Schizoaffective, RDC	0%	0%	45%	N.S.
No relapse in follow-up	50%	31%	52%	N.S.
Follow-up, 2+ years	42%	45%	41%	N.S.
Suicide attempt in follow-up	5%	4%	3%	N.S.
Suicides, follow-up	4%	5%	5%	N.S.
Death, follow-up	10%	14%	5%	N.S.

Table 3. Comparison of nonpsychotic manics, manics with mood congruent and mood incongruent psychotic symptoms

	Nonpsychotic manics	Mood congruent psychotic manics	Mood incongruent psychotic manics	P
N	188	113	88	
Age, median	34	30	31	N.S.
% female	57	50	53	N.S.
Divorced, widowed, separated	22%	23%	27%	N.S.
Hospital >4 wks.	31%	37%	51%	N.S.
Index hospital = first hospital	23%	20%	14%	N.S.
Age first ill, median	31	33	25	N.S.
Ill <1 month at index	37%	46%	51%	N.S.
Previous suicide attempt	12%	15%	17%	N.S.

are the more severely ill group. Response to treatment is no different among the three groups. Patients in the three groups were equally likely to respond to ECT and antidepressant medication. Of course, the mood-incongruent psychotic group was more likely to have antipsychotic drug maintenance, something which is expected. Duration of follow-up was equal among the groups, and there was no significant difference in the number of patients who relapsed. There is a suggestion that the unipolar depressives with congruent psychotic symptoms were more likely to relapse, but this was not statistically significant. There is no significant difference in the number of suicides at follow-up. Deaths from natural causes are less frequent in the mood-incongruent group (5%) than in the other groups (10% and 13%). The mood-incongruent patients were younger at index, which probably accounts for the difference.

Tables 3 and 4 present the comparisons between the nonpsychotic manics, mood-congruent manics, and mood-incongruent manics. Table 3 is quite striking, in that there are no significant differences in age, sex, marital status, length of hospitalization, whether or not the index hospitalization was the first hospitalization, age at first illness, and acuteness of illness. It one compares the acuteness of onset of the manics with onset in the unipolar depressions, the difference is very striking. All manic groups are more likely to have an acute onset (less than a month) before admission.

Mood-incongruent manics are more likely than mood-congruent psychotic manics to have had precipitating events and are more likely to have memory defects or be disoriented. Unlike the differences among unipolars, the mood-congruent psychotic manics and mood-incongruent psychotic manics are equally likely to have hallucinations. Patients in the manic groups are equally likely to have marked improvement with ECT. At hospital discharge, the manic groups show similar improvement regardless of treatment. During the follow-up more attempts at suicide were made among patients in the mood-incongruent group, but there are no significant differences for actual suicides and deaths.

Table 4. Comparison of nonpsychotic manics, manics with mood congruent and mood incongruent psychotic symptoms

	Nonpsychotic manics	Mood congruent psychotic manics	Mood incongruent psychotic manics	P
Precipitating event present	21%	32%	38%	0.01
Organic features present	13%	14%	29%	0.01
Hallucinations present	0%	27%	35%	0.000
Outcome, marked improvement	61%	64%	58%	N.S.
Use of antipsychotic drug	70%	87%	90%	0.001
Marked improvement or improvement, ECT	69%	65%	78%	N.S.
Follow-up, 2 yrs. or more	40%	40%	42%	N.S.
Suicide attempts in follow-up	1%	2%	10%	0.02
Suicide in follow-up	1%	1%	0%	N.S.
Death in follow-up	5%	3%	3%	N.S.

Table 5. Patterns in unipolars vs bipolars, both with mood incongruent psychotic symptoms

	UP	BP
N	60	88
Median, age admission	34	31
% female	73%	53%
First hospitalization = index hospitalization	25%	14%
4-7 + hospitalizations	26%	42%
Age first ill, median	29	25
Ill less than 4 weeks at admission	12%	51%
Previous suicide attempts	35%	17%
Organic features at index	19%	29%
Proportion receiving ECT	50%	10%
Marked improvement with ECT	70%	67%
Proportion receiving lithium	18%	89%
Improvement + marked improvement on lithium	55%	65%
Nonsuppression at 8 AM on dex test ($\geqslant 5$ mg/dl)	28%	9%
Nonsuppression at 4 PM on dex test	53%	56%
Outcome, marked improvement	57%	58%
none or partial improvement	15%	8%
Follow-up $\geqslant 2$ years	41%	42%

Finally, the data lent themselves to a methodology that had not been accomplished before. Mood-incongruent psychotic symptoms in manics and unipolars strongly support the idea of calling them schizoaffective. Thus, one would be able to compare the mood-incongruent unipolars and manics on the basis of variables that ordinarily discriminate between nonpsychotic unipolars and manics. These variables include earlier age of onset in manics, fewer episodes in unipolars, more female unipolars, more nonsuppressors on the dexamethasone suppression test among unipolars, more acute onsets in manics. Table 5 gives us material comparing only the mood-incongruent patients. These expectations remain true in this comparison.

Discussion

The method used in this study is quite different from earlier work. We have presented a continuum of severity going from no psychosis, to congruent psychotic symptoms, to incongruent psychotic symptoms. Because this covers a 10-year period, our sample is substantial.

    The mood-incongruent psychotic unipolars and manics generally fit the concept of the RDC for schizoaffective, depressive, and manic illness. An important clinical point is that schizophrenia is more likely a chronic illness than an affective disorder. It is notable, therefore, that the mood-incongruent depressives are more likely than the nonpsychotic depressives to have been acutely ill (less than 6 months) when admitted. Likewise, few manics in any of the three groups were likely to be ill for longer than 6 months: 16%, 16%, and 15%.

The patients in this study meet the DSM-III criteria for a unipolar or manic syndrome, i.e., major depression or mania. Thus, we have a group of patients who clearly have the syndrome of affective illness, but, in addition, two of the six groups show the presence of clear schizophrenic symptoms, namely mood-incongruent delusions and hallucinations.

The findings were striking. The three groups did not differ substantially from one an other; i.e., nonpsychotic unipolars, mood-congruent psychotic unipolars, and mood-incongruent psychotic unipolars are very similar in terms of treatment response and follow-up. The same is true of the three groups with manic illnesses. Thus, by separating the three groups we have shown the practicality of considering them together in terms of management.

What is the difference between the three groupings? They are obviously different clinically, and one might consider them to be on a continuum of severity. Certainly, the presence of hallucinations in the mood-incongruent psychotic unipolar group supports that possibility.

The major finding is that these groups look rather similar in terms of their prehospitalization background, their treatment results, and their follow-up. In this study, it does not really make any difference in terms of response to therapy and future course that some patients have psychotic symptoms and others do not. There is some reason to believe that those patients with mood-congruent psychotic symptoms are, in fact, the most homogeneous group among the depressives. They fit the concept of "endogenous" depression best of all. The group with no psychotic symptoms probably contains a mixture of some neurotic depressives and some endogenous depressives, and it is entirely possible that the groups of acute onset incongruent psychotic manics and depressives contain a small number of schizophrenics.

On a practical basis, these illnesses are all similar. They respond to treatment well and they have the same quality of follow-up. Of course, as was noted earlier, the diagnosis of schizoaffective disorder depends on the criteria. If there were changes in the criteria, it is quite conceivable that there might be differences in the results.

Conclusions

We compared three groups of unipolar depressives: those who were nonpsychotic, those who had mood-congruent psychotic symptoms, and those who had mood-incongruent psychotic symptoms. We did similar comparisons with a set of manic patients. These separations generally conform to some conceptions of schizoaffective disorder. The acuteness of onset in the three groups of unipolars and three groups of manics is approximately the same. The groups responded equally well to treatment within the manic and unipolar comparisons. The follow-up was very similar. This suggests that for practical management purposes the groups should be considered together. There is one finding of some diagnostic significance: If one simply compares the mood-incongruent unipolars with the mood-incongruent manics, the same pattern of differences is seen as between the nonpsychotic unipolars and the manics. The mood-incongruent manics are younger at onset, have more episodes, have a more acute onset, and are less likely to be women. These findings suggest strongly that the mood-incongruent affective psychoses (schizoaffective disorder, manic or depressive types) are related mainly to ordinary affective disorders.

References

American Psychiatric Association (1987) *Diagnostic and statistical manual of mental disorders*, 3rd edn. DSM-III-R. American Psychiatric Association, Washington, DC

Black D, Winokur G, Nasrallah A (1987a) The treatment of depression: electroconvulsive therapy vs antidepressants, a naturalistic evaluation of 1495 patients. Compr Psychiatry 28:169–182

Black D, Winokur G, Nasrallah A (1987b) Treatment of mania: a naturalistic study of electroconvulsive therapy versus lithium in 438 patients. J Clin Psychiatry 48:132–139

Levinson D, Levitt M (1987) Schizoaffective mania reconsidered. Am J Psychiatry 144: 415–425

Marneros A, Tsuang M (1986) *Schizoaffective psychoses*. Springer, Berlin Heidelberg New York Tokyo, p 319

Spitzer R, Endicott J, Robins E (1978) *Research diagnostic criteria*, 3rd edn. Biometrics Research, New York State Department of Mental Hygiene, New York

Winokur G (1984) Psychoses in bipolar and unipolar affective illness with special reference to schizoaffective disorder. Br J Psychiatry 145:236–242

Winokur G (1985) The validity of neurotic-reactive depression. Arch Gen Psychiatry 42: 116–1122

Winokur G, Kadrmas A, Crowe R (1986) Schizoaffective mania, family history, and clinical characteristics. In: Marneros A, Tsuang M *(eds) Schizoaffective psychoses*. Springer Berlin Heidelberg New York Tokyo pp 115–122

Winokur G, Black D, Nasrallah A (1987) Neurotic depression: a diagnosis based on pre-existing characteristics. Eur Arch Psychiatr Neurol Sci 236:343–348

Winokur G, Black D, Nasrallah A (1988) Depression secondary to other psychiatric disorders and medical illnesses. Am J Psychiatry 145:233–237

The Predictive Value of Grouping Schizoaffective Psychoses Together with Affective Psychoses: Jaspers' Hierarchical Rule Revised

D. von Zerssen,[1] M. Zaudig,[1] C. Cording,[2] H.-J. Möller,[3] and H.-U. Wittchen[1]

Introduction

Subtypes of Functional Psychoses

It is inherent in the nature of mental disorders that a clear grouping according to distinct entities is not possible (see von Zerssen 1986a). This problem is particularly prominent in the area of personality disorders, neuroses, abnormal stress reactions, and other "minor" disorders, but it is also present within the range of functional psychoses. This has implications for research as well as for clinical practice; e.g., how useful is the diagnosis of a special subtype for therapeutic and prognostic purposes?

The Kraepelinean dichotomy of functional psychoses into schizophrenias ("dementia praecox") and affective psychoses ("manic depressive insanity", Kraepelin 1913) seems to be well founded in this respect. It has been empirically validated by genetic investigations, by therapeutic trials (e.g., with respect to the prophylactic value of long-term lithium administration), and by follow-up studies covering up to several decades, starting with the onset of the disorder or with hospital admission and continuing to the final examination.

However, results concerning the Kraepelinean subtypes of schizophrenia (hebephrenic, catatonic, paranoid, and simple types) are much less consistent with respect to clear differences in heredity, therapeutic responsiveness, and long-term course and outcome. Therefore, the clinical relevance of these subtypes has been doubted. From the perspective of long-term course and outcome of a schizophrenic psychosis, other variables such as age at onset, type of onset (acute versus insidious), and premorbid social adjustment proved to be of higher predictive value than the prevalent psychopathology, whether more hebephrenic, catatonic, paranoid, or undifferentiated.

In the area of the affective disorders, the dichotomy of a bipolar manic-depressive vs. a unipolar depressive type (Angst 1966; Perris 1966) has received a lot of empirical support during the past several decades. However, the utility of subtyping bipolar disorders into bipolar I and II (Dunner et al. 1976) and of subtyping unipolar depression into endogenous and psychogenic depression is still a matter of debate (see Zerbin-Rüdin 1988).

---

[1] Max-Planck-Institut für Psychiatrie, Kraepelinstraße 2, 8000 München 40, FRG
[2] Bezirkskrankenhaus Regensburg, Universitätsstraße 84, 8400 Regensburg, FRG
[3] Universitäts-Nervenklinik, Sigmund-Freud-Straße 25, 5300 Bonn 1, FRG

Affective and Schizoaffective Disorders
Edited by A. Marneros and M.T. Tsuang
© Springer-Verlag Berlin Heidelberg 1990

Another controversial issue relates to the boundaries of the main subtypes of functional psychoses, i.e., schizophrenias and affective psychoses. Not only are the "outer" borders ill-defined, i.e., between schizophrenias and similar psychoses (e.g., schizophreniform psychoses and pure paranoid syndromes of unknown origin) on the one hand, and between major depression and other predominantly depressive disorders, such as abnormal reactions with depressed mood, on the other hand; the border between schizophrenias and affective psychoses is also far from being clear. Many acute-onset psychoses display typical schizophrenic and typical manic and/or depressive features either at the same time (Kasanin 1933) and/or in an irregular alternation of predominantly schizophrenic and predominantly affective episodes (Angst 1986). This mixture of the classical features of the two main types of functional psychoses has puzzled researchers as well as clinicians and has led them to look for an adequate classification of this group of so-called schizoaffective disorders (see Marneros and Tsuang 1986). Do they belong to the schizophrenic rather than to the affective group or vice versa? Do they constitute a separate group with a specific heredity, or can they be subdivided into a basically schizophrenic and a basically affective group, and maybe even a third, independent group?

Hierarchical Rules in Psychiatric Diagnostics

All the interpretations given above can be found in the literature. Historically, psychiatrists in Europe and, even more so, in the USA were long of the opinion that the schizophrenic component was more important from a nosological and thus also from a diagnostic point of view. The idea behind this belief was that an affective symptomatology was, in general, less specific for a disorder than were schizophrenic symptoms. This appeared to be particularly true for depressive features which often accompany or initiate other disorders, including otherwise typical schizophrenic psychoses. On the other hand, schizophrenic features are less frequently found in the long-term course of an otherwise typical affective psychosis. This led Jaspers (1972, first published in 1913) to the formulation of his classical hierarchical rule, according to which psychopathological symptoms can be arranged from nosologically nonspecific (such as nervousness, anxious tension, lack of concentration) over more specific (symptoms of typical depression and mania) to highly specific (typical schizophrenic) symptoms. The highest degree of specificity should be reached by typical symptoms of an organic origin (disorders of consciousness, disorientation, memory disturbances, etc.). Their presence would therefore justify the diagnosis of an organic disorder even in the presence of typically schizophrenic and/or manic-depressive and, of course, the still less specific neurotic features. Consequently, it was postulated that schizophrenic symptoms in the absence of organic features indicated a schizophrenic psychosis even when manic-depressive and other less specific features were present, as in the case of a schizoaffective psychosis. On this theoretical basis, the schizoaffective subtype of functional psychoses was incorporated into the group of schizophrenic psychoses in diagnostic schemata, such as the International Classification of Diseases (ICD), up to ICD-9 (World Health Organization

1978), and the first two editions of the Diagnostic and Statistical Manual (DSM) of the American Psychiatric Association (1952, 1968). It is evident that a neurotic disorder can be diagnosed only in the absence of organic, schizophrenic, and typical manic-depressive features. This may become difficult in the case of a depression without clearly psychotic features (delusions, lack of insight); but Jaspers' rule has also been questioned with respect to the hierarchical position of schizophrenic symptoms for several reasons:

1. Symptoms of this kind – even first-rank symptoms according to Kurt Schneider (1959), a follower of Jaspers' hierarchical approach to psychiatric diagnoses – turned out to occur more frequently during manic episodes of an otherwise typical bipolar affective disorder (Pope et al. 1980; Abrams and Taylor 1981) than was originally assumed.
2. In family studies of patients with features of schizophrenic *and* affective psychoses, both types of psychoses were found in a pure form in similar frequency among first- and second-degree relatives (see Zerbin-Rüdin 1986). In some of these studies, the hereditary load with affective disorders even predominated (e.g., Mendlewicz et al. 1979).
3. With one notable exception (Welner et al. 1977), follow-up studies of patients with schizoaffective psychoses demonstrated a more favorable outcome compared with schizophrenics. They rather exhibited an episodic course with symptom-free or almost symptom-free intervals, resembling the course of pure affective disorders. This might indicate a closer relationship of the mixed psychoses to the affective than to the schizophrenic group of functional psychoses.
4. The predominance of females among schizoaffective patients also pointed in the same direction (see von Zerssen 1980; Vogl and Zaudig 1985; Marneros et al. 1988).
5. Similar to the findings in other subgroups of affective psychoses, prophylactic lithium administration proved to be effective in a considerable proportion of schizoaffective but not in purely schizophrenic psychoses (Pope and Lipinski 1978).

It was inferred from these findings that the affective features in schizoaffective psychoses might be of a higher nosological order than the schizophrenic symptomatology. As a consequence of such considerations, the majority of these psychoses were incorporated into the group of affective disorders in the DSM-III and DSM-III-R (American Psychiatric Association 1980, 1987), namely as major depression or mania with mood-incongruent psychotic features. The term "schizoaffective disorder" was reserved for a small group of cases presenting a purely schizophrenic symptom pattern for a certain period of time in addition to periods of mixed schizophrenic and typical affective symptomatology. This group is kept separate from schizophrenia and from affective disorders (= mood disorders in DSM-III-R). It should be noted that the assignment of the majority of schizoaffective psychoses to the affective psychoses is in accord with the British and the Scandinavian tradition and with some German schools of psychiatry.

This classification may be criticized from a genetic point of view because of the increased rate of schizophrenics among first-degree relatives of patients with schizoaffective psychoses compared with those of patients with purely affective psychoses (see Zerbin-Rüdin 1986). In this paper, however, we will deal with the problem of classification only from a clinically more relevant point of view, that is, the prediction of the further course of the psychosis.

Subjects and Methods

Subjects

The data of this study were collected within the framework of the Munich Follow-up Study (MFS) of former inpatients of the Max Planck Institute of Psychiatry (MPIP) ($n = 218$) and subjects of the general population ($n = 483$) who were interviewed 5–8 years after the index investigation (see von Zerssen and Hecht 1987; Möller et al. 1988; Wittchen and von Zerssen 1988). Among the former patients, there were 103 who had received an index diagnosis of a functional psychosis (ICD-9, nos. 295–298). The schizophrenic group ($n = 46$) comprised 43 schizophrenics (no. 295) with the exception of schizoaffectives (no. 295.7) and in addition three patients suffering from purely paranoid psychoses (nos. 297.1/9, 298.3). Schizoaffective psychoses (no. 295.7) formed an additional group ($n = 22$), as did the pure affective disorders (no. 296: $n = 35$, 22 unipolar depressives plus 13 bipolar manic-depressives). The diagnosis had been considered probable or certain at discharge from index hospitalization, which was the first admission in approximately 40%.

The diagnoses were made by experienced psychiatrists according to ICD criteria. The agreement of our clinical diagnoses with operational diagnoses had been checked in other samples and found to be adequate (see Schmid et al. 1982; Zaudig and Vogl 1983; Berger et al. 1984; Vogl and Zaudig 1985).

Assessment

A thorough case history had been filed during index hospitalization. In each case, the psychopathological state had been rated at admission and at discharge by means of self-rating scales (von Zerssen 1976, 1986b) and an observer's rating instrument, the Inpatient Multidimensional Psychiatric Scales (MPS: Lorr and Klett 1967; see also Hiller et al. 1986), by the physician in charge of the patient. At discharge, the same physician had also made a global rating of the patient's mental state on a five-point scale. At follow-up, 5–8 years later, the same scales were again applied, supplemented by other rating devices, among them:

- The Global Assessment Scale (Endicott et al. 1976) of 100 points for evaluating the level of psychosocial functioning during the last week.
- Information about professional efficiency during the last year according to Huber et al. (1979).

- Working incapacity.
- Time spent in psychiatric hospital(s) during the follow-up period.

For this report, we will neglect additional information about social adaptation during the 4 weeks preceding the interviews, which were assessed with the Social Interview Schedule (SIS: Clare and Cairns 1978; German version: Faltermaier et al. 1985; see Hecht et al. 1987); about life events and long-standing social conditions during the follow-up period, assessed with the aid of the Munich Event List (MEL: W. Maier-Diewald et al. unpublished; see Wittchen and von Zerssen 1988; Wittchen et al. 1989); and, finally, information about the occurrence of mental disorders since childhood and their presence during or shortly before the interview, where the Diagnostic Interview Schedule was used (DIS: Robins et al. 1981; German version: H.-U. Wittchen and H.-U. Rupp, unpublished).

Data Handling

For the present analysis, the data obtained at admission and discharge were used to form a set of potential predictors for further course and outcome at follow-up. The criteria for course and outcome were derived from data obtained at follow-up. Thus, we ended up with 16 predictors and six criteria for course and outcome (see Table 1). With two exceptions, the variables were scored so that they predicted (15 variables) or indicated (five variables) an unfavorable course and/ or outcome. One exception was a scale of affective symptomatology at admission (see below) which was scored in the same, i.e., positive, direction as it was at discharge although, according to the literature (see Möller and von Zerssen 1986), the degree of affective symptomatology at admission should predict a favorable course and outcome (see Möller and von Zerssen 1986). As usual, the GAS was scored in such a way that high scores were indicative of a more favorable outcome. For calculating frequencies, the variables which were not binary (e.g., age in contrast to gender) were dichotomized, either according to the median of the total group ($n = 103$), e.g., the new IMPS scores (at three points in time: hospital admission, discharge, follow-up), or to a meaningful cut-off score, e.g., time of working incapacity or time spent in hospital during the follow-up period $>5\%$; GAS score <60, i.e., marked to severe impairment. Two of the predictors were biosocial variables (gender and age at admission), three were psychosocial variables (working difficulties, impaired social adaptability, and lack of constant heterosexual partnership before index admission). The others were related more directly to the mental disorder, four of them to anamnestic characteristics (insidious onset of the disorder and of the index episode, chronic course before admission, and abuse of alcohol and/or other drugs). Four were related to the psychopathological state at admission and discharge (two scores derived from the IMPS for both occasions and a global rating of the mental state at discharge). Finally, two were different diagnostic groupings according to the ICD diagnosis at discharge. The two biosocial, the four psychopathological, and the two diagnostic variables were drawn from a

Table 1. Scales reflecting schizophrenic symptomatology (ScS) and affective symptomatology (AfS), derived from the IMPS

Item no.	Original scale	Abbr.	Content (abbr.)	Scaling
1. Schizophrenic symptomatology (ScS)				
3	Conceptual Disorganization	CNP	incoherent	0 1 2 3 4
6	Motor Disturbances	MTR	posturing	0 1 2 3 4
22	Retardation and Apathy	RTD	speech blocking	0 1 2 3 4
45	Perceptual Distortion	PCP	hears voices	0 1 2 3 4
46	Motor Disturbances	MTR	inadequate giggling	0 1 2 3 4
47	Motor Disturbances	MTR	grimacing	0 1 2 3 4
48	Motor Disturbances	MTR	repetitive movements	0 1 2 3 4
51	Motor Disturbances	MTR	talks to self	0 1 2 3 4
52	Motor Disturbances	MTR	startled glances	0 1 2 3 4
53	Perceptual Distortion	PCP	voices accuse	0 1 2 3 4
56	Perceptual Distortion	PCP	voices order	0 1 2 3 4
57	Perceptual Distortion	PCP	visions	0 1 2 3 4
58	Perceptual Distortion	PCP	other hallucinations	0 1 2 3 4
59	Paranoid Projection	PAR	ideas of reference	0 2
60	Paranoid Projection	PAR	ideas of persecution	0 2
61	Paranoid Projection	PAR	conspiracy	0 2
62	Paranoid Projection	PAR	being controlled by others	0 2
63	Paranoid Projection	PAR	external controlling	0 2
2. Affective symptomatology (AfS)				
a) Depressive symptomatology				
1	Retardation and Apathy	RTD	slowed speech	0 1 2 3 4
13	Retardation and Apathy	RTD	fixed facial expression	0 1 2 3 4
14	Anxious Depression	ANX	blames self	0 1 2 3 4
16	Retardation and Apathy	RTD	slowed movements	0 1 2 3 4
31	Anxious Depression	ANX	guilt	0 1 2 3 4
33	Retardation and Apathy	RTD	whispering speech	0 1 2 3 4
40	Anxious Depression	ANX	suicidal	0 1 2 3 4
83			lack of appetite	0 2
85	Impaired Functioning	IMP	unable to concentrate	0 2
87	Impaired Functioning	IMP	feeling fatigued	0 2
b) Manic symptomatology				
7	Excitement	EXC	unrestrained	0 1 2 3 4
9	Excitement	EXC	hurried speech	0 1 2 3 4
12	Excitement	EXC	elevated mood	0 1 2 3 4
15	Excitement / Grandiose Expansiveness	EXC / GRN	attitude of superiorify	0 1 2 3 4
17	Excitement	EXC	dramatization	0 1 2 3 4
20	Excitement	EXC	speaking loudly	0 1 2 3 4
25	Hostile Belligerence	HOS	irritability	0 1 2 3 4
26	Excitement	EXC	overactive	0 1 2 3 4
35	Excitement	EXC	excess of speech	0 1 2 3 4
37	Excitement	EXC	dominating	0 1 2 3 4

For items 1–45, the original nine-point scale is reduced to a five-point scale by retaining the zero category and making out of each following pair only one category. Binary items are scored as 0 or 2.

data bank (Barthelmes and von Zerssen 1978); the others had to be rated retrospectively on the basis of information stored in the rather elaborate case records.

The IMPS scores were based on two newly constructed scales, a unipolar scale reflecting typical schizophrenic symptomatology (ScS) which contained 18 items and a bipolar scale reflecting typical affective symptomatology (AfS) with a manic and a depressive pole which contained 20 items, ten at each pole. For the present analysis, the ten positive (depressive) and the ten negative (manic) items were all given a positive sign in order to form an additive unipolar scale of affective symptomatology, whether manic or depressive in nature (see Table 1).

The items had been selected in a series of analyses of data from psychiatric inpatients other than those investigated within the MFS. The items had to correlate specifically with one of two higher-order factors composed of primary IMPS scales (see von Zerssen 1985). The first (unipolar) factor comprised the scales Paranoid Projection (PAR), Perceptual Distortion (PCP), Conceptual Disorganization (CNP), Motor Disturbances (MTR), Hostile Belligerence (HOS), and Obsessive-Phobic (OBS). The second (bipolar) factor consisted of the scales Anxious Depression (ANX), Retardation and Apathy (RTD) as well as Impaired Functioning (IMP) versus Excitement (EXC), Hostile Belligerence (HOS), and Grandiose Expansiveness (GRN). Disorientation (DIS) did not achieve loadings >0.40 on one of these two factors. In addition, the items had to constitute two independent factors in principal component analyses with Varimax rotation. The results were cross-validated in an independent sample of psychotics. The scales thus obtained proved to be highly consistent for patients on admission.

The two groupings for predictive purposes of the ICD diagnoses were (a) schizophrenia versus purely affective and schizoaffective psychoses (similar as in DSM-III/DSM-III-R) and, for comparison, (b) schizophrenic and schizoaffective psychoses (according to Jaspers' hierarchical rule) versus purely affective psychoses.

Statistical Data Analyses

Frequency distributions of the primarily binary and the dichotomized variables were computed for the total group ($n = 103$) and the three subgroups of schizophrenic ($n = 46$), schizoaffective ($n = 22$), and affective ($n = 35$) patients and were then compared on the basis of the above-mentioned diagnostic groupings by means of the chi-square test. Furthermore, a correlational analysis was applied to the total set of variables using Pearson's product-moment correlation. Finally, a stepwise multiple regression analysis was carried out for the prediction of each of the six criteria for course and outcome by optimal combinations of variables from the set of 16 potential predictors.

Expectations

It was expected that schizophrenics would exhibit the highest frequencies in the categories of predictors as well as course and outcome criteria reflecting an

Table 2. Frequency distributions of potential predictors and criteria of an unfavorable course and/or outcome

No. Term	Total group of patients (n = 103) %	Diagnostic subgroups			Comparison of schizophr. (n = 46) vs. schizoaffect. + affectives (n = 57) P	Comparison of schizophr. + schizoaffectives (n = 68) vs. affectives (n = 35) P
		schizophr. (n = 46) %	schizoaff. (n = 22) %	affectives (n = 35) %		
Predictors						
1 Male sex	47.6	58.7	31.8	42.9	<0.05	>0.10
2 Young age	49.5	60.9	59.1	28.6	<0.05	<0.01
3 Difficulties at work (including housework)	59.2	69.6	31.8	62.9	<0.05	>0.10
4 Lack of social adaptability	9.7	17.4	4.5	2.9	<0.05	<0.10
5 Lack of constant partnership during the last 6 months	51.5	60.9	68.2	28.6	<0.10	<0.001
6 Insidious onset of disease	8.7	17.4	0.0	2.9	<0.01	>0.10
7 Chronic course until admission	10.7	21.7	4.5	0.0	<0.01	<0.05
8 Chronic abuse of alcohol and/or other drugs	7.8	8.7	9.1	5.7	>0.10	>0.10
9 Insidious onset of the index episode	26.2	41.3	4.5	20.0	<0.01	>0.10
10 ScS at admission above median of total group	49.0	69.6	68.2	8.6	<0.001	<0.001
11 AfS at admission above median of total group	50.0	39.1	77.3	45.7	<0.05	>0.10
12 ScS at discharge above median of total group	28.0[a]	50.0	13.6	8.6	<0.001	<0.01
13 AfS at discharge above median of total group	45.0	54.3	40.9	34.3	<0.10	<0.10
14 Bad psychopathological state at discharge (global rating)	16.5	37.0	0.0	0.0	<0.001	<0.01

15 Diagnosis of schizophrenia vs. schizoaffect. + affect. psychoses at discharge	44.7	100.0	0.0	0.0	—	—
16 Diagnosis of schizophrenia + schizoaff. vs. affective psychoses at discharge	66.0	100.0	100.0	0.0	—	—
Criteria						
a ScS at follow-up above median of total group	26.0[a]	45.7	9.1	11.4	<0.001	<0.05
b AfS at follow-up above median of total group	50.0	56.5	22.7	57.1	>0.10	>0.10
c GAS score <60 (last week before follow-up)	42.7	67.4	18.2	31.4	<0.001	<0.05
d Lack of professional efficiency (last year before follow-up)	45.6	69.6	18.2	31.4	<0.001	<0.05
e Working incapacity during follow-up period >5%	58.3	69.6	50.0	48.6	<0.05	>0.10
f Time in hospital during follow-up >5%	37.9	50.0	31.8	25.7	<0.05	<0.10

[a] Median zero (see Table 3).

unfavorable prognosis, compared with the groups of affectively as well as schizoaffectively ill patients. With respect to the newly developed IMPS scores, it was predicted that, on admission, schizophrenics would receive higher scores on the ScS scale than patients with pure affective psychoses, but not higher scores than patients with schizoaffective psychoses. Furthermore, it was predicted that the scores on the AfS scale of the affectively ill would exceed those of the schizophrenic but not those of the schizoaffective patients. On discharge, higher scores on both scales should be obtained by the schizophrenics than by the two other groups because of the lower remission rate of schizophrenics and the relative nonspecificity of affective symptomatology. A similar constellation was assumed with respect to findings at follow-up. Because of the presumably elevated scores of schizophrenics on both scales at discharge, compared with the other two groups of psychotics, these scores should predict an unfavorable outcome for the total group of patients.

The diagnostic grouping which contrasted schizophrenics with the other two groups of psychotics was expected to predict more of the variance of course and outcome 5–8 years after index hospitalization than the grouping contrasting schizophrenic *and* schizoaffective patients with purely affective psychotics.

Another point of interest was the relative predictive power of the diagnostic and other clinical variables compared with social variables, particularly regarding the prediction of social functioning. In earlier longitudinal studies of schizophrenic patients (Strauss and Carpenter 1974; see Möller and von Zerssen 1986) it was found that social functioning at follow-up was more closely related to the premorbid level of social functioning than to any clinical variable.

Results

The distributions of predictors and indicators of an unfavorable course and/or outcome (Table 2) point to the bad prognosis of schizophrenic psychoses as compared with purely affective and schizoaffective psychoses. The diagnostic combination of schizoaffective psychoses with the affective psychoses – as in DSM-III and DSM-III-R – yields much more statistically significant results in this comparison than the combination of schizoaffective and schizophrenic psychoses – according to ICD-8 and ICD-9. The only exceptions to this rule refer to age and the age-related variable 3 (partnership). As expected, the schizophrenics obtained, on an average, higher scores on the ScS scale at admission and discharge than the affective group; only at discharge are their scores higher than those of the schizoaffective group (Table 3). At admission, the schizoaffectives' scores on the ScS scale equal those of the schizophrenics. On the AfS scale, their scores are even clearly higher than those of the purely affective group. At follow-up, the schizophrenics obtain higher scores on both the ScS and the AfS scales than the two other groups. They are even slightly higher than their own values at discharge 5–8 years earlier.

The correlational analysis of variables (Tables 4–6) reveals several statistically significant associations among the variables. Table 4, which presents the

Table 3. Range and quartiles of ScS and AfS scores (see Table 1)

	Minimum	1st quartile	Median	3rd quartile	Maximum
1. Total group of patients					
ScS at admission	0.00	1.00	5.00	10.00	35.00
AfS at admission	1.00	10.00	17.00	24.00	43.00
ScS at discharge	0.00	0.00	0.00	1.00	9.00
AfS at discharge	0.00	2.00	5.00	8.00	28.00
ScS at follow-up	0.00	0.00	0.00	1.00	14.00
AfS at follow-up	0.00	4.00	7.00	12.00	30.00
2. Diagnostic subgroup of schizophrenics					
ScS at admission	1.00	4.00	8.50	13.25	35.00
AfS at admission	1.00	7.75	15.00	18.25	33.00
ScS at discharge	0.00	0.00	0.50	3.00	9.00
AfS at discharge	0.00	2.75	6.00	10.00	28.00
ScS at follow-up	0.00	0.00	0.00	4.00	14.00
AfS at follow-up	2.00	4.00	8.00	12.00	27.00
3. Diagnostic subgroup of schizoaffectives					
ScS at admission	0.00	3.75	8.50	18.25	29.00
AfS at admission	5.00	17.00	26.50	31.25	42.00
ScS at discharge	0.00	0.00	0.00	0.00	3.00
AfS at discharge	0.00	1.00	4.00	10.25	21.00
ScS at follow-up	0.00	0.00	0.00	0.00	4.00
AfS at follow-up	0.00	0.75	4.00	8.00	16.00
4. Diagnostic subgroup of affectives					
ScS at admission	0.00	0.00	0.00	3.00	6.00
AfS at admission	2.00	11.00	17.00	24.00	43.00
ScS at discharge	0.00	0.00	0.00	0.00	2.00
AfS at discharge	0.00	2.00	4.00	6.00	12.00
ScS at follow-up	0.00	0.00	0.00	0.00	2.00
AfS at follow-up	1.00	5.00	9.00	14.00	30.00

Table 4. Intercorrelations among the 16 predictors

	1	2	3	4	5	6	7	8	9	10	11	12	13	14	15	16
Male sex 1	—															
Young age 2	07	—														
Difficulties at work 3	00	−09	—													
Lack of social adaptability 4	15	13	07	—												
Lack of const. partnership 5	−09	38***	−09	12	—											
Insidious onset (disease) 6	05	11	12	13	03	—										
Chronic course till admiss. 7	17	10	10	42***	08	56***	—									
Chronic abuse 8	30**	00	17	27**	−08	−09	13	—								
Insidious onset (index) 9	10	03	23*	10	00	44***	44***	07	—							
ScS at admission 10	00	07	−09	06	−03	−02	−09	−04	05	—						
AfS at admission 11	−03	−11	−08	00	−14	−11	−13	−14	06	25*	—					
ScS at discharge 12	−04	11	16	−03	17	03	29**	08	00	11	−10	—				
AfS at discharge 13	09	04	23*	14	00	12	15	16	19	18	20*	33***	—			
Bad state at discharge 14	20*	08	26**	30**	07	14	33***	27**	16	05	−07	44***	48***	—		
Diagnosis of schizophrenia vs. schizoaffect. + affect. psychoses at discharge 15	20*	20*	19	23*	17	28**	31**	32***	03	31**	−31**	42***	18	49***	—	
Diagnosis of schizophrenia + schizoaff. vs. affect. psychoses at discharge 16	07	30**	−05	17	33***	15	10	25*	06	54***	−04	28*	22*	32**	64***	—

0. for correlation coefficients omitted. $*P < 0.05$; $**P < 0.01$; $***P < 0.001$.

Table 5. Intercorrelations among the criteria

		a	b	c	d	e	f
ScS at follow-up	a	—					
AfS at follow-up	b	21*	—				
GAS score	c	−52***	−59***	—			
Lack of prof. efficiency	d	35***	38***	−59***	—		
Working incapacity	e	37***	40***	−55***	47***	—	
Time in hospital	f	37***	14	−52***	39***	66***	—

0. for correlation coefficients omitted. $*P < 0.05$; $**P < 0.01$; $***P < 0.001$.

coefficients of correlation among the 16 predictors, contains 38 values which are significant at the 5% level instead of around six as expected by chance. Only one of the correlations, i.e., that between the two different combinations of diagnoses (variables 15 and 16), is spurious; all others are substantial. An argument in favor of the assumption that they indicate real relationships among the variables is the fact that only in one case is the correlation negative (between variables 11 and 15). This is obviously meaningful, because the affective symptomatology at admission (AfS) should be lower in schizophrenics than in manics, depressives, and schizoaffectives. It is also notable that, e.g., an insidious onset of the psychosis (6) and of the index episode (9) and a chronic course until admission (7) are closely interrelated. It has to be mentioned that the combination of schizoaffective psychoses with the purely affective psychoses – compared with schizophrenic psychoses alone – yields more significant associations with data obtained at discharge (namely eight) than their combination with schizophrenic psychoses in comparison with the purely affective psychoses (namely four). Of the 11 variables assessed at admission (1–11), six show a significant association with one or two of the three indicators of a bad short-term outcome at discharge (12–14), namely male sex (3), insidious onset of the index episode (9), a chronic course until admission (7), difficulties at work (3), lack of social adaptability (8), and, amazingly, affective symptomatology at admission (13). This is probably due to components of the IMPS factor RTD in the AfS (see Table 1), which may reflect negative symptoms of schizophrenia.

The correlation coefficients among the six criteria for course and/or outcome (Table 5) are in the expected directions, i.e., they bear positive signs, with the exception of the association with the GAS, which is scored in the direction of a favorable outcome (see section on Data Handling). Remarkably, only two coefficients (17 vs. 18 and 18 vs. 20) are not significant, and in one case (17 vs. 18) this is in accord with the definition of the variables (ScS and AfS) which should reflect relatively independent dimensions of psychopathology (see section on Data Handling). The other insignificant correlation is that between AfS at follow-up and the time spent in psychiatric institutions during the follow-up period. The latter variable (22) is, however, significantly related to the ScS at

Table 6. Correlations between predictors and criteria

		a ScS	b AfS	c GAS	d Lack prof. eff.	e Working incapacity	f Time in hospital
Male sex	1	07	11	-16	22*	05	04
Young age	2	10	-04	-11	15	06	17
Difficulties at work	3	16	03	-12	17	18	14
Lack of social adaptability	4	22*	19	-26**	36***	14	11
Lack of const. partnership	5	23*	-01	-20*	15	29**	31**
Insidious onset (disease)	6	23*	08	-13	20*	12	13
Chronic course till admiss.	7	23*	02	-13	19	10	06
Chronic abuse	8	00	-01	03	17	-06	-09
Insidious onset (index)	9	16	01	-09	12	12	26**
ScS at admission	10	18	-25*	-06	19	05	03
AfS at admission	11	-09	-03	21*	-17	-13	-17
ScS at discharge	12	14	05	-18	16	11	23*
AfS at discharge	13	07	15	-17	19	23*	17
Bad state at discharge	14	20*	18	-41***	43***	38***	30**
Diagnosis of schizophrenia vs. schizoaffect. + affect. psychoses at discharge	15	40***	11	-48***	43***	34***	39***
Diagnosis of schizophrenia + schizoaffect. vs. affect. psychoses at discharge	16	27**	-13	-24*	20*	15	25**

0. for correlation coefficients omitted. $*P < 0.05$; $**P < 0.01$; $***P < 0.001$.

follow-up. On the whole, the correlations among the criteria are more consistent and also higher than those among the predictors.

From the point of view of the long-term prognosis of different forms of functional psychoses, the correlations between predictors and criteria for course and/or outcome are the most important ones (Table 6). Twenty-nine of them reach the 5% level of significance, i.e., almost six times more than the five expected by chance. Furthermore, they are, with only one minor exception, in the expected direction. The exception relates to the negative correlation between ScS at admission and AfS at follow-up.

The significant values are unevenly distributed over the 16 predictors and the six criteria. Among the latter, the AfS score at follow-up is significantly associated with only one predictor, the SfS at admission (see above), whereas the ScS score is correlated significantly with almost every second predictor (seven of 16). The other criteria exhibit six (GAS score and time spent in hospital), five (professional efficiency during the follow-up period), or four (working incapacity during this period) significant correlations with the predictors. Among the predictors, three are not significantly associated with any of the criteria. They are young age (variable 2), difficulties at work (3), and chronic abuse of alcohol and/or other drugs (9). The others correlate significantly with at least one of the criteria. This is true for male sex (1), insidious onset of the psychosis (6) and of the index episode (7), chronic course before hospital admission (8), and the symptom scores at admission and discharge (10–13). The most powerful predictors with six significant out of seven correlation coefficients are the global rating of the psychopathological state at discharge (14) and the diagnostic dichotomy of schizophrenic versus affective and schizoaffective psychoses (15). The diagnostic combination of schizophrenic with schizoaffective psychoses against purely affective psychoses (16) reduces the number of significant correlation coefficients with the criteria by only one, but it also remarkably diminishes the degree of the other significant correlations. On the basis of information on the number and degree of significant correlations with the criteria, it cannot be decided whether the combination of schizoaffective and purely affective psychoses as opposed to schizophrenic psychoses increases the predictive value of the diagnostic dichotomy of functional psychoses compared with the combination of schizoaffective and schizophrenic psychoses only because of the favorable psychopathological outcome of schizoaffective psychoses at discharge from index hospitalization. According to the frequency distributions of predictors (Table 3) and their intercorrelations (Table 5), this might be the case.

In order to explore this question more thoroughly, a stepwise multiple regression analysis was performed. The resulting optimal combinations of predictors per criterion for course and/or outcome (Table 7) clearly indicate the predictive power of the diagnostic dichotomy into schizophrenic vs. schizoaffective and purely affective psychoses: This and only this – not the alternative dichotomy into schizophrenic and schizoaffective vs. purely affective psychoses alone – enters into the multiple regression equations for the prediction of four of the six predictors, once alone and three times in combination with other vari-

Table 7. Multiple regression analysis

Predictors[a] No. Term	beta weight	Criterion[a] Code Term	% variance explained by the combination of predictors
15 Diagnosis of schizophrenia vs. schizoaffect. + affect. psychoses at discharge	0.40	a ScS at follow-up above median	15.23
10 ScS at admission	−0.26	b AfS at follow-up above median	8.54
4 Lack of social adaptability	0.20		
15 Diagnosis of schizophrenia vs. schizoaffect. + affect. psychoses at discharge	−0.37	c GAS score <60 (last week before follow-up)	25.62
14 Bad psychopathological state at discharge	−0.23		
14 Bad psychopathological state at discharge	0.24	d Lack of professional efficiency (last year before follow-up)	27.52
15 Diagnosis of schizophrenia vs. schizoaffect. + affect. psychoses at discharge	0.26		
4 Lack of social adaptability	0.23		
14 Bad psychopathological state at discharge	0.36	e Working incapacity during follow-up >5%	19.93
5 Lack of constant partnership	0.27		
15 Diagnosis of schizophrenia vs. schizoaffect. + affect. psychoses at discharge	0.34	f Time in hospital during follow-up >5%	19.46
5 Lack of constant partnership	0.25		

[a] See Table 2.

ables. The latter are lack of partnership before index admission (once), the global rating of the psychopathological state at discharge (twice), and lack of social adaptability before index admission (once, in addition to the mental state at discharge). The mental state at discharge also enters into another equation, this time together with a lack of partnership before index admission. Neither the diagnostic dichotomy of schizophrenic vs. schizoaffective and purely affective psychoses nor the mental state at discharge before index hospitalization are among the predictors of one dependent variable, i.e., AfS at follow-up. This outcome criterion is only poorly predictable by two other independent variables, namely lack of social adaptability before and a low ScS score at index admission. The other criteria's variations, which are explained by the combination of predictors in the respective equations, range from 15% (for ScS at follow-up) to 28% (for professional efficiency during the last year before follow-up and the time spent in psychiatric hospitals during the follow-up period). The diagnostic dichotomy of functional psychoses into schizophrenic vs. schizoaffective and purely affective psychoses is among the predictors of the three criteria (c, d, and f), more than 25% of whose variance can be explained.

Discussion

In our analysis of data from a follow-up study of 103 former inpatients with an index diagnosis of a functional psychosis, the predictive value of grouping schizoaffective psychoses together with purely affective psychoses clearly exceeded that of including the schizoaffective in the schizophrenic group. The larger resemblance of schizoaffective and affective than of schizoaffective and schizophrenic psychoses was evident in the frequency distribution of most of our 16 variables serving as predictors and the six variables serving as criteria of an unfavorable – or, in one instance (the GAS at follow-up) of a favorable – course and/or outcome. On the whole, the schizophrenics could be distinguished from the two other groups of psychotics as the most disadvantaged group (see also Möller et al. 1988).

Remarkably, at admission the schizoaffective group obtained not only high scores on the additive scale reflecting schizophrenic symptomatology (ScS), but even the highest scores on the scale measuring affective symptomatology (AfS). This indicates that they indeed displayed a schizo*affective* symptom pattern and that the diagnosis was not only based on data concerning the previous course (acute onset, no chronicity, etc.) and the favorable short-term course during the index hospitalization documented by the global ratings of their mental state at discharge. At follow-up, the schizophrenics received the comparatively highest scores on both the AfS and, in particular, the ScS scales. This is concordant with the higher values they obtained in the other four criteria for an unfavorable course and/or outcome and could be expected beforehand.

In complete agreement with the distributions of scores of predictors and criteria, the correlational analysis of these variables yielded a closer relationship of the diagnostic dichotomy of schizophrenic vs. affective and schizoaffective psychoses to other potential predictors of an unfavorable course and/or outcome than that of schizophrenic plus schizoaffective vs. purely affective psychoses. Above all, the first dichotomy proved to be most closely associated with the different criteria for an unfavorable course and/or outcome, followed by the global rating of the mental state at discharge from index hospitalization and by the second diagnostic dichotomy. Among the other predictors, only two social variables, lack of social adaptability and lack of partnership before index admission, correlated significantly with more than one or two of the criteria. However, the more powerful predictors were the clinical variables, diagnosis, and psychopathological state at discharge.

In a stepwise multiple regression analysis, only the first diagnostic dichotomy, the mental state at discharge, and the two social variables just mentioned, entered more than once into the equations for predicting criteria of course and/or outcome. The ScS score at admission, combined with lack of social adaptability, was the best predictor of the AfS score at follow-up. However, this prediction can be disregarded because it explained less than 10% of the variance of the outcome criterion. With one exception (ScS score at follow-up), the other criteria were predictable to at least one fifth and up to more than one fourth of their variance.

Apparently, clinical variables other than diagnosis and mental state at discharge did not enter into the regression equations because of their redundancy: They were taken into account in making the diagnosis and partially (namely the symptoms still present at discharge that were added up to the ScS and the AfS scores) in rating the patients' psychopathological state at discharge globally.

The fact that both diagnosis *and* state at discharge were represented in the same equations indicates that they carried, in part, independent information: The predictive value of combining the schizoaffective with the purely affective psychoses in the first diagnostic dichotomy cannot be entirely explained by their more favorable short-term outcome during index hospitalization compared with schizophrenic psychoses. In view of the high ScS and AfS scores of schizoaffective patients at admission, it should be possible to diagnose these disorders before the remission has taken place by the end of hospitalization. There may be differences between these psychotic subtypes with respect to course and outcome over a longer period of time than in our study. Even for a follow-up period of similar length, the prognosis of schizoaffective psychoses would probably be less favorable if the previous course of the disorder and the tendency to clinical and social remission during the index episode were not taken into account when making the diagnosis. Furthermore, there are apparent differences in the genetic background of affective and schizoaffective disorders; this is more homogeneous in the former than in the latter (see Zerbin-Rüdin 1988). Therefore, it would be appropriate to specify the schizoaffective subtype in diagnostic schemata more clearly than in the DSM-III and DSM-III-R. Nonetheless, from the point of view of short-term prognosis and the prediction of course and outcome for several years, it is apparently justified to group the schizoaffective psychoses together with the affective and not with the schizophrenic psychoses (as in ICD-9). Consequently, Jaspers' hierarchical rule should no longer serve as a guideline in the diagnostic grouping of endogenous psychoses.

References

Abrams R, Taylor MA (1981) Importance of schizophrenic symptoms in the diagnosis of mania. Am J Psychiatry 138:658–661

American Psychiatric Association (1952) Diagnostic and statistical manual: mental disorders (DSM), 1st edn. American Psychiatric Association, Washington DC

American Psychiatric Association (1968, 1980, 1987) Diagnostic and statistical manual of mental disorders, 2nd edn (DSM-II); 3rd edn (DSM-III); 3rd edn revised (DSM-III-R). American Psychiatric Association, Washington DC

Angst J (1966) Zur Ätiologie und Nosologie endogener depressiver Psychosen. Springer, Berlin Heidelberg New York

Angst J (1986) The course of schizoaffective disorders. In: Marneros A, Tsuang MT (eds) Schizoaffective psychoses. Springer, Berlin Heidelberg New York Tokyo, pp 63–93

Barthelmes H, von Zerssen D (1978) Das Münchener Psychiatrische Informationssystem (PSYCHIS München). In: Reichertz PL, Schwarz B (eds) Informationssysteme in der medizinischen Versorgung. Schattauer, Stuttgart, pp 138–145

Berger M, Wittchen H-U, von Zerssen D (1984) Versuche der Typisierung von Subgruppen depressiver Erkrankungen anhand multivariater statistischer Analysen von Selbst- und Fremdbeurteilungsskalen sowie operationaler Diagnosekriterien. In: Wolfersdorf MG, Straub R, Hole G (eds) Depressiv Kranke in der Psychiatrischen Klinik. Roderer, Regensburg, pp 390–402

Clare A, Cairns VE (1978) Design, development and use of a standardized interview to assess social maladjustment and dysfunction in community studies. Psychol Med 8:589–604

Dunner DL, Gershon ES, Goodwin FK (1976) Heritable factors in the severity of affective illness. Biol Psychiatry 11:31–42

Endicott J, Spitzer RL, Fleiss JL, Cohen J (1976) The Global Assessment Scale: a procedure for measuring overall severity of psychiatric disturbances. Arch Gen Psychiatry 33:766–771

Faltermaier T, Wittchen, H-U, Ellmann R, Lässle R (1985) The Social Interview Schedule (SIS): content, structure and reliability. Soc Psychiatry 20:115–124

Hecht H, Faltermaier A, Wittchen H-U (1987) Social Interview Schedule (SIS): halbstrukturiertes Interview zur Erfassung der aktuellen sozialpsychologischen Situation. Roderer, Regensburg

Hiller W, von Zerssen D, Mombour W, Wittchen H-U (1986) IMPS: Inpatient Multidimensional Psychiatric Scale (Deutsche Bearbeitung). Beltz Test, Weinheim

Huber G, Gross G, Schüttler R (1979) Schizophrenie. Springer, Berlin Heidelberg New York

Jaspers K (1972) General psychopathology. Manchester University Press, Manchester

Kasanin J (1933) The acute schizoaffective psychoses. Am J Psychiatry 90:97–126

Kraepelin (1913) Psychiatrie, 8th edn, vol 3, pt 2. Barth, Leipzig

Lorr M, Klett CJ (1967) Inpatient Multidimensional Psychiatric Scale (IMPS), rev edn. Consulting Psychologists, Palo Alto CA

Marneros A, Tsuang MT (eds) (1986) Schizoaffective psychoses. Springer, Berlin Heidelberg New York Tokyo

Marneros A, Deister A, Rohde A, Jünemann H, Fimmers R (1988) Long-term course of schizoaffective disorders, pt 1: definitions, methods, frequency of episodes and cycles. Eur Arch Psychiatry Neurol Sci 237:264–275

Mendlewicz J, Linkowski P, Wilmotte J (1979) Relationship between schizoaffective illness and affective disorders or schizophrenia: morbidity risk and genetic transmission. In: Obiols J, Ballus C, Gonzalez Monclus E, Pujol J (eds) Biological psychiatry today, vol A. Elsevier, Amsterdam, pp 406–411

Möller H-J, von Zerssen D (1986) Der Verlauf schizophrener Psychosen unter den gegenwärtigen Behandlungsbedingungen. Springer, Berlin Heidelberg New York Tokyo

Möller H-J, Schmid-Bode W, Cording-Tömmel C, Wittchen H-U, Zaudig M, von Zerssen D (1988) Psychopathological and social outcome in schizophrenia versus affective/schizoaffective psychoses and prediction of poor outcome in schizophrenia: results from a 5–8 year follow-up. Acta Psychiatr Scand 77:379–389

Perris C (1966) A study of bipolar (manic-depressive) and unipolar recurrent depressive psychoses. Acta Psychiatr Scand [Suppl] 194:1–89

Pope HG jr, Lipinski JF (1978) Diagnosis in schizophrenia and manic-depressive illness: a reassessment of the specificity of "schizophrenic" symptoms in the light of current research. Arch Gen Psychiatry 35:811–828

Pope HG jr, Lipinski JF, Cohen BM, Axelrod DT (1980) "Schizoaffective disorder": an invalid diagnosis? A comparison of schizoaffective disorder, schizophrenia, and affective disorder. Am J Psychiatry 137:921–927

Robins LN, Helzer JE, Croughan J, Ratcliff KS (1981) National Institute of Mental Health Diagnostic Interview Schedule: its history, characteristics, and validity. Arch Gen Psychiatry 38:381–389

Schmid W, Bronisch T, von Zerssen D (1982) A comparative study of PSE/CATEGO and DiaSika: two psychiatric computer diagnostic systems. Br J Psychiatry 141:292–295

Schneider K (1959) Clinical psychopathology. Grune and Stratton, New York

Strauss JS, Carpenter WT (1974) The prediction of outcome in schizophrenia. II. Relationships between predictor and outcome variables: a report from the WHO International Pilot Study of Schizophrenia. Arch Gen Psychiatry 31:37–42

Vogl G, Zaudig M (1985) Investigation of operationalized diagnostic criteria in the diagnosis of schizoaffective and cycloid psychoses. Compr Psychiatry 26:1–10

von Zerssen D (1976) Klinische Selbstbeurteilungs-Skalen (KSb-S) aus dem Münchener Psychiatrischen Informations-System (PSYCHIS München). Manuale. Beltz Test, Weinheim

von Zerssen D (1980) Konstitution. In: Kisker KP, Meyer J-E, Müller C, Strömgren E (eds) Psychiatrie der Gegenwart, vol I/2, 2nd edn. Springer, Berlin Heidelberg New York, pp 619–705

von Zerssen D (1985) Psychiatric syndromes from a clinical and a biostatistical point of view. Psychopathology 18:88–97

von Zerssen D (1986a) Diagnose; Nosologie; Syndrom; Typus. In: Müller C (ed) Lexikon der Psychiatrie, 2nd edn. Springer, Berlin Heidelberg New York Tokyo, pp 194–198, 474–477, 662–664, 696–699

von Zerssen D (1986b) Clinical Self-Rating Scales (CSRS) of the Munich Psychiatric Information System (PSYCHIS München). In: Sartorius N, Ban TA (eds) Assessment of depression. Springer Berlin Heidelberg New York Tokyo, pp 270–303

von Zerssen D, Hecht H (1987) Gesundheit, Glück, Zufriedenheit im Licht einer katamnestischen Erhebung an psychiatrischen Patienten und gesunden Probanden. Psychother Psychosom Med Psychol 37:83–96

Welner A, Croughan J, Fishman R, Robins E (1977) The group of schizoaffective and related psychoses: a follow-up study. Compr Psychiatry 18:413–422

Wittchen H-U, von Zerssen D (1988) Verläufe behandelter und unbehandelter Depressionen und Angststörungen. Springer, Berlin Heidelberg New York Tokyo

Wittchen H-U, Essau CA, Hecht H, Teder W, Pfister H (1989) Reliability of life event assessments: test-retest reliability and fall-off effects of the Munich Interview for the assessment of A Life Events and Conditions. J Affective Disord 16:77–91

World Health Organization (1978) Mental disorders: glossary and guide to their classification in accordance with the ninth revision of the International Classification of Diseases. World Health Organization, Geneva

Zaudig M, Vogl G (1983) Zur Frage der operationalisierten Diagnostik schizoaffektiver und zykloider Psychosen. Arch Psychiatr Nervenkr 233:385–396

Zerbin-Rüdin E (1986) Schizoaffective and other atypical psychoses: the genetical aspect. In: Marneros A, Tsuang MT (eds) Schizoaffective psychoses. Springer, Berlin Heidelberg New York Tokyo, pp 225–231

Zerbin-Rüdin E (1988) Beiträge der genetischen Forschung zur Klassifikation affektiver Störungen. In: von Zerssen D, Möller H-J (eds) Affektive Störungen. Springer, Berlin Heidelberg New York Tokyo, pp 29–45

Schizoaffective Disorders in Clinical Routine: Symptomatology, Etiology, and Course

R.-D. STIEGLITZ and H. HELMCHEN[1]

Introduction

In 1933, Kasanin introduced the concept of "schizoaffective psychoses" (SAP) to describe a group of young patients with a seemingly normal premorbid personality, who present a sudden onset of the disorder with both schizophrenic as well as affective symptoms and who have a good prognosis. This group of psychotic disorders has met with increasing interest ever since. This refers both to theoretical considerations about the development of nosological concepts (see Pichot 1986) as well as a great number of empirical research activities on various levels (see Brockington and Meltzer 1983; Clayton 1982; Hilz 1987; Procci 1976; Tsuang and Marneros 1986).

The status of this group of disorders remains unclear in spite of intensive research efforts, which have increased in the past 15–20 years. This is reflected, for example, in the revised version of the DSM-III (DSM-IIIR, APA 1987), ". . . one of the most confusing and controversial concepts in psychiatric nosology . . ." (p. 208).

In particular, the relationship to the schizophrenic and the affective disorders has not been clarified to date. As in the DSM-III (APA 1980), the SAP are assigned to the "psychotic disorders not elsewhere classified" in the revised version (DSM-IIIR, APA 1987). In the ICD-10, currently in preparation by the WHO in Geneva, the SAP are located among the mood (affective) disorders in the draft of April 1987 but are again among the schizophrenic disorders in the draft of April 1988, as was already the case in the ICD-9; the definition of the schizoaffective disorders has remained more or less unchanged in the ICD-10 compared with the ICD-9 (Albus et al., in press). Viewed from the standpoint of classification (Angst et al. 1983; Brockington and Meltzer 1983. Kendell 1986) the foremost task is to delimit the SAP from the schizophrenic and affective psychoses and to assign them to one of the two groups, or to arrange them along a continuum (see also Crow 1986) between the two poles. Based on Jaspers' hierarchical principle, clinicians seem more likely to see the SAP as a variant of schizophrenia (Sprock 1988). However, the research results are very mixed when a great number of characteristic features are considered (among others, course). This may depend on – among other things – the great number of competing definitions of SAP (Maier et al. 1986; Berner and Lenz 1986) and on

[1] Freie Universität Berlin, Abteilung für Psychiatrie, Eschenallee 3, 1000 Berlin (West) 19, FRG

Affective and Schizoaffective Disorders
Edited by A. Marneros and M.T. Tsuang
© Springer-Verlag Berlin Heidelberg 1990

methodological problems (Angst 1980). There is also disagreement about whether a subclassification of the SAP is possible and meaningful (e.g., Tsuang and Simpson 1984) or not (e.g., McGlashan and Williams 1987), and whether a multiaxial classification is necessary (Maj and Perris 1985).

At present, there is no generally accepted definition whose validity has been adequately proven (e.g., with respect to course, therapy response). The position of the SAP in relation to the schizophrenic and affective psychoses is likewise the object of a series of follow-up studies, taking the outcome in particular into consideration (see Coryell and Zimmerman 1988). Here, too, the results are rather heterogeneous. While some authors perceive a greater similarity to the schizophrenic psychoses (Williams and McGlashan 1987), others stress greater similarity with the affective psychoses (Möller et al. 1988) or postulate an intermediate position (Harrow and Grossman 1984).

In a series of studies, an attempt was made to describe the course of SAP in a differentiated form with respect to the stability or the change of the psycho-pathological picture (Winokur et al. 1985; Marneros et al. 1988a). However, in this regard as well, many questions remain (Angst 1986).

According to Marneros and Tsuang (1986), there is agreement only about the fact that the SAP refer to a heterogeneous group of disorders, contingent not only on differing nosological concepts, and that presently one cannot do without the diagnosis of SAP. In this situation, further empirical studies using a large population seem appropriate to examine both the relationship of the SAP to schizophrenic and to affective psychoses as well as the possibility of their subdivision into homogeneous subgroups. However, future research should start with a broad definition of the SAP (Kendell 1986). Here, the classification in the ICD-9 can be regarded as a relatively broad concept of the SAP. These clinical diagnoses still have a value in research and practice (Pietzcker 1988; Huber et al.

Table 1. ICD-9 final diagnosis (1981–1988)

ICD-9 category	Subgroups	No. of cases[a]
Schizophrenic psychoses	295.3: paranoid type	1303
	295.7: schizoaffective type	340
Affective psychoses	296.0: manic-depressive psychosis, manic type	31
	296.1: manic-depressive psychosis, depressed type	685
	296.2: manic-depressive psychosis, circular type but currently manic	163
	296.3: manic-depressive psychosis, circular type but currently depressed	225

[a] Including repeated admissions.

1989), despite existing criticism (for instance, that they are less reliable than operationalized diagnoses).

The following questions were the object of the study presented here:
1. What picture do the SAP present in the clinical routine?
2. In what relation do the SAP stand to the schizophrenic and affective psychoses?
3. Can homogeneous subgroups be formed within the SAP?

The description of the SAP on the basis of anamnestic, psychopathological, and somatic variables is effected using the AMDP (Arbeitsgemeinschaft für Methodik und Dokumentation in der Psychiatrie) system (AMDP 1981; Guy and Ban 1982; see below). According to an inquiry made by Emrich and Hippius (1984), the ICD-9 and the AMDP are the diagnostic and documentational procedures most frequently used in research and practice in German-speaking countries.

Subjects and Methods

Subjects

The AMDP data at the time of admission and discharge served as the starting point for the following analyses. In addition, the admission and final diagnoses were based upon the ICD-9 (Table 1) for all patients with an SAP, and the following diagnostic groups served as comparisons:

- Schizophrenic psychoses:
  295.3: paranoid type (abbr.: SPP)
- Affective psychoses:
  296.0: manic-depressive psychosis, manic type (abbr.: MT)
  296.1: manic-depressive psychosis, depressed type (abbr.: DT)

Table 2. Features of study population (ICD-9: 295.7 schizoaffective disorder, $n = 207$)

Sex Female ($n = 115$)	55.6%
Male ($n = 92$)	44.4%
Ratio	1.25:1
Age of onset (years)	
Mean	26.8
SD	9.7
Range	13–64
Age of study (years)	
Mean	39.6
SD	11.7
Range	21–76
Number of episodes	458
Number of first manifestations	32

296.2: manic-depressive psychosis, circular type but currently manic (abbr.: MCT)

296.3: manic-depressive psychosis, circular type but currently depressed (abbr.: DCT).

There were more women than men in the group of SAP (Table 2). The mean age at first manifestation was about 26.8 years, the age at the time of the study about 39.6 years. For 32 patients it was a matter of first manifestation. Unless otherwise mentioned, the patients were entered into the following analyses only once.

Instrument of Evaluation

The AMDP system was used to describe the patients (AMDP 1981; Guy and Ban 1982). It is a documentation system that contains predominantly general information and data recorded using ratings at the start of treatment. Through repeated use, one can illustrate – for example – the course of the treatment.

The system consists of the following parts, ready for electronic data processing:

1. Anamnesis 1: demographic data (e.g., education, level of employment)
2. Anamnesis 2: life events (e.g., death of spouse/partner, shop/business defunct)
3. Anamnesis 3: psychiatric history (e.g., birth and childhood, previous psychiatric episodes)
4. Psychopathological symptoms: 100 items
5. Somatic signs: 40 items.

A manual (AMDP 1981; Guy and Ban 1982) with explanations of the anamnestic sheets and definitions of the psychopathological symptoms and somatic signs is available as an aid to the user. A test manual (Baumann and Stieglitz 1983) summarizes the empirical studies concerning the AMDP system.

Since its publication, a number of studies have been performed using the AMDP system, dealing mainly with the system evaluation (reliability and validity; see Baumann and Stieglitz 1983, 1989) in the context of studies of psychotropic drugs (Bobon et al. 1983). A review by Stieglitz et al. (1987) indicates the various diagnostic uses of the system. Most of the information contained in the AMDP system can be assigned in the manner of a multiaxial classification to the areas of symptomatology, etiology, and time (Stieglitz et al. 1988; Table 3). This classification also serves as the basis for the following analyses.

Empirical studies about SAP using the AMDP system are clearly underrepresented in comparison to those relating to the schizophrenic and affective psychoses. Most still refer to the AMP system, the forerunner of the AMDP system (Fähndrich and Helmchen 1983; Baumann and Stieglitz 1983). They deal mainly with the distinction of SAP from other groups (Baumann 1974; Angst and Scharfetter 1980; Sulz-Blume 1980; Sulz 1981) and with classification problems in this connection (Angst et al. 1983; Brauchli 1981).

Table 3. Axes of the AMDP system

Axis I Symptomatology[a]	Axis II Etiology	Axis III Time
Paranoid-hallucinatory syndrome (PARHAL)	22[b] Precipitating factors – answered by patient – answered by psychiatrist – divergency between patient and psychiatrist	24 Present illness – First manifestation – Age at first manifestation
Psycho-organic syndrome (PSYORG)	23 Life events	25 Characteristics of previous illness – Course since first manifestation – intermittent or chronic – full or partial remission – Severity (increased, decreased, constant, or fluctuating) – Changes in symptomatology
Manic syndrome (MANI)	23 Other current illnesses	
Depressive syndrome (DEPRES)	26 Present episode – Somatic problems – Psychological problems	26 Present episode – Duration of present episode
Hostility syndrome (HOST)	27 Birth and childhood – Pathological pregnancy and/or birth – Motor and/or speech delay – Childhood neurotic symptoms	31 Suicide attempts (patient) – The number of confirmed attempts – The time in relation to the present admission
Apathy syndrome (APA)	28 Family psychiatric history	32 Previous psychiatric episodes
Autonomic syndrome (AUT)		33 Number of previous psychiatric admissions

[a] Syndromes of Gebhardt et al. (1983), Pietzcker et al. (1983).
[b] Item number (see AMDP 1981; Guy and Ban 1982).

Table 4. Definitions of schizoaffective episodes

SAP episodes[a]	Corresponding AMDP syndromes[b]
Schizophrenic	Paranoid-hallucinatory syndrome
Depressive	Depressive syndrome and/or apathy syndrome
Manic	Manic syndrome
Manic-depressive mixed	Manic syndrome and depressive syndrome and/or apathy syndrome
Schizodepressive	Paranoid-hallucinatory syndrome and depressive syndrome and/or apathy syndrome
Schizomanic	Paranoid-hallucinatory syndrome and manic syndrome
Schizomanic-depressive mixed	Paranoid-hallucinatory syndrome and manic syndrome and depressive syndrome and/or apathy syndrome
Not definable	

[a] According to Marneros et al. (1988a).
[b] Gebhardt et al. (1983); Pietzcker et al. (1983); see Table 3.

Definitions

Episode

Unlike the definition given by Marneros et al. (1988a), an episode is to be understood as the cross-sectional picture upon admission to the clinic. Analogous to Maneros et al. (1988a), one can differentiate between eight types of SAP based upon logical combinations and corresponding with the predominant psychopathological picture of an episode (Table 4): schizophrenic, depressive, manic, manic-depressive mixed, schizomanic, schizodepressive, schizomanic-depressive mixed, and not definable.

At admission, the individual episode is to be characterized by the prominence of the corresponding AMDP syndromes (Gebhardt et al. 1983; Pietzcker et al. 1983). The following were taken into account: paranoid-hallucinatory syndrome (PARHAL), depressive syndrome (DEPRES), manic syndrome (MANI), and apathy syndrome (APA). In various studies (see review in Baumann and Stieglitz 1983, 1989), these have proven to be important in the description of endogenous depression (ICD 296.1 and 296.3: DEPRES; APA) and mania (ICD 296.0 and 296.2: MANI), as well as paranoid schizophrenia (ICD 295.3: PARHAL). Each episode was classified according to the above-mentioned division, if it fell at least within the range of mean – standard deviation of the corresponding reference group in one or more syndromes.

Example. For the total sample of depressive patients, there emerged a mean (M) of 15.62 (SD = 6.50) in the depressive syndrome. Accordingly, an episode of SAP was classified as "depressive" if the raw score in the depressive syndrome was greater than 9 (15.62 − 6.50 = 9.12).

Outcome

To describe the outcome, several variables were considered that are included in the AMDP system, or else can be computed on the basis of those that are included:

1. Short-term (index episode)
   - length of hospital stay
   - psychopathology at discharge
2. Long-term (course of illness up to the index episode)
   - course of first manifestation
   - severity of previous illness in relation to the degree at first manifestation
   - changes in symptomatology.

Statistics

The analysis was made using the SPSS program procedures. It was nonparametrical since the assumptions for the corresponding parametrical procedures were not fulfilled.

Results

Symptomatology

AMDP Syndromes

One-way analyses of variance (Kruskal-Wallis one-way analysis of variance) show significant differences between the groups (Table 5; $P < 0.01$).
    Subsequent selected contrasts (Mann-Whitney U test, $P < 0.05$; Table 6) show the following differences for the SAP:

Table 5. One-way analysis of variance (Kruskal-Wallis, K-W) of the ICD-9 diagnostic groups on axis I (symptomatology) subaxes at admission

AMDP syndromes[a]	K-W P[b]	ICD-9					
		295.3	295.7	296.0	296.1	296.2	296.3
PARHAL	**	61.6	55.9	47.8	46.7	47.8	45.8
PSYORG	**	50.2	48.8	50.4	49.0	46.2	49.6
MANI	**	51.7	58.4	65.8	47.4	68.2	48.2
DEPRES	**	49.1	51.6	52.8	60.5	48.9	59.7
HOST	**	55.3	53.8	57.0	46.7	57.6	48.0
AUT	**	46.1	45.7	45.4	52.5	45.3	48.6
APA	**	53.1	49.4	43.7	56.8	42.3	57.8

[a] For abbreviations see Table 3.
[b] **$\chi^2 \geqslant 15.08$, df $= 5$, $P \leqslant 0.01$.

Table 6. Selected contrasts of the AMDP syndromes (Mann-Whitney U test, $P < 0.05$; ICD-9 295.7 versus 295.3, 296.0, 296.1, 296.2, 296.3) at admission

AMDP syndromes[a]	ICD-9				
	295.3	296.0	296.1	296.2	296.3
PARHAL	<[b]	>	>	>	>
PSYORG					
MANI	>	<	>	<	>
DEPRES	>		<		<
HOST			>	<	>
AUT			<		<
APA	<	>	<	>	<

[a] For abbreviations see Table 3.
[b] >, SAP significantly higher than comparison group; <, SAP significantly lower than comparison group.

1. Compared with the SPP, lower scores for the paranoid-hallucinatory and apathy syndrome and higher scores for the manic and depressive syndrome.
2. Compared with the MT and MCT, higher scores for the paranoid-hallucinatory and apathy syndrome and lower scores for the manic syndrome as well as with the MCT for the hostility syndrome.
3. Compared with the DT and DCT, higher scores for the paranoid-hallucinatory, manic, and hostility syndromes, lower scores for the depressive, apathy, and autonomic syndromes.

The results show that the SAP can be delimited on the syndrome level. They are most often located between the schizophrenic and affective psychoses (manic and/or depressive patients).

Further Symptom Areas

In addition to a description and a differentiation of the SAP on the syndrome level, one finds references in the literature to the consideration of additional psychopathological phenomena:

1. Psychotic productive symptoms (delusions and/or hallucinations; Marneros et al. 1988b).
2. Formal disorders of thinking (Clayton 1982; Shenton et al. 1987).
3. Schneiderian first-rank symptoms (Levitt and Tsuang 1988).
4. Suicidal tendencies (Angst 1980; Clayton 1982; Marneros et al. 1988d).

Table 7 contains the percent frequencies for the occurrence of these symptoms.

Table 7. Comparison of frequencies of the ICD-9 diagnostic groups on selected psychopathological aspects

	Percentage present at admission ICD-9						P^a
	295.3	295.7	296.0	296.1	296.2	296.3	
Delusions	80	64	29	20	27	16	**
Hallucinations	63	31	19	4	6	2	**
Delusions or hallucinations	86	68	33	21	28	17	**
Formal disorders of thought	90	94	91	86	87	87	ns
First-rank symptoms	74	48	19	7	13	4	**
Suicidal tendencies	17	25	5	37	8	47	**

[a] **, $\chi^2 \geqslant 15.08$; df $= 5$, $P \leqslant 0.01$; ns, not significant.

Table 8. Selected contrasts of special psychopathological aspects (Mann-Whitney U test, $P < 0.05$; ICD-9 295.7 versus 295.3, 296.0, 296.1, 296.2, 296.3)

	ICD-9				
	295.3	296.0	296.1	296.2	296.3
Delusions	$<^a$	>	>	>	>
Hallucinations	<		>	>	>
Delusions and hallucinations	<	>	>	>	>
Formal disorders of thought					
First-rank symptoms	<	>	>	>	>

[a] >, SAP significantly higher than comparison group; <, SAP significantly lower than comparison group.

Significant differences (χ^2, df $= 5$, $P < 0.01$) emerge in all of the comparisons except the formal disorders of thinking as defined in the AMDP. As expected, the greatest differences appear between the schizophrenic and the affective psychoses (exception: suicidal tendencies). The SAP occupy an intermediate position between the two, tending toward a somewhat greater similarity to the schizophrenic psychoses. The picture is confirmed by additional comparisons of means concerning the sum values of the individual areas (Kruskal-Wallis' one-way analyses of variance and subsequent pair comparisons using the Mann-Whitney U test; Table 8). Here, significant differences emerge in all of the comparisons (Kruskal-Wallis, $P < 0.01$).

With regard to delusions and hallucinations, the SAP occupy an intermediate position between the schizophrenic and the affective psychoses. They are altogether different from the groups of affective psychoses (exception: hallucinations in comparison with MT) and the schizophrenic patients. The like holds true for Schneider's first-rank symptoms.

For disorders of thinking, no significant difference arises between the groups when the frequencies are compared, but there is a significant difference when means are compared. The SAP occupy an intermediate position here, too, but they do not differ significantly from any other comparison group.

Etiology

The results concerning the AMDP variables presented in Table 9 are those that can be summarized with regard to etiology. With the exception of two variables (other current illnesses, psychological problems) significant differences appear in the frequency comparisons between the groups (χ^2, df = 5, $P < 0.05$).

Stress in the sense of life events in recent years is approximately equally frequent in the SAP as in the SPP, MT, and MCT. Illnesses among family members due to psychiatric disorders are just as frequent in the SAP as in the DCT.

If one looks more closely at only the schizophrenic and affective disorders of the first-degree relatives (without regard to the MT, since no disorders in the family were specified there), the SAP for both illness groups regarding frequency are located in an intermediate position with 4.1% and 8.2%:

Table 9. Comparison of frequencies of the ICD-9 diagnostic groups on axis II (etiology) subaxes

	Percentage present ICD-9						P^a
	295.3	295.7	296.0	296.1	296.2	296.3	
Life-event (in recent years)	71	70	67	47	72	60	**
Other current illnesses	32	25	24	27	31	33	ns
Family psychiatric history	14	22	0	17	13	24	*
Precipitating factors: patient	45	47	43	60	61	52	**
Precipitating factors: psychiatrist	64	60	71	74	66	64	**
Precipitating factors: divergency between patient and psychiatrist	67	61	71	77	70	67	**
Somatic problems	8	16	26	19	2	11	**
Psychological problems	52	63	50	47	63	49	ns
Pathological pregnancy and/or birth	11	4	0	5	9	3	**
Motor and/or speech delay	8	2	5	2	0	0	**
Childhood neurotic symptoms	22	19	10	12	11	11	**

[a] $*\chi^2 \geqslant 11.07$, df = 5, $P \leqslant 0.05$; $**\chi^2 \geqslant 15.08$, df = 5, $P \leqslant 0.01$; ns, not significant.

- Schizophrenic psychoses in the family: 296.3: 0% – 295.3: 6.1%.
- Affective psychoses in the family: 295.3: 2.6% – 296.3: 16.3%.

The agreement with the schizophrenic and the bipolar-depressive psychoses is the greatest with reference to the influences assumed by the psychiatrist and by the patient to promote the illness (precipitating factors).

Somatic problems before the onset of the episode are significantly different between the groups, but the SAP are not particularly striking here.

Regarding developmental disturbances, one finds that childhood neurotic symptoms in particular appear more frequently in the schizophrenic group and in the SAP than in the other groups. With reference to the other two variables, the SAP are different from the schizophrenic psychoses but concur with at least one group of the affective psychoses.

Time

Course

The age at the time of the first manifestation in the five groups differs significantly in the comparison of the analyses of variance (Kruskal-Wallis one-way analysis of variance, $P < 0.05$).

The SAP have a mean age at first manifestation of $M = 26.8$ years ($SD = 9.7$), which lies in the same order of magnitude as that of the SPP ($M = 26.2$, $SD = 8.9$) and MCT ($M = 26.9$, $SD = 10.1$).

It differs significantly (Mann-Whitney U test, $P < 0.05$) from the MT ($M = 40.1$, $SD = 14.0$), DT ($M = 50.1$, $SD = 16.2$), and DCT ($M = 34.5$, $SD = 13.0$).

A significant difference emerges between the groups (χ^2, df = 5, $P < 0.01$) regarding the definite suicide attempts of the patients in the past. The SAP ($= 34\%$) agree most with the MCT ($= 33\%$) and differ from the SPP ($= 23\%$), MT ($= 5\%$), and DT ($= 24\%$) through a greater frequency of suicide attempts and from the DCT ($= 41\%$) through a lesser frequency.

For those patients whose history showed an attempted suicide, differences between the groups emerge with regard to the time interval (χ^2, df = 4, $P < 0.01$). These are frequently further in the past (more than 1 month) for the SAP and the MCT than for the two groups of depressive patients. There is no information for the unipolar manic patients.

Significant differences between the groups appear for the duration of the present episode (χ^2, df = 5, $P < 0.01$). For the SAP, shorter intervals of time emerge more frequently (less than 1 month) between the beginning of the present manifestation and admission; for the two groups of depressive patients, the intervals are more frequently longer (longer than 1 month).

Outcome

Short-term

The groups are significantly different (Kruskal-Wallis one-way analysis of variance; $P < 0.05$) with regard to the length of hospital stay (number of days in the hospital).

Table 10. Selected contrasts of AMDP syndromes (Mann-Whitney U test, $P < 0.05$; ICD-9 295.7 versus 295.3, 296.0, 296.1, 296.2, 296.3) at discharge

AMDP syndromes[a]	ICD-9				
	295.3	296.0	296.1	296.2	296.3
PARHAL	<[b]		>		
PSYORG	<		<		
MANI	>		>		>
DEPRES	<		<		<
HOST	<		>		
AUT	<		<		
APA	<				

[a] For abbreviations see Table 3.
[b] >, SAP significantly higher than comparison group; <, SAP significantly lower than comparison group.

The SAP (M = 68.1, SD = 55.3) are located in the same range as the DT (M = 71.1, SD = 50.9) and DCT (M = 73.6, SD = 43.4). They differ significantly from the MCT (M = 45.8, SD = 35.9) and the MT (M = 41.0, SD = 31.1), but not from the SPP (M = 59.1, SD = 42.2). A significant relationship does emerge for the length of hospital stay and the number of episodes ($r = -0.16$, $P < 0.01$), but the numerical level of the correlation is low.

In addition, significant differences appear in all of the AMDP syndromes at the time of discharge (Kruskal-Wallis one-way analyses of variance, $P < 0.05$). The SAP differ from the schizophrenic patients (Mann-Whitney U test, $P < 0.05$), showing lower scores in all but one of the syndromes (exception: manic syndrome). In comparison with the DT, they have lower scores in the depressive, psycho-organic, and autonomic syndromes and higher scores in the paranoid-hallucinatory, manic, and hostility syndromes. Compared with the DCT, the SAP have lower scores in the depressive and higher scores in the manic syndrome. There are no differences in relation to the MT and MCT (Table 10).

According to Angst et al. (1988), a series of AMDP symptoms can additionally be interpreted as negative symptoms, some of which enter into the apathy syndrome (Gebhardt et al. 1983). At the time of discharge, significant differences appear between the groups (Table 11) in eight of the 14 negative symptoms (χ^2, df = 5, $P < 0.01$).

No symptom occurs more frequently in the SAP; some symptoms do not occur at all (inhibited thinking, blocking, mutism). As expected, negative symptoms are found most frequently among the schizophrenic patients and most rarely in the two groups of manic patients.

When one looks at the SAP particularly in relation to the schizophrenic patients and to both groups of depressive patients the significant differences in frequency are found (a) between schizophrenics and at least one group of

Table 11. Negative symptoms in the AMDP system according to Angst et al. (1988)

	Percentage present at discharge ICD-9						P^a
	295.3	295.7	296.0	296.1	296.2	296.3	
Concentration	49	38	29	26	27	26	**
Inhibited thinking	3	0	0	5	0	4	ns
Retarded thinking	23	10	5	17	6	9	**
Blocking	4	0	0	0	0	0	ns
Incoherence	10	4	5	0	1	0	**
Restricted thinking	14	9	5	16	5	11	ns
Feeling of loss of feeling	2	2	0	6	0	6	ns
Blunted affect	27	18	5	15	7	15	**
Parathymia	19	5	0	0	1	2	**
Affective rigidity	15	10	0	9	8	8	**
Lack of drive	35	16	19	23	12	19	**
Mutism	3	0	0	1	0	0	ns
Reduced social contact	32	12	19	18	5	17	**
Decreased libido	5	5	5	7	0	7	ns

^{a} ** $\chi^2 \geqslant 15.08$, df $= 5$, $P \leqslant 0.01$; ns, not significant.

depressive patients in the symptoms concentration, retarded thinking, incoherence, blunted affect, parathymia, and affective rigidity; (b) below the schizophrenic patients and the two depressive groups in the symptoms lack of drive and reduced social contact.

Long-term

In assessing the long-term outcome, those patients of all of the diagnostic groups of schizophrenic and affective psychoses studies here were taken into consideration for whom one could assuredly assume four previous psychiatric episodes ($n = 197$). Due to the small number of cases, it was not possible to include the MT in the following.

There were no differences between the groups in relation to severity of illness since first manifestation regarding the variables "decreased" and "constant" (χ^2, df $= 4$, $P < 0.05$). On the other hand, differences do emerge for the variables "increased" and "fluctuating" (χ^2, df $= 4$, $P < 0.05$). Here, an increase in the degree of severity is most rarely shown in the SAP and fluctuation most rarely in the DT.

Changes in symptomatology are – as expected – most frequently observed in the SAP and in the two groups of bipolar affective psychoses (χ^2, df $= 4$, $P < 0.05$).

Significant differences do not exist for the course variable "intermittent" (χ^2, df = 4, n.s.). For 13.3% of the SPP and 5% of the DT the course was rated as chronic; this was not the case for any patient in the other groups (χ^2, df = 4, $P < 0.05$).

Significant differences emerge between the groups with regard to remission (χ^2, df = 4, $P < 0.01$). A full or partial remission is most frequently indicated for the SAP. In reference to the differences between full and partial remission, a full remission is observed most frequently in the groups of affective patients. Here, the SAP are located between the schizophrenic and the affective psychoses.

Classification

Clinical Diagnosis

An SAP, as defined by the ICD-9, was diagnosed at discharge in 340 cases from 1981 through 1988 (see Table 1). They are relatively equally distributed over these years (1981: 5.0%, 1982: 5.3%, 1983: 6.7%, 1984: 5.5%, 1985: 7.1%, 1986: 5.2%, 1987: 7.4%, 1988: 7.0%).

Of these 340 cases, 102 had a different diagnosis at admission. Most frequently ($n > 5$) this was:
– Schizophrenic psychosis, paranoid type (295.3: $n = 39$).
– Manic-depressive psychosis, depressed (296.1: $n = 13$).
– Manic-depressive psychosis, circular type but currently manic (296.2: $n = 6$).

Conversely, SAP was diagnosed 288 times at admission. This was changed in 50 cases, most frequently ($n \geqslant 5$) into:
– Schizophrenic psychosis paranoid type (295.3: $n = 11$).
– Manic-depressive psychosis, circular type but currently manic (296.2: $n = 6$).
– Residual schizophrenia (295.6: $n = 5$).

For 18 (= 56%) of the 32 first manifestations it was possible to make the diagnosis within the first episode, for an additional 13 within the second or third episode. This was not possible until the sixth episode for just one patient.

Syndrome Diagnosis

When one examines the psychopathological picture of the SAP cross-sectionally and in terms of course according to the classification into types of episodes (see above) the first manifestations are to be investigated first, and then all episodes together.

First Manifestations

For 32 patients diagnosed as schizoaffective in the first or a subsequent episode it was the first manifestation. For 15 patients (= 47%), psychic stress preceded the first episode.

For the majority of the patients ($n = 13$) a schizodepressive syndrome was apparent at the first hospitalization (Table 12). Other syndromes followed, but

Table 12. Schizoaffective disorder: first manifestation, first episode, course, and type

	n
First manifestation	32
First episode	
schizodepressive	13
depressive	5
other	14
Course (after at least 3 episodes, $n = 14$)	
monomorphous	2
polymorphous	12
Type	
bipolar	7
depressive	7

were by far more infrequent, being found in at most five patients (depressive syndrome). When the course of the first manifestations is further pursued for those who had at least three episodes ($n = 14$, M $= 3.46$, SD $= 0.85$, range 3–6), the results show a polymorphous course for 12 patients ($= 86\%$) and a monomorphous course for only two (only schizodepressive episodes). Here we refer to the differentiation made by Marneros et al. (1988d) into polymorphous (at least one syndrome shift) and monomorphous courses (no syndrome shift).

Among the patients with a polymorphous course, the following data appear:
– Two patients had only schizoaffective episodes.
– Nine patients had purely schizophrenic and/or affective episodes in addition to schizoaffective episodes.
– One patient had only schizophrenic or affective episodes.

When one attempts a further subdivision with respect to bipolar type (current or previous manic syndrome) vs. depressive type (no current or previous manic syndrome; see also DSM-IIIR 1987), seven patients each are alloted to the two types.

All Episodes

For the 207 SAP, there are a total of 458 episodes (Table 13), 42 ($= 9.2\%$) of which could not be definitely assigned to one particular type. Most of the episodes are schizomanic (19%) or purely manic (18.6%). These are followed by the schizodepressive (15.7%), the schizomanic-depressive mixed (13.3%), and the depressive (12%) episodes. Manic-depressive mixed (8.5%) and purely schizophrenic (3.7%) episodes are the rarest.

Depressive episodes appear more frequently among men (18.3% vs. 8.1%) as do schizodepressive episodes (18.8% vs. 13.7%). On the other hand, manic episodes are seen more frequently in women (20.8% vs. 14.8%) as are schizo-

Table 13. Schizoaffective disorder: episodes (total, $n = 458$)

SAP episodes	Male		Female		Total	
	n	%	n	%	n	%
Not definable	10	5.7	32	11.3	42	9.2
Schizophrenic	8	4.6	9	3.1	17	3.7
Depressive	32	18.3	23	8.1	55	12.0
Manic	26	14.8	59	20.8	85	18.6
Schizodepressive	33	18.8	39	13.7	72	15.7
Schizomanic	24	13.7	63	22.2	87	19.0
Manic-depressive mixed	16	9.1	23	8.1	39	8.5
Schizomanic-depressive mixed	26	14.8	35	12.3	61	13.3
Total	175	38.2	283	61.7	458	100

manic episodes (22.2% vs. 13.7%). The other syndrome configurations are approximately equally frequent.

Sociodemographic Variables

With regard to sex distribution (see also Table 1), more women than men receive the diagnosis of an SAP (1.25:1). Most of the patients are single ($n = 78$, 37.6%), married ($n = 73$, 35.2%), or divorced ($n = 43$, 20.7%). Only very few are widowed ($n = 5$, 2.4%) or separated ($n = 7$, 3.3%). There is no information for one patient.

Of the 207 patients, 183 have a school diploma, 19 have none, and two are still attending school. There is no information on this item for three patients. Elementary school, high school, and college diplomas are equally frequent (61 vs. 58 vs. 60). Four patients have certificates from schools for special education. For the other patients, education is still unfinished or they did not graduate. With respect to the kind of employment (classifications where >5%), most of the patients are employed as white-collar workers (38%), blue-collar workers (13%), or civil servants (8%); 12% are housewives. With regard to present employment status, 24 (12%) are unemployed, and 29 (14%) no longer work in their trained profession. Moreover, 48 are retired, seven of these prematurely.

Conclusions and Discussion

As a whole, the results show that the SAP represent a group of disorders which can be distinguished from the schizophrenic and the affective psychoses with regard to most of the AMDP variables studied here (particularly for the areas of symptomatology and course). The SAP are – for the most part – located between these two groups, i.e., they occupy an intermediate position and cannot be assigned to one of the two groups.

From the viewpoint of classification, it also seems possible to form subgroups of the SAP in accordance with the psychopathology in the course (polymorphous vs. monomorphous, or bipolar vs. depressive type).

However, one must take into account that the present investigation deals with a natural, descriptive study of heterogeneous patients (first manifestations, readmissions). The sources of information are likewise heterogeneous. Their main emphasis is on current assessments at the time of clinic admission and discharge (e.g., psychopathology), but there are also retrospective evaluations (e.g., assessments of previous manifestations of the illness). Subgroups were formed, taking into consideration what can be logically combined. Their formation was then based upon pragmatic criteria concerning division.

As in most other studies (Angst 1986), this study also covers only a small section and not the entire course of the illness. First manifestations whose course could be followed are in the minority here, too.

Therefore, the results of these first analyses need to be cross-validated by successively enlarging the sample (particularly by including all of the first manifestations) and to be extended through studies in the following directions:

1. Formation of subgroups by means of multivariate statistical methods based upon the cross-sectional and longitudinal psychopathological data (types of episodes, etc.) and additional items of the previous course of the illness (outcome, etc.).
2. Identification of prognostically relevant variables for response to therapy and the course within these subgroups (e.g., predictive significance of psychopathology at discharge for the future course).
3. Separation of the SAP subgroups from comparison groups of schizophrenic and affective psychoses (e.g., schizomanic vs. manic vs. schizophrenic) using discriminant analysis.
4. Analysis of the decision-making process in diagnosis aided by an expert system (with the goal of differentiating between relevant and irrelevant variables).

References

Albus M, Strauß A, Stieglitz RD (1990) Schizophrenia, schizotypical, and delusional disorders (section F2): results of the ICD-10 field trial. Pharmacopsychiatry (in press)
AMDP (1981) Das AMDP-System. Springer, Berlin Heidelberg New York
Angst J (1980) Verlauf unipolar depressiver, bipolar manisch-depressiver und schizoaffetiver Erkrankungen und Psychosen. Ergebnisse einer prospektiven Studie. Fortschr Neurol Psychiatr 48:3–30
Angst J (1986) The course of schizoaffective disorders. In: Marneros A, Tsuang MT (eds) Schizoaffective psychoses. Springer, Berlin Heidelberg New York Tokyo, pp 63–93
Angst J, Scharfetter C (1980) Depressive symptoms in functional psychoses based on the AMP-system. In: Achte K, Aalberg V, Lönnquist J (eds) Psychopathology of depression. Psychiatr Fenn [Suppl] 55–61

Angst J, Scharfetter C, Stassen HH (1983) Classification of schizo-affective patients by multidimensional scaling and cluster analysis. Psychiatria Clin 16:254–264

Angst J, Stassen HH, Woggon B (1988) Effect of neuroleptics on positive and negative symptoms and the deficit state. Paper presented at the Clozapine (Leponex/Clozaril) scientific update meeting, October 31–November 1, 1988, Montreux, Switzerland

APA (American Psychiatric Association) (1980) DSM-III: Diagnostic and statistical manual of mental disorders, 3rd edn. American Psychiatric Association, Washington, DC

APA (American Psychiatric Association) (1987) DSM-IIIR: Diagnostic and statistical manual of mental disorders, 3rd edn, revised. American Psychiatric Association, Washington DC

Baumann U (1974) Diagnostische Differenzierungsfähigkeit von Psychopathologie-Skalen. Arch Psychiatr Nervenkr 219:89–103

Baumann U, Stieglitz RD (1983) Testmanual zum AMDP-System. Springer, Berlin Heidelberg New York

Baumann U, Stieglitz RD (1989) Evaluation des AMDP-Systems anhand der neueren Literatur (1983–1987). Fortschr Neurol Psychiatr 57:357–373

Berner P, Lenz G (1986) Definitions of schizoaffective psychosis: mutual concordance and relationship to schizophrenia and affective disorder. In: Marneros A, Tsuang MT (eds) Schizoaffective psychoses. Springer, Berlin Heidelberg New York Tokyo, pp 31–49

Bobon D, Baumann U, Angst J, Helmchen H, Hippius H (eds) (1983) AMDP-system in pharmacopsychiatry. Karger, Basel

Brauchli B (1981) Zur Nosologie in der Psychiatrie. Enke, Stuttgart

Brockington IF, Meltzer HY (1983) The nosology of schizoaffective psychosis. Psychiatr Dev 4:317–338

Clayton PJ (1982) Schizoaffective disorders. J Nerv Ment Dis 170:646–650

Coryell W, Zimmerman M (1988) Diagnosis and outcome in schizo-affective depression: a replication. J Affective Disord 15:21–27

Crow TJ (1986) The continuum of psychosis and its implication for the structure of the gene. Br J Psychiatry 149:419–429

Emrich HM, Hippius H (1984) Die Bedeutung diagnostischer Kriterien für biologisch-psychiatrische Untersuchungen. In: Hopf A, Beckmann H (eds) Forschungen zur biologischen Psychiatrie. Springer, Berlin Heidelberg New York, pp 43–49

Fähndrich E, Helmchen H (1983) From AMP to AMDP. In: Bobon D, Baumann U, Angst J, Helmchen H, Hippius H (eds) AMDP-system in pharmacopsychiatry. Karger, Basel, pp 10–18

Gebhardt R, Pietzcker A, Strauss A, Stoeckel M, Langer C, Freudenthal K (1983) Skalenbildung im AMDP-System. Arch Psychiatr Nervenkr 233:223–245

Guy W, Ban T (1982) The AMDP-system. Springer, Berlin Heidelberg New York

Harrow M, Grossman LS (1984) Outcome in schizoaffective disorders: A critical review and reevaluation of the literature. Schizophr Bull 10:87–108

Hilz MJ (1987) Schizoaffektive Psychosen und ihre Stellung in der Systematik psychiatrischer Krankheitsbilder. Nervenheilkunde 6:164–170

Huber G, Gross G, Klosterkötter J (1989) Konzepte und Kriterien affektiver Psychosen. Nervenarzt 60:90–94

Kasanin J (1933) The acute schizoaffective psychoses. Am J Psychiatry 8:97–123

Kendell RE (1986) The relationship of schizoaffective illnesses to schizophrenic and affective disorders. In: Marneros A, Tsuang MT (eds) Schizoaffective psychoses. Springer, Berlin Heidelberg New York Tokyo, pp 18–30

Levitt JJ, Tsuang MT (1988) The heterogeneity of schizoaffective disorder: implications for treatment. Am J Psychiatry 145:926–936

Maier W, Philipp M, Schlegel S, Heuser I, Buller R, Frommberger U, Wetzel H, Wilhelmi D, Wittenborg A, Demuth W (1986) Operational diagnoses for schizophrenic and schizoaffective disorders. I. Interrater reliability. Pharmacopsychiatry 19:178–179

Maj M, Perris C (1985) An approach to the diagnosis and classification of schizoaffective disorders for research purposes. Acta Psychiatr Scand 72:405–413

Marneros A, Tsuang MT (1986) Schizoaffective disorders: present level and future perspectives. In: Marneros A, Tsuang MT (eds) Schizoaffective psychoses. Springer, Berlin Heidelberg New York Tokyo, pp 309–318

Marneros A, Deister A, Rohde A (1988a) Syndrome shift in the long-term course of schizo-affective disorders. Eur Arch Psychiatry Neurol Sci 238:97–104

Marneros A, Deister A, Rohde A, Jünemann H, Fimmers R (1988b) Long-term course of schizoaffective disorders. Part I. Definitions, methods, frequency of episodes, and cycles. Eur Arch Psychiatry Neurol Sci 237:264–275

Marneros A, Deister A, Rhode A, Jünemann H, Fimmers R (1988c) Long-term course of schizoaffective disorders. Part II. Length of cycles, episodes, and intervals. Eur Arch Psychiatry Neurol Sci 237:276–281

Marneros A, Deister A, Rohde A, Jünemann H, Fimmers R (1988d) Long-term course of schizoaffective disorders. Part III. Onset, type of episodes, and syndrome shift, pre-cipitating factors, suicidality, seasonality, inactivity of illness, and outcome. Eur Arch Psychiatry Neurol Sci 237:283–290

McGlashan TH, Williams PV (1987) Schizoaffective psychosis. II. Manic, bipolar, and de-pressive subtypes. Arch Gen Psychiatry 44:138–139

Möller HJ, Schmid-Bode W, Cording-Tömmel C, Wittchen HU, Zaudig M, Zerssen D v (1988) Psychopathological and social outcome in schizophrenia versus affective/ schizoaffective psychoses and prediction of poor outcome in schizophrenia. Acta Psychiatr Scand 77:379–389

Pichot P (1986) A comparison of different national concepts of schizoaffective psychosis. In: Marneros A, Tsuang MT (eds) Schizoaffective psychoses. Springer, Berlin Heidelberg New York Tokyo, pp 8–17

Pietzcker A (1988) Hat die klinische ICD-Diagnostik noch eine Bedeutung für die biologisch-psychiatrische Forschung? In: Beckmann H, Laux G (eds) Biologische Psychiatrie. Synopsis 1986/87. Springer, Berlin Heidelberg New York Tokyo, pp 94–97

Pietzcker A, Gebhardt R, Strauss A, Stöckel M, Langer C, Freudenthal K (1983) The syndrome scales in the AMDP-system. In: Bobon D, Baumann U, Angst J, Helmchen H, Hippius H (eds) AMDP-system in pharmacopsychiatry. Karger, Basel, pp 88–99

Procci WR (1976) Schizo-affective psychosis: fact or fiction? Arch Gen Psychiatry 33: 1167–1178

Scharfetter C (1971) Das AMP-System. Springer, Berlin Heidelberg New York

Shenton ME, Solovay MR, Holzman P (1987) Comparative studies of thought disorders. II. Schizoaffective disorder. Arch Gen Psychiatry 44:21–30

Sprock J (1988) Classification of schizoaffective disorder. Compr Psychiatry 29:55–71

Stieglitz RD, Fähndrich E, Helmchen H (1987) Applications du système AMDP dans le diagnostic et la prédiction. Acta Psychiatr Belg 87:117–140

Stieglitz RD, Fähndrich E, Helmchen H (1988) AMDP in multiaxial classification. In: Mezzich JE, von Cranach M (eds) International classification in psychiatry: unity and diversity. Cambridge University Press, Cambridge, pp 180–204

Sulz KD (1980) Schizoaffektive Psychose: eine multivariate Analyse von Psychopathologie und nosologischer Einordnung. Dissertation, Universität München

Sulz-Blume B (1980) Der Beitrag anamnestischer Merkmale zur diagnostischen Differen-zierung depressiver Syndrome. Dissertation, Universität München

Tsuang MT, Marneros A (1986) Schizoaffective psychosis: questions and directions. In: Marneros A, Tsuang MT (eds) Schizoaffective psychoses. Springer, Berlin Heidelberg New York Tokyo, pp 1–7

Tsuang MT, Simpson JC (1984) Schizoaffective disorder: concept and reality. Schizophr Bull 10:14–25

Williams PV, McGlashan TH (1987) Schizoaffective psychosis. I. Comparative long-term out-come. Arch Gen Psychiatry 44:130–137

Winokur G, Scharfetter C, Angst J (1985) Stability of psychotic symptomatology (delusions, hallucinations), affective syndromes, and schizophrenic symptoms (thought disorder, incongruent affect) over episodes in remitting psychoses. Eur Arch Psychiatry Neurol Sci 254:303–307

Cycloid and Affective Disorders: Reproduction, Motherhood, Postpartum Psychoses, and Offspring Characteristics

T.F. McNeil[1]

Considerable demands are typically placed on a woman physically, mentally, and psychosocially throughout pregnancy, labor and delivery, the postpartum period, and early motherhood. Women with a history of serious mental disorder appear to experience especially many difficulties during this period (McNeil et al. 1983a, 1984a; McNeil 1986; Persson-Blennow et al. 1986). The question of the similarities and differences between cycloid and affective psychoses may possibly be illuminated by viewing these mental disorders within the context of the special set of conditions represented by reproduction and motherhood. Furthermore, the investigation of the early-life characteristics of the offspring of women with these psychoses may yield evidence of (dis)similarities in the effects of both genetic and environmental influences on the offspring, associated with the different types of maternal psychoses. The similarities and differences between reproducing cycloid and affective women and their offspring is the central theme of this chapter.

The Project

The opportunity to make comparisons of reproducing cycloid and affective women and their offspring is found within a study conducted by the author and colleagues in southern Sweden (McNeil et al. 1983b). In the early 1970s, we began a prospective, longitudinal investigation of the offspring of 88 pregnant index women who had been hospitalized for psychoses of a nonorganic nature, i.e., schizophrenic, cycloid, affective, and other psychoses. A sample of control offspring of 104 pregnant women with no history of hospitalization for psychosis was also studied, for comparison purposes. Controls were matched with index cases on prenatal clinical status, parity, maternal age, social class, and marital status at confirmation of pregnancy. Almost all of the index cases (93%) and controls (98%) who were asked to participate in the study accepted the invitation to do so.

In order to minimize possible researcher bias, all research personnel who actively studied the mothers and offspring were without knowledge of both the index/control status of the mothers and the psychiatric diagnosis of any apparent index case. In the first phase of this study, the women and their offspring were

---

[1] Department of Psychiatry, University of Lund, Malmö, Sweden

Affective and Schizoaffective Disorders
Edited by A. Marneros and M.T. Tsuang
© Springer-Verlag Berlin Heidelberg 1990

studied prospectively from pregnancy until the child was 2 years of age. The women were interviewed during pregnancy, and the author personally observed the labor and delivery. A major subset of cases were also investigated concerning the neurological and somatic condition of the offspring at 3–4 days after birth, mother-infant interaction at six ages during the first year of life, and the offspring's fear of strangers, attachment to the mother, and exploratory behavior at 1 year of age.

In the second phase of the study, the cases were followed up in their homes when the offspring were about 6 years of age. The offspring were investigated using a number of different methods (McNeil and Kaij 1987) which were integrated into a summary evaluation of the mental status of the child.

The study data presented here concerning the mothers represent perhaps a unique cross-sectional descriptive study of the current demographic, life-situational, and health characteristics of a small number of women who developed a cycloid or affective psychosis and who later became pregnant and gave birth. While these two diagnostic groups are comparable with one another in this respect, they may well not be representative of all individuals with cycloid psychosis or affective illness. Furthermore, these index samples were defined in a diagnostically restrictive manner, and thus may not be representative of cases defined as having cycloid or affective disorders in other diagnostic or research contexts.

Diagnostic Criteria

The goal in sample selection was to choose index cases in such a manner that maternal psychiatric diagnosis would infer an increased risk (and especially genetic risk) for serious psychopathology among the offspring. Sample selection was done in 1973–1977, at which time a very broad definition of schizophrenia was specified by DSM-II (APA 1968). Thus we chose to use our own diagnostic system (McNeil et al. 1983b) for the project. Psychotic cases were excluded if there were signs of an organic component (alcohol or drug abuse, clear somatic disease or injury, or mental retardation). Clouding of consciousness and psychosis associated with childbirth were not necessarily regarded as reflecting an organic factor.

"Nonorganic" cases were classified on the basis of their total illness history up to the time of the diagnostic evaluation as representing cycloid psychosis ($n = 15$), affective illness ($n = 15$), and schizophrenia ($n = 17$). These three categories constituted "endogenous psychoses." Psychogenic psychoses ($n = 6$), post-partum psychoses only ($n = 18$), and "other psychoses" ($n = 17$) were identified as being "nonendogenous psychoses." The cases were later also diagnosed using the Research Diagnostic Criteria (RDC; Spitzer et al. 1978), for comparison purposes. Each diagnostic group was assigned its own demographically matched control group.

In this project the diagnostic criteria for inclusion as *cycloid psychosis* were (a) acute onset, (b) recurrent course (at least two episodes) and complete recovery between episodes, (c) homotypical heredity (i.e., similar disease in first- or second-degree biological relatives), and (d) all of the following symptoms: prominent mood disturbances, clouding of consciousness, and nonmood-related hallucinations and/or delusions. This definition of cycloid psychosis, excluding the homotypical heredity criterion, corresponds to a high degree to both Legrain's criteria for "bouffée délirante" (Pull et al. 1983; Pichot 1986) and Kasanin's (1933) definition of schizoaffective psychosis. However, as pointed out by Perris (1986), cycloid psychosis is not synonymous with schizoaffective disorder, and patients with cycloid psychosis do not necessarily meet modern diagnostic criteria for schizoaffective disorder (when schizoaffective disorder is defined by positive criteria, rather than representing only a residual diagnostic category).

In the current sample, cycloid psychosis only partially overlapped with an RDC diagnosis of schizoaffective psychosis: ten of the 15 project cycloid psychosis cases were classified according to RDC as having schizoaffective disorder, while the remaining five were classified as having either schizophrenia (three cases) or affective disorder (two cases; McNeil et al. 1983b). In contrast, four other index cases fulfilling RDC criteria for schizoaffective disorder were excluded from the cycloid group because they lacked homotypical heredity (these cases were included in the project's nonendogenous group, see below).

The project's criteria for *affective illness* represented the typical symptoms of serious mood disorder, and both bipolar and unipolar forms were accepted. Emphasis was again placed on homotypical heredity. In the presence of homotypical heredity (in first- or second-degree relatives), the criterion for inclusion was at least two depressive episodes or one manic episode. In the absence of homotypical heredity, at least three depressive episodes, or two manic episodes, or one manic episode and one depressive episode were required for inclusion. Clouding of consciousness or the occurrence of every episode in association with obvious psychic trauma represented exclusion criteria for endogenous affective illness. All of the 15 cases diagnosed as affective illness according to these project criteria were classified as bipolar depression or major depressive disorder according to RDC. Twelve of the 15 cases were bipolar.

On the other hand, ten additional index cases meeting RDC criteria for serious affective disorders (manic disorder, bipolar depression with mania, or major depressive disorder) did not fulfill the project criteria for affective illness; nine of the ten cases were postpartum psychoses.

As defined by project criteria, cycloid and affective disorders were similar to one another with respect to the presence of affective symptomatology, recurrent course (at least two episodes), and the requirement or tendency to have homotypical heredity. The two diagnoses differ most clearly from one another regarding nonmood-related hallucinations/delusions (required for cycloid psychosis) and clouding of consciousness, the latter representing an inclusion criterion for cycloid psychosis and an exclusion criterion for affective illness.

Schizophrenia was defined in a restrictive manner, based on Bleuler's "primary symptoms" (1911). The criteria for schizophrenia were (a) insidious onset;

(b) autism; (c) splitting of affect, thought, and/or volition; (d) flattening of affect; (e) loosening of associations and formal thought disorder; and (f) disturbances in perception including deshabituation. A majority of the 17 cases also had hallucinations and delusions. Clouding of consciousness was a criterion for exclusion from schizophrenia.

In total, almost one-half of the cases diagnosed as nonorganic psychoses did not meet the restrictive project criteria for one of the endogenous psychoses (cycloid psychosis, affective illness, or schizophrenia). These remaining cases were relegated to the "nonendogenous psychoses" ($n = 41$), which were further subdivided into psychogenic ($n = 6$), postpartum ($n = 18$), and other psychoses ($n = 17$). A majority of the nonendogenous cases were nevertheless diagnosed as having schizophrenic, schizoaffective, or affective disorders on the basis of the RDC, observing the strictness of the project criteria for the "endogenous psychoses." The use of both narrower and broader diagnostic criteria on the same sample yields the opportunity to test the practical effectiveness of these criteria, when evaluated against results such as the frequency of postpartum psychoses (McNeil 1986) or the development of disturbances in the offspring (McNeil and Kaij 1987). Furthermore, the existence of six different diagnostic groups within the total index sample yields the opportunity to determine whether the notable characteristics of the patients with cycloid and/or affective disorder are descriptive only of these particular diagnostic groups or of index cases in general.

Results

Sample Characteristics

Relationship to Project, Sample Attrition

Among the different diagnostic and control groups asked to participate in the study, the rejection rate was highest among the patients with cycloid disorder (17%), and somewhat lower among those with affective disorder (12%). The cycloid patients were one of the two groups that were most frequently reserved in their emotional contact with the interviewer during pregnancy (40%); reservedness was seldom noted among those with affective disorder (7%). Among all the different diagnostic groups, the affective patients were the most consistent in their contact with the interviewer, and their degree of evenness (93%) paralleled that for control cases; in contrast, 33% of the cycloid patients evidenced either worsening of contact during discussion of loaded topics or "cyclic" changes in contact, seemingly unrelated to the topic under discussion. Furthermore, over the 6-year interval from giving birth to the follow-up when the child was 6 years of age, 40% of the cycloid but only 13% of the affective patients dropped out of the study. Thus, these two diagnostic groups showed consistent differences in their relationship to the project.

Psychiatric History and Clinical Characteristics

The psychiatric records of the women were used to obtain information regarding psychiatric history and clinical characteristics. Most (69%) of the cycloid patients (with available information) were described as having had normal mental adjustment prior to the onset of the disorder during adulthood (at 16 years or older), and only one cycloid patient (8%) was known to have been deviant prior to 13 years of age. In contrast, more than one-half (54%) of the affective patients were reported to have been mentally deviant before adulthood, 31% developing some abnormality during childhood, and 23% evidencing mental disturbance during early adolescence (13–15 years).

The age of onset of the current mental disorder was somewhat lower among affective than cycloid patients. Onset occurred before age 21 in 53% of the affective, as compared with 33% of the cycloid patients (median, 19 and 22 years, respectively). A longer time had passed from onset of illness until the project delivery among the affective (9.1 years) than cycloid (5.8 years) patients. The affective patients were the youngest among all diagnostic groups at onset of illness, and they had the longest interval from onset of illness to project delivery.

According to the diagnostic definition, all cycloid and affective patients had a recurrent disease course, and equally high proportions of both groups (73%) had had four or more disease episodes prior to the current pregnancy. Most of the affective patients (86%) were known to be mentally normal (i.e., classed at level 1–2 on the 7-point scale of severity of psychopathology, Table 1) at their healthiest time between episodes; in contrast, this was true of only 57% of the cycloid patients, and the remaining cycloid patients (43%) were classified as being "mildly disturbed" (level 3) at their healthiest.

The cycloid patients were also more seriously disturbed than the affective patients during the illness episodes. A disturbance at severity level 7 at the worst time ever was found for 73% of the cycloid but only for 33% of the affective patients, whereas a greatest severity level 5 was found for only 7% of the cycloid but for fully 33% of the affective patients. Furthermore, the total length of all

Table 1. Abridged version of the General Psychopathology Scale

Category 1. "Healthy": no known symptoms; functions well in all respects

Category 2. Functions well and without symptoms, but when stressed, shows occasional isolated signs of disturbance

Category 3. Mild symptoms in nonstressing situations, or many symptoms in stressing situations

Category 4. In nonstressing situations shows symptoms that are troublesome; is sometimes considered deviant or sick by those around him/her; more or worse symptoms than in category 3

Category 5. Clear mental symptoms serious enough to occupy a dominant place in person's life; normal functions interfered with or thrust aside

Category 6. Grave psychiatric disturbances that completely dominate life for the present; cannot adequately care for self

Category 7. Very seriously ill, insight lacking, out of contact psychiatric hospitalization(s) up to the time of project delivery was approximately twice as long for cycloid patients (mean 49 and median 31 weeks) as for affective patients (mean 25 and median 15 weeks). The cycloid patients were the most seriously ill among all diagnostic groups, in terms of both severity of active disturbance and length of hospitalization.

Demographic Characteristics

The affective patients were generally slightly older than the cycloid patients at the current delivery (mean 29.5 vs 27.8 years, and median 30 vs 29 years, respectively). On the average, the affective patients already had twice as many children as did the cycloid patients (mean 1.2 and 0.6, respectively). Fully one-half (53%) of the cycloid, as compared with only one-fourth (27%) of the affective patients, were now having their first child. The 0-parae among cycloid patients were found in all age categories (up to 34 years), whereas the 0-parae among the affective patients were almost exclusively limited to the youngest age category (up to 24 years), suggesting a basic difference in the reproductive rates of the two groups.

Social class, defined by the parents' occupations, was generally higher among cycloid than affective patients, patients in the upper classes being more frequent among those with cycloid (20%) than those with affective (7%) disorder, and lower class patients being more frequent among those with affective (60%) than those with cycloid (33%) disorder. The cycloid patients were even somewhat higher in social class, and the affective patients somewhat lower in social class than were random population control cases.

Equally high proportions of cycloid (67%) and affective (73%) patients were formally married by the time of the delivery. Identical proportions of both groups (93%) were cohabiting, and only one woman in each group had no partner at that time. By the arbitrary time of fall, 1980, an equal number of cycloid and affective patients (71% each) had been married once only; somewhat more cycloid than affective patients (21% vs 7%) had never been married, and somewhat more affective than cycloid patients (21% vs 7%) had been married twice. About one-half of the patients (46% cycloid, 54% affective) who had ever married had also divorced at least once. The rate of marriages ending in divorces was 42% for cycloid and 50% for affective patients. These divorce rates were much higher than those in the matched control groups (17% and 6%, respectively), and represented the highest divorce rates among all different diagnostic and control groups.

Maternal Characteristics

Life Situation and Experience of Pregnancy

The women were interviewed after quickening during pregnancy concerning their life situation and experience of pregnancy (McNeil et al. 1983a). Equally small proportions of both groups were not currently living with the father of the coming child, and both groups reported similar rates of material-situational problems. Dissatisfaction with housing was more common among cycloid (40%) than affective (0%) patients. Interpersonal problems were reported by more cycloid than affective patients, while both groups tended to have more problematic relationships with their partners than did control women. The cycloid patients had differentially increased rates of problematic relationships with their own mothers, and their own parents were much more often negative toward the pregnancy than was the case for affective patients. The pregnancy was somewhat more frequently unplanned and initially undesired among the affective patients (53% vs 33% cycloids); however, no difference between groups was found in the frequency of negative long-term attitudes toward the pregnancy. The cycloid patients and controls were similar with regard to the total amount of reported physical health problems during pregnancy, including the frequency of specific symptoms such as nausea, fatigue, headache, fainting tendency, etc; the affective patients reported fewer such symptoms than did their controls. The cycloid patients reported greater fears concerning maldevelopment in the child and being a good mother than did their controls; the affective patients reported notably fewer such fears. No difference was found between cycloid and affective patients concerning fear of the coming delivery. In total, the two diagnostic groups were similar to one another in many respects concerning life situation and experience of pregnancy, but the cycloid patients tended to experience more housing difficulties, interpersonal problems, and fears concerning the child's health and mothering.

Mental Health During Pregnancy

Most index women (including 53% of the cycloid and 60% of the affective patients) were not in contact with a psychiatrist during the current pregnancy. Equal proportions of cycloid and affective patients (40%) had prescriptions for psychopharmaceutical drugs covering the pregnancy period.

When the women were blindly interviewed by the author during pregnancy (McNeil et al. 1984a), the cycloid patients were judged to be significantly more frequently mentally disturbed than were controls, while the affective patients were not significantly different from controls. Only 27% of the cycloid but fully 60% of the affective patients showed no currently active disturbance (i.e., they were classified at level 1–2 on the 7-point scale). Among the six different diagnostic groups, the affective patients had the lowest rate of mental disturbance, while the cycloid patients had the second highest rate; those with cycloid disorder (53%) were most frequently rated as evidencing "mild mental disturbance" (level 3).

The cycloid patients had many more (mean 3.1) of the 13 different symptoms/mental characteristics that were assessed than did the affective patients (mean 1.4), who differed little from control women (mean 1.0). The most frequently noted characteristics for cycloid patients were seldom chosen to describe affective patients, i.e., tense-anxious (60% cycloid vs 7% affective), withdrawn (40% cycloid vs 7% affective), emotionally labile (33% cycloid vs 13% affective), and suspicious (27% cycloid vs 7% affective).

On the other hand, maternal reports of the effect of the pregnancy on mental health were very similar for cycloid and affective patients (McNeil et al. 1984b). Quite similar proportions of both groups reported better mental health (40% cycloid vs 33% affective) and worse mental health (20% cycloid vs 20% affective) associated with this pregnancy. Among all the diagnostic groups, more improvement than worsening was reported only by the cycloid and the affective patients.

Labor and Delivery Experiences

As observed by the author and midwives attending the labor and delivery, no difference was found between the cycloid and affective patients concerning attitude toward or use of analgesics and anesthetics, and the two diagnostic groups received approximately the same degree of help and attention from the midwives. In general, the cycloid patients tended to be more "extreme" in their behavioral characteristics, while the affective patients scored more in the middle of the scales. A withdrawn or demanding style of relating to the other people present was equally frequent among cycloid (60%) and affective (55%) patients; the cycloid patients tended more often to be cooperative (30% cycloid vs 18% affective), while the affective patients' style of relating was more frequently characterized as "neutral" (10% cycloid vs 27% affective). Cycloid patients were more often unusually near or distant in their contact with the observer (38% cycloid vs 0% affective), while the affective patients were grouped in the middle of the nearness-distance scale (91%). As assessed by the midwife, the cycloid patients were more frequently extremely anxious, 33% of the cycloid patients (vs 0% affective) being rated at the highest category of anxiety; the affective patients tended to be rated as just "somewhat more anxious than usual" (25% cycloid vs 58% affective). No notable difference was found between the two diagnostic groups on degree of control over their own behavior during labor/delivery, or on their view of the labor/delivery at 2 h postpartum. The maternal response to the newborn child was more often reserved or quiet among cycloid (25%) than affective (8%) patients.

More notable differences were found between the diagnostic groups on the behavior of the partners of the women. The partners attended the labor/delivery more often in the cycloid (67%) than the affective (46%) group. The attending partners of the cycloid patients were more frequently highly emotionally engaged in the labor/delivery (29% cycloid vs 0% affective), and their partners were more frequently described as very unusually fearful regarding the mother (57% cycloid vs 17% affective). The partners of the cycloid patients were also much more often ineffective in assisting the mother (71% cycloid vs 17% affective). The amount of body contact between the woman and partner during labor was highly discriminative of the two diagnostic groups. A very low degree of body contact was found only among cycloid patients (71% cycloid vs 0% affective), while some body contact beyond just holding hands was found almost exclusively among affective patients (14% cycloid vs 67% affective). The partners of the cycloid patients more frequently responded in a positive manner to the newborn infant (50% cycloid vs 29% affective), while the partners of the affective patients were more often reserved, quiet, unsure, or negative toward the newborn (25% cycloid vs 57% affective).

Mothering Characteristics in Mother-Infant Interaction

Mother-infant interaction was observed during feeding and in an unstructured play situation on six occasions during the first year, i.e., at the maternity ward at 3 days postpartum, and then in the home at 3 and 6 weeks and 3.5, 6, and 12 months (Persson-Blennow et al. 1984, 1986; Näslund et al. 1985; McNeil et al. 1985). A number of operationally defined maternal behaviors were studied, such as various forms of social and physical contact with the infant, consideration for the infant's needs, tension, and uncertainty.

Significant differences on maternal behaviors were found between cycloid patients and their controls at all six ages. For example, at 3 days postpartum, the cycloids were characterized by significantly poorer harmony in feeding, poorer synchronization to the infant's pace of eating, less vocal contact with the infant, a greater discrepancy between intonation and content of vocal contact, and more expressed uncertainty regarding the infant's needs. At 6 weeks, the cycloid patients showed significantly less social contact (both visually and verbally) with the infant and evidenced more tension in interaction. At 3.5 months, the cycloid patients again had less social contact (visually and verbally and smiled less at the infant), evidenced poorer synchronization to the infant's pace of eating, and showed less consideration for the infant's needs in play. Even at 1 year, the cycloid patients evidenced greater tension and uncertainty in interaction, showed less social contact toward the infant, expressed more uncertainty regarding the infant's needs, and also demonstrated greater discrepancy between verbal intonation and content. The cycloid patients deviated from controls more than did any other diagnostic group.

In contrast, the affective mothers showed no significant differences from their controls in observations at 3 days, 3 weeks, 6 weeks, or 6 months. The affective patients were significantly different from their controls on only one variable at 3.5 months (less physical contact during play) and at 1 year (less vocal contact with the infant). The affective patients were outstanding in comprising the one index diagnostic group that was most like the control mothers in interaction with their infants.

Postpartum Psychotic Episodes

Psychiatric records provided information about the occurrence of postpartum psychotic episodes (PPPs) and their clinical characteristics (McNeil 1986). Current PPP episodes were independently diagnosed in accordance with the RDC by a psychiatrist (L.G. Nordström), who had access only to the case notes for this particular PPP episode.

While none of the 104 control cases developed a PPP following the current delivery, PPPs were found with a frequency of 28% following the 88 index births. The rates were highest among both cycloid (47%) and affective (47%)

patients, somewhat lower among schizophrenics (24%), other psychotics (24%), and women in the postpartum psychosis diagnostic group (i.e., those with only PPPs earlier; 17%), and zero among the six cases with psychogenic psychosis.

The nonendogenous cases fulfilling the broader RDC criteria for affective disorder had a much lower rate of PPPs (10%) than did the more strictly defined project-criteria endogenous affectives (47%); and those fulfilling the broader RDC criteria for schizoaffective disorder had a lower rate of PPPs (20%) than did the strictly defined project-criteria cycloid patients (47%). In contrast, nonendogenous cases fulfilling the broader RDC criteria for schizophrenia had a higher rate of PPPs (36%) than did project-criteria schizophrenics (24%). Thus, narrower definitions of affective and schizoaffective/cycloid disorders yielded higher rates of PPPs, while a narrower definition of schizophrenia yielded a lower rate of PPPs.

The PPPs of the cycloid patients were blindly diagnosed as affective disorders in four cases, unspecified functional psychosis in two cases, and schizophrenia in one case; confusion was evident in three of the seven PPPs. The PPPs of the affective patients were blindly diagnosed as affective disorders in four cases, a schizoaffective disorder in one case, and unspecified functional psychosis in the two remaining cases; two of the seven affective patients evidenced confusion. Confusion was found even in some PPPs of the other diagnostic groups.

Notably, all of the seven cycloid patients and five of the seven affective patients with PPPs had onset of symptoms within the first 2 weeks postpartum; in contrast, a concentration of schizophrenics was found among cases with onset of PPP after 3 weeks postpartum. In both the cycloid and affective groups, six of the seven PPP cases were hospitalized. The latency between onset of symptoms and hospitalization was 0 to 2 days for four of the six hospitalized cycloid patients, and 1 week at the most for the remaining two cases; the latency for affective patients was 3 days in two cases, 1 week in three cases, and unspecifiable in the remaining case. The longest mean hospitalizations in the total index group were found among the cycloid patients (mean 10.5 weeks) and other psychoses (11.0 weeks), while the affective patients had the shortest hospitalization times of any diagnostic group (5.0 weeks). The severity rating for the PPPs also tended to be somewhat higher among cycloid than affective patients.

Offspring Characteristics

Characteristics at Labor and Birth

While most of the offspring of the affective patients (93%) were delivered at term, those of the cycloid patients had the highest rate of nonterm deliveries among all diagnostic groups, with 20% being delivered postterm and 13% preterm. The offspring of cycloid and affective patients did not differ from one another with regard to birth weight, body length, or body size relative to gestational age. Fetal distress (bradycardia/tachycardia and/or meconium staining of amnionic fluid) occurred more often among the offspring of cycloid (47%) than affective (21%) patients. Nevertheless, most women in both groups (87%

cycloid vs 93% affective) had spontaneous vaginal deliveries. No differences were observed between the two offspring groups concerning Apgar scores, amount of postnatal stimulation received, or frequency of abnormalities noted at immediate postnatal examination. The offspring of affective patients were much more often sleepy or drowsy (i.e., arousal state 1–3 on the 6-point Prechtl/ Beintema scale; Prechtl and Beintema 1964) during the first 45 min after delivery than were the offspring of cycloid patients (54% affective vs 18% cycloid), and the offspring of affective patients were outstanding in this respect within the entire sample.

Neonatal Neurological Characteristics

A neonatal neurological assessment was performed on the third-fourth day post-partum. Clear neurological abnormality was relatively uncommon (10%) in the combined index and control sample. The offspring of cycloid patients more frequently showed clear abnormality (25% vs 9% in offspring of affective patients), a high total number of deviation points accumulated across different neurological items (50% vs 9% affective), abnormally increased or decreased muscle tone (42% vs 9% affective), and deviation on one or more of the simple reflexes (33% vs 0% affective). The abnormalities found among the offspring of cycloid patients were described in terms of hyperexcitability, jitteriness, apathy, and unusual wakefulness; the one abnormal case among the offspring of affective patients was not describable in terms of any known neurological pattern or syndrome. The offspring of cycloid patients had the highest rate of neurological abnormality among any diagnostic group, and the offspring of the affective patients showed the lowest rates of neurological abnormality among all groups.

Infant Behaviors in Mother-Infant Interaction

The infants were observed concerning sucking ability, crying, visual and vocal contact with the mother, motor activity, and smiling and wakefulness as shown during mother-infant interaction at the six different ages (Persson-Blennow et al. 1984, 1986; Näslund et al. 1985; McNeil et al. 1985). Considerably fewer statistically significant index-control differences were found in the infant behaviors than in the maternal behaviors (presented above), but clear differences were found between the offspring of cycloid and affective patients, especially with regard to the age at which the deviations appeared. The offspring of cycloid patients differed significantly from controls at every observation age up to and including 3.5 months. At 3 days of age, the offspring of the cycloid patients were significantly more often deviant on several different variables (with trends toward poorer continuity of eating, poorer sucking ability, and less wakefulness during feeding); at 3 weeks, they showed significantly less vocal contact, and at 6 weeks less social contact toward the mother; at 3.5 months they smiled less at the mother. The offspring of cycloid patients showed no significant differences from controls at 6 or 12 months. In contrast, the offspring of affective patients showed no differences from controls during the first 6 months, but did evidence deviance at 12 months, at which time they showed less total social contact, including significantly reduced visual contact toward the mother. The offspring of cycloid patients were the most deviant among all the groups of offspring during the early period but not later, while the offspring of affective patients were deviant only at the 1-year observation.

Infant Attachment, Fear of Strangers, and Exploratory Behavior at 1 Year of Age

Infant attachment to the mother, fear of strangers (FOS), and exploratory behavior were studied in standardized test situations in the home in association with observation of mother-infant interaction at 1 year of age. Attachment was characterized as representing secure attachment (type B), anxious avoidant attachment (type A), or anxious ambivalent attachment (type C), according to Näslund et al. (1984a). The results were quite similar for the offspring of cycloid and affective patients. While the offspring of schizophrenics and women in the total nonendogenous group had more anxious attachment (types A and C) than did their controls, the offspring of cycloid and affective patients had rates of anxious attachment that were similar to or lower than those for their controls (22% cycloid vs 22% control; 17% affective vs 28% control).

In contrast, the results for FOS indicated differences between these two offspring groups (Näslund et al. 1984b). The failure to show FOS was considered to represent deviation. Fewer of the offspring of affective patients showed deviation (25%) than did their controls (33%). In contrast, offspring of the cycloid patients had a significantly more frequent total absence of FOS (67%) than did their controls (22%); the offspring of cycloid patients were similar to the offspring of schizophrenics (70%) in this respect.

The results for exploratory behavior were again different for the two offspring groups (Näslund et al. 1984c). The offspring of affective mothers showed a singularly high rate of deviance (86%) on exploration (representing both extremes in leaving or not leaving the mother to go to a new toy). In contrast, the rate of deviance found among the offspring of cycloid mothers (38%) was quite similar to that for both controls (36%) and the other diagnostic groups.

Mental Disorder in the Children at 6 Years of Age

The children were followed up in their homes at about 6 years of age. The mothers were interviewed by one researcher, and the children were independently assessed by another researcher, using a battery of instruments and techniques (McNeil and Kaij 1987). The information obtained at this follow-up was used to summarize the current mental status of the offspring, expressed on the basis of the Children's Global Assessment Scale (CGAS; Shaffer et al. 1983). The CGAS ranges from 1 to 100 points, with scores of 70 or lower indicating "mental disturbance," and a score of 100 points indicating optimal mental functioning and adjustment.

The total index of the children of these patients had a significantly lower (poorer) mean CGAS score than did that of controls (McNeil and Kaij 1987), but considerable differences were found among the various diagnostic groups.

The children of schizophrenic mothers and those of the nonendogenous groups had lower mean scores than did controls. The mean for the children of cycloid mothers (71.67) was only minimally and not significantly lower than that for their controls (mean 75.94), while the mean score for the offspring of affective mothers (81.15) was considerably higher than that for their controls (70.94); the offspring of the affective mothers had the second highest mean score among all diagnostic and control groups. Almost one-half (46%) of the affective mothers' offspring had CGAS scores of 81–100, and almost one-third (31%) were placed at the highest interval of mental functioning (CGAS, 91–100).

When expressed in terms of rates of mental disturbance (CGAS ≤ 70), the children of the total index patients showed significantly more frequent mental disturbance than did that of controls (50% vs 28%, respectively). The offspring of schizophrenic mothers showed the highest disturbance rate (82%), while the offspring of cycloid mothers (56% disturbance) were rather typical for the total index group. In contrast, the offspring of the affective mothers had a very low disturbance rate (15%), well below that of even the total *control* group.

A broadening of the strict project criteria for schizophrenic, cycloid, and affective disorders, to include nonendogenous cases defined as schizophrenic, schizoaffective, and affective disorders in accordance with the RDC, led to some attenuation of the great differentiation in disturbance rates among the groups of offspring. However, even with the inclusion of RDC-defined cases, differences were still evident between offspring of more broadly defined schizophrenic (73% disturbance) and affective mothers (23%). The disturbance rate for offspring of the broader group of cycloid/schizoaffective patients (50%) was exactly halfway between the rates for the offspring of schizophrenic and affective patients.

Summary of (Dis)Similarities Between Cycloid and Affective Cases

The two diagnostic groups, cycloid and affective disorders, showed both similarities to and differences from one another across the large number of comparisons available within the extensive project data. However, in general, the two groups were more frequently different from one another than similar to one another, especially concerning their outstanding characteristics within the total index sample.

Similarities

The cycloid and affective patients were notably similar to one another on characteristics such as their number of prior illness episodes, current marital status, high rate of divorce, attitude toward the current pregnancy and reported physical symptoms in the pregnancy, the reported effect of the pregnancy on their mental health, the high risk for PPPs with early onset postpartum, and the relatively low rate of anxious attachment of their offspring to the mother. These two diagnostic groups were outstanding within the total index group on several of these characteristics, i.e., their high divorce rates, their experiences of improvement in mental condition during pregnancy, and their high rates of PPP episodes.

Dissimilarities

The differences between the two diagnostic groups were far more frequent and covered all areas of the study. As compared with the affective patients, the cycloid patients showed psychiatric histories characterized by more normal premorbid adjustment prior to illness onset at a higher age, more (mild) mental disturbance between illness episodes, and more severe disturbance and longer psychiatric hospitalizations during illness episodes (including the current PPPs). At the current pregnancy, the cycloid patients had lower parity, higher social class, more housing difficulties and interpersonal problems (especially with their own parents), and more fears regarding the child and mothering; the cycloid patients showed more mental disturbance during this pregnancy, and had a poorer relationship to the project, with greater sample attrition over time. At labor/delivery, the cycloid patients were more extreme in their behavior, and their partners had greater problems dealing with the delivery, but were more positive toward the newborn. The cycloid patients were more deviant with regard to mothering characteristics during the whole first year of the infant's life. The offspring of the cycloids showed more nonterm gestational age, more neonatal neurological abnormality, more early behavioral deviation in interaction with the mother, more deviation on fear of strangers and less deviation on exploratory behavior at 1 year, and more frequent mental disturbance at 6 years of age.

The *outstanding differential characteristics of the cycloid patients*, as compared with all other diagnostic groups, were their great severity of mental illness, their notable reservedness in relation to the interviewer, their high rate of nonterm delivery, their high frequency of deviant mothering characteristics, their offspring's high rate of neonatal neurological abnormality, and the presence of early behavioral deviance in their offspring during mother-infant interaction.

The *outstanding differential characteristics of the affective patients*, as compared with all other diagnostic groups, were their young age at onset of illness, their even and open relationship to the interviewer, their low rate of mental disturbance during the current pregnancy, their great nondeviance and similarity to control women on mothering characteristics, their offspring's drowsiness/ sleepiness soon after birth, their offspring's low rate of neonatal neurological abnormality, their offspring's deviance on exploratory behavior at 1 year, and their offspring's notably low rate of mental disturbance and high rate of superior mental adjustment at 6 years of age.

The cycloid and affective patients thus appear not only to differ from one another but even to be diametrically opposite to one another with regard to their relationship to the interviewer and the project, their mental characteristics during pregnancy, their mothering behaviors, their offspring's neonatal neurological status, and their offspring's early behavior in interacting with the mother.

The deviations observed among the offspring of the cycloid patients represented gestational, neonatal neurological, early behavioral, and later mental abnormalities that were generally absent among the offspring of the affective mothers. These abnormalities among the cycloid patients' offspring would appear to have a biological origin, as they existed from the time of birth or the first few days postpartum.

Across most project data analyzed to date, the cycloid mothers and their children appear to be the most clearly disturbed diagnostic group, and the group that was most similar to the schizophrenics on characteristics such as rates of mental disturbance during pregnancy, poor mothering, and offspring deviations on neonatal neurological status and fear of strangers, etc. The cycloid mothers and their children were in many study areas not just "halfway" between the affective patients and the schizophrenics (as "schizoaffectives" are often observed to be; Marneros and Tsuang 1986) but rather they were more deviant than schizophrenics in many areas (e.g., mothering characteristics, offspring neonatal neurological abnormality). The affective mothers, on the other hand, tended to be the most nondeviant of all diagnostic groups, generally being most similar to the "postpartum diagnostic group" (interestingly, this was the other group including the most cases of RDC-defined affective disorder) and to controls.

If affective and cycloid disorders do have anything in common beyond their general mental disorder status, their affective symptomatology, and their episodic disease course, the current data might suggest that the communality is reflected in the effect of pregnancy and the postpartum period on the mother's mental condition. Beyond that, the current results obtained on these small samples of reproducing women appear to suggest that cycloid and affective disorders (as currently defined) represent two quite different types of disturbances, and further that cycloid psychosis is a disorder that is separate and different from the other diagnostic categories included in this study.

Acknowledgements. This work was supported by grants no. 3793 and 6214 from the Swedish Medical Research Council, by grant no. MH18857 from the PHS, DHEW, U.S.A., and by the Grant Foundation Inc., U.S.A.

References

American Psychiatric Association (1968) DSM-II: diagnostic and statistical manual of mental disorders, 2nd edn. American Psychiatric Association, Washington
Bleuler E (1911) Dementia Praecox oder die Gruppe der Schizophrenien. In: Aschaffenburg G (ed) Handbuch der Psychiatrie. Deuticke, Leipzig
Kasanin J (1933) The acute schizoaffective psychoses. Am J Psychiatry 13:97–126
Marneros A, Tsuang MT (eds) (1986) Schizoaffective psychoses. Springer, Berlin Heidelberg New York
McNeil TF (1986) A prospective study of postpartum psychoses in a high-risk group. I. Clinical characteristics of the current postpartum episodes. Acta Psychiatr Scand 74:205–216
McNeil TF, Kaij L (1987) Swedish high-risk study: sample characteristics at age 6. Schizophr Bull 13:373–381

McNeil TF, Kaij L, Malmquist-Larsson A (1983a) Pregnant women with nonorganic psychosis: life situation and experience of pregnancy. Acta Psychiatr Scand 68:445–457

McNeil TF, Kaij L, Malmquist-Larsson A, Näslund B, Persson-Blennow I, McNeil N, Blennow G (1983b) Offspring of women with nonorganic psychoses. Development of a longitudinal study of children at high risk. Acta Psychiatr Scand 68:234–250

McNeil TF, Kaij L, Malmquist-Larsson A (1984a) Women with nonorganic psychosis: mental disturbance during pregnancy. Acta Psychiatr Scand 70:127–139

McNeil TF, Kaij L, Malmquist-Larsson A (1984b) Women with nonorganic psychosis: pregnancy's effect on mental health during pregnancy. Acta Psychiatr Scand 70:140–148

McNeil TF, Näslund B, Persson-Blennow I, Kaij L (1985) Offspring of women with nonorganic psychosis: mother-infant interaction at three-and-a-half and six months of age. Acta Psychiatr Scand 71:551–558

Näslund B, Persson-Blennow I, McNeil T, Kaij L, Malmquist-Larsson A (1984a) Offspring of women with nonorganic psychosis: infant attachment to the mother at one year of age. Acta Psychiatr Scand 69:231–241

Näslund B, Persson-Blennow I, McNeil T, Kaij L, Malmquist-Larsson A (1984b) Offspring of women with nonorganic psychosis: fear of strangers during the first year of life. Acta Psychiatr Scand 69:435–444

Näslund B, Persson-Blennow I, McNeil TF, Kaij L, Malmquist-Larsson A (1984c) Deviations on exploration, attachment, and fear of strangers in high-risk and control infants at one year of age. Am J Orthopsychiatry 54:569–577

Näslund B, Persson-Blennow I, McNeil TF, Kaij L (1985) Offspring of women with nonorganic psychosis: mother-infant interaction at three and six weeks of age. Acta Psychiatr Scand 71:441–450

Perris C (1986) The case for the independence of cycloid psychotic disorder from the schizoaffective disorders. In: Marneros A, Tsuang MT (eds) Schizoaffective psychoses. Springer, Berlin Heidelberg New York

Persson-Blennow I, Näslund B, McNeil TF, Kaij L, Malmquist-Larsson A (1984) Offspring of women with nonorganic psychosis: mother-infant interaction at three days of age. Acta Psychiatr Scand 70:149–159

Persson-Blennow I, Näslund B, McNeil TF, Kaij L (1986) Offspring of women with nonorganic psychosis: mother-infant interaction at one year of age. Acta Psychiatr Scand 73:207–213

Pichot P (1986) A comparison of different national concepts of schizoaffective psychosis. In: Marneros A, Tsuang MT (eds) Schizoaffective psychoses. Springer, Berlin Heidelberg New York

Prechtl HFR, Beintema D (1964) The neurological examination of the full-term new-born infant. Heinemann, London (Little club clinics in developmental medicine, no 12)

Pull CB, Pull MC, Pichot P (1983) Nosological position of schizo-affective psychosis in France. Psychiatr Clin 16:141–148

Shaffer D, Gould MS, Brasic J, Ambrosini P, Fisher P, Bird H, Aluwahlia S (1983) A children's global assessment scale (CGAS). Arch Gen Psychiatry 40:1228–1231

Spitzer RL, Endicott J, Robins E (1978) Research diagnostic criteria (RDC) for a selected group of functional disorders. Biometrics Research division, New York State Psychiatric Institute, New York

The Course of Juvenile Schizoaffective and Schizophrenic Psychoses: The Use of Pattern Analysis for Classifying the Development of Schizophrenia-Like Illnesses

D. Bunk and C. Eggers[1]

Introduction

The use of current research methods for the study and analysis of records deriving from longitudinal studies of patients' illnesses gives rise to a number of problems for which there are no simple satisfactory solutions. In the process of diagnosis one is faced with a range of events and symptoms that appear during the course of the illness. The methods used to construct different classes of symptoms from separable events during the course of the illness result sometimes in precise and at other times in rather crude descriptions. In part, precision depends on the degree to which the particular diagnostic criteria used can differentiate between features of the illness. In part, the separability of periods of illness depends on the duration of the symptoms, that can themselves vary during the period.

There are also problems of a more epistemological nature. One can look at sequential events from two points of view. According to constructivist theories (von Foerster 1985; Maturana and Varela 1987), there is a basic assumption that, at a given moment in time, every phenomenon is rigidly dependent on the previous one. (The point can be summarized in the formula, $\text{Phenomenon}_{t0} = f(\text{Phenomenon}_{t0-1})$; $t0 = $ time of observation, $t0 - 1 = $ previous time of observation.) Here causal relations (or more likely effects) between the two phenomena are presumed to exist. A clinician may accept this point of view in order to help him understand better a particular event. However, from another point of view one may wish to ask what phenomenological similarities there are between two individuals. Then one must look for commonalities in the courses of their illness. This in turn means that one must find some regular features in the duration of the illness just to enable a comparison between the two courses. (One can express these commonalities as a rule: $\text{Phenomenon}_{t0} = \text{Phenomenon}_{t0-c}$; $c = $ a constant for the rate at which periods of the illness follow each other.)

Investigations into the developmental course of an illness that can be traced back to childhood or adolescence are relevant not only for the prescription of therapeutic measures but also for assessing the likely prognosis in individual

---

[1] Klinik für Kinder- und Jugendpsychiatrie an der Rheinischen Landes- und Hochschulklinik, Hufelandstraße 55, 4300 Essen 1, FRG

Affective and Schizoaffective Disorders
Edited by A. Marneros and M.T. Tsuang
© Springer-Verlag Berlin Heidelberg 1990

cases. The range of schizophrenic/schizophreniform illnesses are among the more serious of mental illnesses whose treatment is both complex and long-term. Studies of the development of the psychoses are particularly important for the early recognition of features that may point to the onset of the illness in a chronic form.

The frequency of schizophrenia-like illness between the ages of 10 and 14 makes up about 4%–5% of the total incidence of schizophrenia (Eggers 1986). Little is known about the incidence of subgroups of schizophrenia in this age group. Longitudinal studies of symptom development over many years are very rare. In 1973, Eggers described a group of 57 patients retrospectively diagnosed to have a schizophrenia-like illness with an acute onset between the ages of 8 and 14. For these cases there exist well-documented cases histories covering a period of 8–54 years (mean 16 years). These case histories were reanalyzed by Eggers (1986) using more modern research diagnostic criteria (RDC) and the international classification of diseases (ICD-9). The main purpose of the study was the separation of schizoaffective from other schizophrenia-like illnesses by means of a comprehensive description of the typical clinical characteristics, the course of the illness, the premorbid state, and the degree of mental impairment and structural deficits of the personality at the end of the documented period. Eggers was able to show that schizoaffective psychoses in juveniles could be separated from "pure" schizophrenic illness by the occurrence of frequent short (<6 months) periods of exacerbated symptoms. In contrast, those with schizophrenia had a more remarkable premorbid phase. Indeed, the schizoaffectives with a more unusual premorbid period were also those who showed postpsychotic existential changes (e.g., "dynamic insufficiency" and "deformed personality", Janzarik 1968). Overall, those with a straightforward schizoaffective course had a better prognosis. Eggers found the coincidence of manic-depressive and schizophrenic features in the same psychotic period or the successive appearance of schizophrenic, schizoaffective, manic, and depressive (or manic-depressive) periods typical for juvenile schizoaffective illness. The appearance of individual Schneiderian first-rank symptoms (e.g., voices express the subject's thoughts aloud, comment on or address him/her; influenced by external forces that may control his/her thoughts and feelings) in themselves did not allow a prognosis to be made with confidence.

Eggers' study (1986) raises three major questions for the longitudinal evaluation of the developmental course of psychiatric illness:

1. How can the course of illness best be represented in order to facilitate comparative investigations?
2. What methods are best suited to describe features common to the development of illnesses and to characterize different courses?
3. What types of correlation exist between the different characteristics of the course of illness and the degree of eventual remission or a residual personality defect?

Methods

Subjects

Of the 57 patients in Eggers' study (1986), the records of 16 with schizoaffective and 41 with a diagnosis of pure schizophrenia were available for analysis. The type and duration of each period of illness, the duration of illness ("Di" in years) and the frequencies of episode alternations ("Ae") were precisely recorded. Degree of remission was assessed on a 3-point scale (0 = no schizophrenic defect, 1 = mild defect, 2 = severe defect). Periods of illness with the following features were delineated, and the duration was measured in months (see Table 1):

1. Without psychotic symptoms
2. Pure schizophrenic illness
3. Schizoaffective illness
4. Manic phase
5. Depressive phase.

According to DSM-III time criteria, we classified the length of the periods into two categories: longer than 6 months and shorter than 6 months.

Table 1. Codes for periods within the course of schizophrenic and schizoaffective illness

Period	Duration < 6 months	Duration > 6 months
Schizophrenic	A	B
Schizoaffective	C	G
No psychotic symptoms	E	F
Manic	M	*
Depressive	D	*

* Pure depressive or manic periods lasting longer than 6 months were not observed.

Analysis

Each individual course of illness was represented by a series of code letters (Table 2). Patterns of code letters common to all individuals in the two groups were sought. For this purpose we used the "pattern-analysis" method of filtering for redundancy from information theory. The repetition of a given series of letters, of a given length, for each patient represents a pattern or "concept" basic to the diagnostic category of the patients studied.

Pattern analysis is an appropriate method of searching for sequences of periods that might be typical for a given illness and thus to uncover "concepts" relevant for the putative diagnostic categories under investigation. An example for the previous use of this method in information theory is provided by Eisenecker's (1987) computer analysis of language structures. The author was able to show that linguistic concepts could be revealed by filtering redundant patterns

Table 2. Code sequences and degree of remission (defect)

Schizoaffective group

Subject no.		Defect
1	CFCECFDECFCE	1
2	DFAFAFBF	2
3	DFCECECFCF	1
4	CEDFDFDFCF	0
5	DFAEAFCDFDECEGE	2
6	CECFCECECME	0
7	CBECEBE	2
8	BFDFDECF	1
9	DFDECFBEBE	1
10	AEAEAFAFCEAFDF	0
11	DECFCFCE	1
12	DEMDECECFCF	1
13	CFCEAFCAECECEAECECFAECE	0
14	CECECECECECECECFCFGF	0
15	DEGFCFCE	1
16	DEDECEB	2

Schizophrenic group

Subject no.		Defect	Subject no.		Defect
17	AF	0	38	AF	0
18	AF	1	39	AEAEAF	0
19	AF	0	40	AEAF	0
20	AFAFAFAFAEAF	2	41	AEAEAEAF	1
21	AF	0	42	AFAEAEAEAEAF	1
22	AF	0	43	AEAEAEAEAEAEAFAEAFAFAEAFAF	1
23	AF	2	44	AFAEAFAE	2
24	AEAEBFBF	2	45	AFAFAF	1
25	AFAECECF	2	46	BFBFBFB	2
26	AFAEAEAEAEAEAEB	2	47	AF	2
27	AEAEAEAEAEAF	1	48	AF	2
28	AEAF	0	49	AFB	2
29	BF	2	50	AFAEAFAFAFAEAEAEB	2
30	AEBF	2	51	AFAEAEAEAF	2
31	BF	2	52	BEAAFAAF	2
32	BFBEF	2	53	AFAEB	2
33	BFAEBFAF	0	54	AEAEAEBEAFAEAEAEAEAFAEAFAEAFAF	2
34	BFAF	1	55	AFBEAEB	2
35	BFBFBFAE	1	56	BFA	1
36	AEAEAF	0	57	BFBEAEAEAFAF	1
37	AF	0			

from a series of letters coding language features, as long as the sequence was nonrandom. This procedure operates according to the so-called pregnancy principle, whereby the longest and most frequent chain of letters in one case is sought among all the other examples. By applying this procedure to the encoded periods of the course of illness of our schizophrenic and schizoaffective patients, we hoped to answer our second question above, namely to describe the features of these illnesses that are common to the one but different to the other diagnostic category.

Our procedure consisted first of encoding the periods of illness and second, of the pattern analysis. From this we determined the frequency of specific periods and the derived "concepts." For futher correlation analysis two formal parameters of the courses of the two groups were calculated and compared, e.g., the duration of illness (Di, in years) and the frequency of episode alternation (Ae; this is the length of the code sequences shown in Table 2). To answer the third question in our study (see above), correlations between the degree of remission, the incidence of periods and "concepts" and the formal parameters were calculated separately for each group with the Spearman rank correlation.

In this retrospective study the two groups were not randomly selected but separated by diagnostic criteria referring to the occurrence of different periods of the illness. Because of the different length of the courses in our sample we assume that the observed frequency of periods in each case is positively related to the duration of illness. Furthermore, the group selection criteria (periods with defined symptoms) are connected to time. This influences the probability for the occurrence of other periods. For example, in a schizoaffective course of a certain duration the probability of the occurrence of schizophrenic periods decreases if the frequency of schizoaffective periods increases, and vice versa. Because of the depending variances on period frequencies it is not possible to compute statistical tests on group differences for these variables.

Results

Duration of Illness, Frequency of Episode Alternation

Tables 3 and 4 show descriptive statistics and t test results for the variables Di and Ae. Schizophrenics in our sample had a significantly longer duration of illness then the schizoaffective group but showed a significantly lower mean frequency of episodes.

As the standard deviation of the duration of illness for the schizophrenics is relatively high compared with that for the schizoaffectives, we repeated the computation after excluding the four subjects in the schizophrenic group with a Di longer than 40 years (nos. 21, 39, 47, and 57; see Table 2). The results of the revised sample are shown in Tables 5 and 6. The difference in the Di was now nonsignificant, but the difference in the mean frequency of episodes remained unchanged.

This last result indicates that the number of episodes is not dependent on the length of illness. This result is supported by a nonsignificant correlation

Table 3. t test for duration of illness (Di) in years: complete data set

Group	No. of cases	Mean	Standard deviation	Median	Range
Schizoaffective	16	12.1563	5.156	13.0	2.0–21.6
Schizophrenic	41	17.7732	10.827	15.6	6.0–54.0

F value	2-Tail probability	Pooled variance estimate			Separate variance estimate		
		t value	Degrees of freedom	2-Tail probability	t value	Degrees of freedom	2-Tail probability
4.41	0.003	−1.98	55	0.053	−2.64	52.61	0.011

Table 4. t test for frequencies of episode alternation (Ae): complete data set

Group	No. of cases	Mean	Standard deviation	Median	Range
Schizoaffective	16	11.5625	4.926	10	7–23
Schizophrenic	41	7.0732	6.133	6	2–29

F value	2-Tail probability	Pooled variance estimate			Separate variance estimate		
		t value	Degrees of freedom	2-Tail probability	t value	Degrees of freedom	2-Tail probability
1.55	0.361	2.61	55	0.012	2.88	33.98	0.007

Table 5. t test for duration of illness (Di) in years: schizophrenics with Di >40 years omitted

Group	No. of cases	Mean	Standard deviation	Median	Range
Schizoaffective	16	12.1563	5.156	13	2.0–21.6
Schizophrenic	37	14.5865	4.456	15	6.0–22.0

F value	2-Tail probability	Pooled variance estimate			Separate variance estimate		
		t value	Degrees of freedom	2-Tail probability	t value	Degrees of freedom	2-Tail probability
1.34	0.461	−1.74	51	0.088	−1.64	25.16	0.114

Table 6. t test for frequencies of episode alternation (Ae): schizophrenics with Di > 40 years omitted

Group	No. of cases	Mean	Standard deviation	Median	Range
Schizoaffective	16	11.5625	4.926	10	7–23
Schizophrenic	37	7.2432	6.296	6	2–29

F value	2-Tail probability	Pooled variance estimate			Separate variance estimate		
		t value	Degrees of freedom	2-Tail probability	t value	Degrees of freedom	2-Tail probability
1.63	0.309	2.44	51	0.018	2.69	36.16	0.011

Table 7. Pregnant patterns and single episodes, schizoaffective group

	n	Mean	SD	MD	Min	Max
Pattern						
CE	16	1.7	2.0	1.0	0.0	8.0
CF	16	1.1	0.9	1.0	0.0	3.0
Episodes						
E	16	3.1	2.1	3.0	0.0	8.0
F	16	2.4	1.2	3.0	0.0	4.0
C	16	2.5	2.1	2.0	0.0	8.0
B	16	0.4	0.7	0.0	0.0	2.0
A	16	0.8	1.6	0.0	0.0	5.0

Table 8. Pregnant patterns and single episodes, schizophrenic group

	n	Mean	SD	MD	Min	Max
Pattern						
AE	41	1.4	2.2	1.0	0.0	9.0
AF	41	1.3	1.3	1.0	0.0	5.0
Episodes						
E	41	1.3	1.8	1.0	0.0	8.0
F	41	1.8	1.2	1.0	1.0	5.0
A	41	2.4	2.0	2.0	0.0	8.0
B	41	0.6	0.9	0.0	0.0	4.0

between Di and the Ae for both groups of the unrevised sample (schizoaffective: $R_{Di/Ae} = 0.11$; $P = 0.67$; schizophrenic: $R_{Di/Ae} = 0.12$; $P = 0.44$).

Pattern Analysis (Mean Frequencies of Pattern and Single Episodes)

The mean frequencies of the "concepts" that emerged from the pattern analysis were calculated for each patient and are shown in Tables 7 and 8.

Patterns of "Pregnant" Episode Sequences. For the schizoaffective group the longest and most frequent pattern was the sequence CE (mean, 1.7/patient). The second most frequent "pregnant concept" was the sequence CF (mean, 1.1/patient). This means that the course of illness for the group typically alternated between short schizoaffective periods (<6 months) and symptom-free periods that could last more or less than 6 months. Depressive periods (not shown in Table 7) followed by shorter or longer periods free of symptoms occurred with a mean frequency of 0.6/patient. The number of manic and schizoaffective periods (code M and G) lasting longer than 6 months was so small as not to warrant further analysis. There were two main "pregnant concepts" in the course of illness of the schizophrenic group (AE and AF, Table 8). This means that the course was characterized by short schizophrenic periods followed by shorter or longer periods free of symptoms (respective mean frequencies, 1.4 and 1.3/patient). In contrast, longer periods of schizophrenic symptoms were relatively seldom followed by shorter or longer symptom-free periods (code BE, 0.1/patient and BF, 0.4/patient; not shown in Table 8).

Patterns of Longer "Nonpregnant" Episode Sequences. These concepts are non-pregnant because they do not occur in each case. The sequence of short C (schizoaffective) – E (short symptom free) – C (schizoaffective) periods occurred on average with a frequency of 1.0/patient in the schizoaffective group. The sequence CFC occurred with a frequency of 0.6/patient.

There were no comparable patterns in the group of schizophrenic patients. Here the most frequent sequence was of A (short schizophrenic) – E (short symptom-free) – A (short schizophrenic) periods (1.2/patient). The sequence B (long schizophrenic) – F (long symptom-free) – B (long schizophrenic) was rare (0.2/patient). Long recurring schizophrenic periods with short intervening symptom-free periods were not observed.

Frequencies of Single Periods. The main interest in this analysis lay with the incidence of shorter and longer schizophrenic periods (i.e., A and B). Shorter schizophrenic periods (A, <6 months) had a mean frequency of 2.4/patient in the schizophrenic group (Table 8). In contrast, the incidence in the schizoaffective group was only 0.8/patient (Table 7). Longer periods of schizophrenia (B, >6 months) were rare in both groups of patients (0.6/schizophrenic patient and 0.4/schizoaffective patient, Tables 7 and 8). There was a similar incidence of longer and shorter symptom-free periods (E and F) for schizophrenic patients (E 1.3 and F 1.8/patient, Table 8). The frequency of longer and shorter symptom free-periods for schizoaffective patients was respectively E, 3.1 and F, 2.4/ patient. It may be noted that this group also showed an incidence of 3.1 short schizoaffective periods per patient (Table 7).

Correlations of Course Characteristics with Remission

The frequency of periods and "concepts" during the course of illness were the two main variables for which we sought correlations with the degree of schizophrenic defect shown separately by the schizophrenic and schizoaffective patients in remission. These correlations were sought in order to see if there were grounds for making a prognosis on the basis of the characteristics of the developmental course of the two illnesses. Duration of illness (Di) and the frequency

Table 9. Spearman correlation coefficients: defect with patterns, episodes, episode alternation (Ae) and duration of illness (Di): schizoaffective group

	R	P
CE	−0.53080	0.0344 s.
CF	−0.44821	0.0817 n.s.
E	−0.28184	0.2903 n.s.
F	−0.32449	0.2201 n.s.
C	−0.24171	0.3671 n.s.
B	0.57418	0.0200 s.
A	−0.06209	0.8193 n.s.
Ae	−0.61987	0.0104 s.
Di	−0.00789	0.9769 n.s.

P, two-tailed probability.
s., significant; n.s., not significant.

Table 10. Spearman correlation coefficients: defect with patterns, episodes, episode alternation (Ae) and duration of illness (Di): schizophrenic group

	R	P
AE	0.08688	0.5891 n.s.
AF	−0.01664	0.9177 n.s.
E	0.10832	0.5002 n.s.
F	0.25085	0.1137 n.s.
A	0.05574	0.7292 n.s.
B	0.40731	0.0082 s.
Ae	0.27409	0.0829 n.s.
Di	−0.21841	0.1701 n.s.

P, two-tailed probability.
s., significant; n.s., not significant.

of episode alternation (Ae) were included in the correlation analysis (Tables 9 and 10). The only significant correlation in the schizophrenic group was that between the amount of defect shown in remission and the frequency of longer schizophrenic periods (B) during the illness (R = 0.40, P = 0.008; Table 10). This means that when there were relatively frequent long schizophrenic periods during the illness, then defect symptoms were more apparent in remission. Neither Di nor Ae seems to cause a personality defect.

One of three significant correlations in the schizoaffective group was a negative relationship between the defect symptoms in remission and the "concept" CE (R = −0.53, P = 0.03; Table 9). This means that when the short schizoaffective episodes followed by short symptom-free periods were frequent (with respect to other periods) then defect symptoms were less apparent in remission. The high positive relation between defect and long schizophrenic episodes (B, R = 0.57, P = 0.02) supports the assumption, as in the schizophrenic group, that only schizophrenic episodes lasting longer than half a year are probably responsible for residual defects. The significant negative correlation of defect with the frequency of episodes (R = −0.61, P = 0.01; Table 9) seemed very strange to us at first. An inspection of the raw data set revealed the following result. There are four subjects in the schizoaffective group (nos. 2, 7, 9, and 16; see Table 2) who had one long schizophrenic episode lasting over more than 4 years. These patients show either a severe or a slight defect in remission. They have a relatively long course but only a small number of episode alternations. The probability of further episodes decreases if the length of one or more episodes increases (see also "Methods"). We interpret these findings in this way: the more "vivid" a developmental course of illness – with respect to short non-schizophrenic episodes and the absence of long schizophrenic episodes – the lower the probability of defect.

Discussion

We will first assess a few crucial points in our methodology. In encoding the periods of illness we arbitrarily divided their duration into periods shorter or longer than 6 months. In fact, some of these periods lasted as long as several years (see B for the schizophrenic group in Table 2). Interpretation of the results should take into consideration that the sum of the periods does not correspond to the actual duration of the course. Thus, although the number of longer schizophrenic periods is relatively small, their duration exerts a proportionately greater influence on the postpsychotic personality changes. This is indicated by the high positive correlation between defect and long schizophrenic episodes. The question remains open as to whether the same results would be achieved using a different criterion for the length of the periods of illness. However, if one divided phase duration into four categories, the number of varieties of "concepts" would increase considerably. From a clinical point of view, it is questionable whether such an analysis would yield meaningful results. Another effect of the lack of correspondence between the number of periods and the duration of illness, also found by Marneros et al. 1988, is that one cannot make statistical comparisons between the mean values for periods and "concepts." Such a procedure would lead to a considerable underestimate of the clinical importance of the rare long periods.

We studied the records of 57 patients with a schizophrenia-like illness that showed an onset in early adolescence or preadolescence. One of us (C.E.) diagnosed the subgroups of schizophrenia and schizoaffective illness. Unusual for clinical psychiatric research, typical characteristics for the course of each illness were sought with the technique of pattern analysis and compared, for the purposes of prognosis, with the severity of defect shown in remission. Typical for the schizoaffective course was a recurring sequence of short periods of affective illness with short symptom-free periods (CE). If a course of illness showed this pattern relatively frequently, then the probability of developing severe symptoms of defect seemed to be small. Indeed, schizoaffective patients had more symptom-free periods lasting at least 6 months than did the schizophrenic group. This, in itself, points to the increased likelihood of this group developing less severe signs of defect. The major feature of the schizophrenic course was a similar alternation between short periods with and short periods without schizophrenic symptoms (AE). But this pattern did not seem to be related to the degree of defect shown in remission. The alternation of short periods of illness (<6 months) appeared to have little prognostic value. The degree of defect shown by schizophrenics at the end of the observed course seemed to be related only to the occurrence of schizophrenic periods lasting longer than 6 months. The same applies to the schizoaffective group when long schizophrenic episodes appear. However, in general, the results of the pattern analysis indicate that there are only short "concepts" (2-code episode sequences) typical for the separate groups. This implies that there is a marked variety of symptoms and heterogeneity of course shown by these two subgroups (see Eggers 1986). Nevertheless, it is sensible to attempt to seek features of the course common to different patients in order to achieve a greater insight into the nature of the illness than that which is possible to derive from a cross-sectional analysis.

There is a sense in which our results seem trivial. They confirm the original diagnosis into schizophrenic and schizoaffective subgroups. But this itself supports the way in which the borders between these two forms of illness were drawn. For example, let us take the patterns AF and AE that were found to be typical for the schizophrenic course. It would seem from the courses shown in Table 2 that subjects 2 and 10 from the schizoaffective group show course features more typical of the schizophrenic group. The correlation with later remission status and the frequency of period sequences and single periods shows no conflict with studies of the development of the course of illness in patients whose onset occurred later, in adulthood (Marneros et al. 1988). In both instances it was observed that a proportional increase in the duration of schizophrenic periods is related to increasing severity of defect shown in remission, but that an increased proportion of schizoaffective periods provides for an improved prognosis.

Crow (1980) suggested dividing schizophrenic psychoses into two types. The an increased incidence of premorbid abnormalities and more cognitive disturbance than those with positive, or type-I, features. Although the two groups did not differ in the age of onset of the illness, type-II subjects had spent much more time in the hospital. More recently, Carpenter et al. (1988) compared patients with and without symptoms of defect along the lines described by Crow. Patients with schizophrenic defect scored worse on scales evaluating prognosis, premorbid adaptability, and duration of institutionalization. Indeed, the main reason for hospitalization turned out to be the presence of type-II symptoms. Carpenter et al. suggest that the two types of syndrome should be viewed as poles at opposite ends of a continuum.

We regard our results to be partially consistent with the findings from the groups of Crow, Andreasen, and Carpenter. Patients in our sample with long schizophrenic episodes (B) and a severe defect in personality structure could probably be classified as type-II subjects retrospectively. This is of interest when one considers that the records for our patients go back to the 1950s and earlier. With changes in diagnosis and treatment since then this woud not necessarily be expected. But through these reports we should qualify our assessment in one respect. We categorized certain periods in our retrospective analysis as being free of symptoms. It remains open to question whether these periods really were free of clinically relevant symptoms or merely were free of acute symptoms warranting hospitalization, but it should be emphasized that our analysis consisted of individually based reinvestigations. These included interviewing relatives of the patients and inquiring about the incidence of even mild psychotic symptoms. Thus, it does not seem likely that relevant periods of illness went unnoticed (Eggers 1973).

We want to point out the interaction of diagnostic processes, the fact of hospitalization, the variety of new treatment methods and concepts, and the developmental course of the individual schizophrenic disorder. The frequency and duration of hospitalization is relevant insofar as social integration on remission is the more difficult to achieve, the longer the patient remains in the clinic. On the other hand, for an inpatient, reciprocal interactions between the type of symptoms shown and his or her environment could influence both the devel proposal was based on studies of structural changes in the brain, numbers of dopamine receptors assessed post mortem, and clinical features. Subjects with type-I psychosis show many features typical of acute schizophrenia, especially positive symptoms such as hallucinations, delusions, and thought disorders. There is a good chance that such patients will respond to neuroleptic treatment and show a good prognosis with respect to cognitive abilities. Increased numbers of dopamine receptors are predicted for this group. Type-II subjects are characterized by flat affect, poverty of speech, and apathy. There is a strong tendency for the illness to become chronic. Symptoms of defect are more common, and structural changes may be present in the brain. Andreasen and Olsen (1982) found evidence for both syndromes in a popuation of 52 adult schizophrenics (DSM-III). Further, they report that their negative, or type-II, subjects showed opmental course and treatment strategies for schizophrenic psychoses in different hospitals. All this may contribute to the marked inter- and intraindividual variability of the developmental course of psychoses.

References

Andreasen NC, Olsen S (1982) Negative and positive schizophrenia. Arch Gen Psychiatry 39:689–794

Carpenter WT, Douglas WH, Wagman AM (1988) Deficit and nondeficit forms of schizophrenia: The concept. Am J Psychiatry 145:578–583

Crow TJ (1980) Molecular pathology of schizophrenia: more than one desease process? Br Med J 12:66–68

Eggers C (1973) Verlaufsweisen kindlicher und präpuberaler Schizophrenien. Springer, Berlin Heidelberg New York

Eggers C (1986) Schizoaffective psychoses in children and juveniles. In: Marneros A, Tsuang MT (eds) Schizoaffective psychoses. Springer, Berlin Heidelberg New York Tokyo

Eisenecker U (1987) Künstliche Intelligenz und Musteranalyse. Heise, Hannover

Janzarik W (1968) Schizophrene Verläufe. Springer, Berlin Heidelberg New York Tokyo

Marneros A, Deister A, Rohde A, Jünemann H, Fimmers F (1988) Long-term course of schizoaffective disorders. Part I, II, III. Eur Arch Psychiatry Neurol Sci 237:264–290

Maturana H, Varela F (1987) Der Baum der Erkenntnis. Scherz, Bern

von Foerster H (1985) Sicht und Einsicht. Braunschweig, Vieweg

Schizoaffective Disorders in the Elderly

B. Pitt[1]

In his classic monographs on *The significance of affective symptoms in old age* (1962) and *Persistent persecutory states of the elderly* (1966) Felix Post found that 38% of elderly depressives occasionally exhibited paranoid symptoms, and that 58% of late paraphrenics had at some time or other depressive admixtures. In a subsequent (1971), far less frequently cited paper (Post 1971) he addressed the problem of schizoaffective symptomatology in late life.

For 5 years all in-patients over 60 under his care at the Bethlem and Maudsley hospitals were earmarked when they presented a problem of differential diagnosis between paraphrenic and affective illnesses on admission or later. (Paraphrenia is the most common form in which schizophrenia presents for the first time in late life; other presentations, though not unknown, are extremely rare.) This was the case in only about 4% of cases, so the study yielded only 29 patients for whom the diagnosis of schizoaffective disorder seemed justified.

Post then tested the hypothesis that, given time, these patients would exhibit affective or paraphrenic symptoms only. (The climate of the Maudsley Hospital at the time did not favour the diagnosis of "schizoaffective disorder," it being felt that the label could be avoided by a more rigorous diagnostic approach and follow-up.) They were followed up for not less than 3 and an average of 4.5 years. The hypothesis was not confirmed. Almost half the patients developed a lasting mixed paraphrenic/affective clinical picture, while the rest exhibited this mixture over briefer periods, or affective and paraphrenic symptoms in succession, at different times.

Post then went on to compare this consecutive series of 29 schizoaffective patients with consecutive elderly depressives (100) and paraphrenics (93), all treated in the same unit. The schizoaffective patients were intermediate between the other two groups in respect of sex distribution, family history of affective disorder, history of unsatisfactory sexual adjustment, marriage rate, social class, psychological disturbances and more definite psychiatric illness before the age of 50 and recent disturbing life events. Differences significant at the 5% level are listed in Table 1.

There were also a number of attributes which the schizoaffective patients exhibited more frequently than either the depressives or the paraphrenics,

---

[1] Department of Psychiatry of Old Age, St. Mary's and the Royal Postgraduate Hospital Medical Schools, London, England

Affective and Schizoaffective Disorders
Edited by A. Marneros and M.T. Tsuang
© Springer-Verlag Berlin Heidelberg 1990

Table 1. Characteristics of patients in three groups compared by Post (in percent)

	Depressives	Schizoaffective	Paraphrenic
Female sex	53*	72*	86
Sexual maladjustment	40*	60*	77
Low social class	13*	49*	62
Psychological disorder before 50	47	38*	16*
Life event	60*	21*	0*

* 5% significance level.

Table 2. Differences between schizoaffectives, depressives and paraphrenics

	Schizoaffectives	Depressives	Paraphrenics
Total psychiatric heredity	76	62*	40*
Abnormal personality	86*	63*	68
Cerebral pathology	41	30*	17*
Disabled during most of observation period	48	34	33

* 5% significance level.

namely frequency in family history of all types of psychiatric disorder, abnormal personality traits and the incidence of cerebral disorder (Table 2).

Compared with 3% of the depressives and none of the paraphrenics, 17% of the schizoaffectives had a family history of schizoaffective disorder. Only one schizoaffective and one depressive, compared with five paraphrenics, had a family history of schizophrenia. And 24% of schizoaffectives, compared with 32% of depressives and 17% of paraphrenics, had a family history of affective disorder.

One initially paraphrenic patient only had a "cerebral disorder" – myxoedema. Three initially depressed patients had such disorders: one temporal lobe epilepsy, two transient cerebrovascular insufficiency. But eight (two-thirds) of the patients with "cerebral disorders" were initially schizoaffective: two were myxoedematous, consistent with Asher's (1949) "myxoedematous madness", four became demented, one developed carcinomatosis and one had transitory cerebrovascular deficiency.

During follow-up, only one schizoaffective patient remained symptom free, compared with 26% of the depressives and a surprising 57% of paraphrenics, though all groups received comparable treatment. This is in complete contrast to the findings of Vaillant (1964) and Stephens et al. (1966) that the affective features improved the prognosis of schizophrenia in younger patients. Even allowing for the high incidence of "cerebral disorder" among the elderly schizoaffectives, they fared strikingly poorly. Nor did the depressives do all that well, consistent with Murphy's (1983) finding that only a third of depressives remained symptom free in the first year after referral to a psychogeriatric service. The comparatively good prognosis for the paraphrenics, on the other hand, suggests that the condition may be rather distantly related to schizophrenia in younger patients.

Unfortunately, the topic of schizoaffective disorder in the elderly has apparently been neglected since Post's study. A subsequent Maudsley Hospital study (Brockington and Leff 1979) omitted patients over 65, and a recent review (Levitt and Tsuang 1988) makes no mention of the elderly. The follow-up study by Jorgensen and Munk-Jorgensen (1985) of 106 patients over 60 admitted to the Aarhus Hospital, Denmark, with paranoid disorders (excluding affective psychosis and dementia) found five with depressive delusions, while in the ensuing 5–15 years (average 10) the diagnosis was changed to affective psychosis in five cases. This writer (Pitt 1988) presented at a symposium data on patients referred to the Claybury Hospital psychogeriatric service: 71 of 500 (14%) were referred because of paranoia. Paranoid personality accounted for only four of these, confusional states for 17, and paraphrenia, paranoid states and paranoid schizophrenia for 43; seven patients (1.4% of all the referrals) were significantly depressed as well as paranoid and could (retrospectively) be classified as schizoaffective.

Following in Post's footsteps, Holden (1987) used the Camberwell Register and the Maudsley Hospital Case Register to identify 47 patients with paranoid psychosis occurring for the first time after the age of 60, who were followed up for 10 years or until death. They were divided into six subgroups: five patients whose paranoia was secondary to depression were designated "affective," and five with at least one subsequent episode diagnosed as affective disorder, "schizoaffective." In five "symptomatic" patients the mental state appeared to have an association with chronic physical illness. Thirteen patients who progressed to dementia were designated "organic." The remaining 19 patients were then divided according to the presence or absence of Schneiderian first-rank

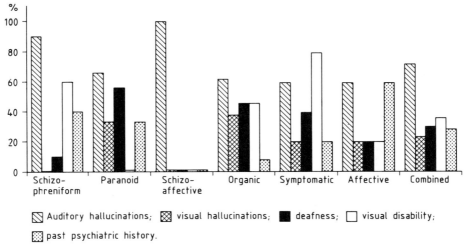

Fig. 1. Characteristics of subgroups at presentation. (From Holden 1987)

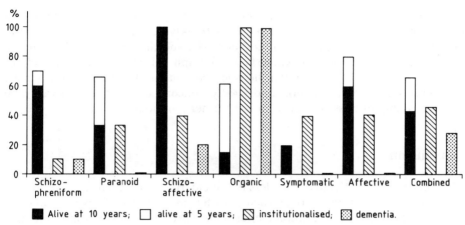

Fig. 2. Outcome of subgroups during the 10-year follow-up. (From Holden 1987)

symptoms into a "schizophreniform" (ten cases) or a "paranoid" group (nine cases).

Compared with the other groups at presentation (Fig. 1), the schizoaffective patients lacked any previous psychiatric history, were neither deaf nor visually impaired and had no visual hallucinations, though they all heard voices. Affective patients, on the other hand, had a strong previous psychiatric history, and one fifth were deaf, visually impaired or visually hallucinated. While a family history (a third schizophreniform) was reported in 42% of the functional groups (and only 23% of the "organic"), separate statistics for the schizoaffectives are not given.

The outcomes are interesting, though the numbers within the subgroups are, of course, small (see Fig. 2). All the schizoaffective patients survived the 10 years, but two of the five were in institutions, and one had developed dementia. These outcomes were less good than those of the "schizophreniform" group, except that the latter did not survive as long: only one patient was in an institution and one was demented (of ten). Survival in the affective group was less, but none became demented; the same proportion were in institutions.

All these "post-Post" studies have looked at affective disorders in the setting of paraphrenia and other paranoid psychoses of late life. This paper does not review any recent studies of paranoid or schizophrenic symptoms in the affective context. Such phenomena, however, are not rare, and they are by no means always mood congruent (Pitt 1986). Paranoid delusions may at first seem appropriate to severe depression and guilt: e.g. "Everyone is talking about me and I am being followed by the police because I have defrauded the state by claiming more benefits than I am entitled to, and paying too little tax, and deserve severe punishment." At a later stage, though, when the depression and guilt have largely lifted as a result of antidepressant therapy, the delusions and hallucinations may persist but the patient no longer feels that they are deserved, but that they are rather persecutory: "They are waiting for me outside the hospital, I hear the other patients and some of the staff saying bad things about me and I'm afraid, but I've done nothing wrong." Here, the addition of a neuroleptic is usually effective. Sometimes frankly depressive episodes are followed by bouts of paraphrenia (Logsdail 1984), and the writer recalls a woman who was always abrasive, but when she was paraphrenic she blamed her landlord for all her woes (e.g. alleging that he released rats into her flat), and when she was depressed she was hypochondriacally concerned about her bowels and would irritably dismiss reference to her former paranoia.

Conclusion

The topic of schizoaffective disorders in the elderly has been largely overlooked since Post's (1971) study, though such disorders are not rare. They may take the form of (a) psychoses with simultaneous schizophrenic (mainly paraphrenic) and affective features of equal prominence, which persist until treated and do not resolve into one disorder or the other; (b) primarily paraphrenic disorders with prominent affective features; (c) primarily affective disorders with prominent mood-incongruent paranoid features; or (d) paraphrenic and affective episodes in the same patient. Post differentiated schizoaffective subjects from affective and paraphrenic by the richness of the family history of psychiatric (including schizoaffective) illness, abnormal previous personality, associated cerebral pathology and (unlike younger schizoaffectives) a poor prognosis. The time is ripe for further and confirmatory research in this neglected area.

References

Asher R (1949) Myxoedematous madness. Br Med J 2:555–559
Brockington IF, Leff JP (1979) Schizo-affective psychosis: definitions and incidence. Psychol Med 9:91–99
Holden NL (1987) Late paraphrenia or the paraphrenias? A descriptive study with a 10-year follow-up. Br J Psychiatry 150:635–639
Jorgensen P, Munk-Jorgensen P (1985) Paranoid psychosis in the elderly: a follow-up study. Acta Psychiatr Scand 72:358–363
Levitt JL, Tsuang MT (1988) The heterogeneity of schizoaffective disorder: implications for treatment. Am J Psychiatry 145:926–936
Logsdail S (1984) Affective illness changing to paranoid state: report on three elderly patients. Br J Psychiatry 144:209–210
Murphy E (1983) The prognosis of depression in old age. Br J Psychiatry 141:135–142
Pitt B (1986) Characteristics of depression in the elderly. In: Murphy E (ed) Affective disorders in the elderly. Churchill Livingstone, London
Post F (1962) The significance of affective symptoms in old age. Maudsley Monograph 10. Oxford University Press, London
Post F (1966) Persistent persecutory states of the elderly. Pergamon, Oxford
Post F (1971) Schizo-affective symptomatology in late life. Br J Psychiatry 118:437–445
Stephens JH, Astrup C, Mangrum JC (1966) Prognostic factors in recovered and deteriorated schizophrenias. Am J Psychiatry 122:1116–1121
Vaillant GE (1964) Prospective prediction of scizophrenic remission. Arch Gen Psychiatry 122:811–828

Life Events in Affective and Schizoaffective Disorders

E.S. PAYKEL[1]

Methodological Requirements

Modern empirical research into the relationship between life events and psychiatric disorders has been undertaken for longer than 20 years. Acceptable research has depended on adequate methodology. The key issue is that of reliable and valid life-event ascertainment.

The earliest studies employed information obtained from case records, or self-report questionnaires (Holmes and Rahe 1967), but later studies have moved towards semi-structured interviews of the subjects (e.g. Brown and Birley 1968; Paykel et al. 1969). This move was a response to recognition of the problems inherent in retrospective reporting of events. An event can only be reported after it has happened. The inaccuracies of recall which all subjects experience may be compounded in the psychiatric patient by distortions due to illness. In addition, "effort after meaning" in attempts to explain illness in terms of preceding stress may lead to events being over-reported or exaggerated, both by patients and by relatives.

Self-report questionnaires preclude detailed factual checking and they also encounter ambiguities and misinterpretations of what is meant by any specific event. Moreover, they fail to tackle the problem of accurate recall of the time of occurrence of an event. In our own experience using semi-structured interviews, it has been necessary to give frequent reminders of the time period in question in order to avoid a tendency in subjects to report events outside the study period. Use of life events recorded in routine case records presents similar problems compounded further by vagaries in selection of events for enquiry and recall.

Several semi-structured interview schedules are available. Among these, Brown's (Brown et al. 1973a; Brown and Harris 1978) is the most detailed, involving a lengthy and comprehensive interview with tape recording, and later full rating of events and their qualities. Our own (Paykel 1983) is shorter, taking between a half and one and a quarter hours to administer. It covers 64 events and makes judgements of two central aspects, independence and objective negative impact.

Events do not occur in a vacuum, and the individual may bring about his own events. Illness itself can create events, for example the loss of a job, and it is

---

[1] Department of Psychiatry, University of Cambridge, Addenbrooke's Hospital, Cambridge CB2 2QQ, England

Affective and Schizoaffective Disorders
Edited by A. Marneros and M.T. Tsuang
© Springer-Verlag Berlin Heidelberg 1990

therefore important to separate out those events which are consequences of illness from those which might be causative. One step towards eliminating illness-caused events is to interview in detail to establish timing of symptom onset, and to confine attention to time periods preceding it. Brown et al. (1973a) introduced a further concept of the "independent" event into life-event research. They pointed out that with detailed scrutiny of circumstances it is possible to isolate events which are unlikely to have been produced by illness and are therefore of particular importance as possible causative factors.

A way of assessing the amount of stress associated with different events also needs to be found. Various methods which have been used effectively for this purpose (Paykel 1983) include an additive scale with consensus weighting (Holmes and Rahe 1967) and contextual judgements by raters of threat of an event to the average person in the same situation (Brown et al. 1973a). We have made use of a similar rating, objective negative impact, but have also found it useful to categorise events into different types, such as exists and entrances, undesirable and desirable (Paykel et al. 1969, 1975, 1976). One method which should usually be avoided in life-event research is the subjective personal judgement of stress. If a patient has experienced a psychiatric disorder soon after a life event has taken place, it is understandable to regard the event as stressful, even if this would not be the case in other circumstances.

The timing of the interview also matters. We have found it best to delay data collection until acute psychiatric disturbance has diminished, in order to avoid reporting directly distortions due to illness.

The ultimate aims are reliability and validity. A review of reliability studies (Paykel 1983) has shown that self-report inventories tend to give low reliability, whilst studies employing interview methods tend to lead to moderately high reliability. Validity in life-event research can be tested by comparing the information gained from the patient with information gained from another informant, usually a close relative. Generally, much higher agreement has been found when interview methods have been employed (Paykel 1983).

The findings of studies of life events and psychiatric disorders should always be interpreted in the light of the attention which has been given to these methodological issues in data collection.

Life Events and Onset of Depression

Life events have been studied most extensively with respect to onset of depression. This review will focus on samples receiving psychiatric treatment, since studies of milder disorders in the community raise additional issues as to whether a qualitatively different disturbance is being studied.

Table 1 summarises findings of 27 published retrospective comparisons (one employing two comparison groups) of psychiatrically treated depressed patients with control groups. Fifteen studies, from the USA, England, Ireland Italy, Spain, Poland, Kenya and India, employed general population controls, including one study of elderly patients (Murphy 1982). All found more events reported prior to depressive onset, although in one study with small numbers the difference did not reach significance. Two studies compared depressives with medical patient controls. Both found more events reported by depressives but the differences were not very striking or clearly attributable to causes rather than to effects of depression.

Comparisons of depressives and other psychiatric patients were also summarised in the table. Depressives have been found to report more events than schizophrenics, indicating in the retrospective frame greater causative effects. In one study (Leff and Vaughn 1980) differences for independent events were suggestive but not significant and there was no difference for undesirable events. Two additional studies not shown in the table failed to find differences between depressives and schizophrenics, but life-event methodologies were limited (Eisler and Polak 1971; Lahniers and White 1976). A third study (Harder et al. 1980) did not clearly separate depressives and neurotics.

Some comparisons with mixed psychiatric patients have also suggested greater effects in depressives, but not fully consistently. On the other hand, three comparisons of suicide attempters with depressives found more events in suicide attempters.

Some other studies using different designs or samples are not shown in the table. In a small study (Paykel 1974) using patients as their own controls, we found that event rates in depressives dropped on follow-up, but not fully to the general population level. One study has shown heroin addicts with secondary depression to have more stressful events than those without depression (Prusoff et al. 1977), while another study obtained similar findings for depressed compared with nondepressed schizophrenics (Roy et al. 1983), as did a questionnaire study of secondarily depressed and nondepressed alcoholics (Fowler et al. 1980). A follow-up study of addicts found events to be associated with continuing depression and failure of recovery, as measured by the Beck Depression Inventory, although the direction of causation was not clear (Kosten et al. 1983).

A specific hypothesis would suggest that depression, and only depression, is induced by certain types of events. Most prominent in the literature is the role of loss. The concept of loss is somewhat diffuse, including interpersonal separations and deaths, loss of self-esteem, and other kinds of losses.

Interpersonal losses of various kinds have received the most study. Findings from the studies are summarised in Table 1. Twenty studies have reported specifically on recent separations. In 11, depressives reported more separations than the controls, which included both subjects from the general population and other psychiatric patients, suggesting some specificity. There was, however, no excess over medical patients. Two studies found not only that exit events were related to depression but also that their converse, entrance events, were not (Paykel et al. 1969; Fava et al. 1981). However, one study (Slater and Depue 1981) found that primary depressives who made a suicide attempt had experienced more exits than those who did not, indicating a greater relationship to the attempt. Some additional studies, not shown in the tables, have found a relationship between depression and recent deaths (Paykel 1982).

Table 1. Controlled comparisons of effects of life events on onset of clinical depression

Nature of controls	Authors	Excess any events	Excess separations	Excess other types of events
General population	Paykel et al. (1969)	Yes	Yes	Various, especially undesirable events
	Thomson and Hendrie (1972)	Yes	Not reported	More stress overall
	Cadoret et al. (1972)	Suggestive	Suggestive	Not reported
	Brown et al. (1973b)	Yes	Not reported	Markedly and moderately threatening events
	Fava et al. (1981)	Yes	Yes	Undesirable, negative impact
	Vadher and Ndetei (1981)	Yes	Yes	Suggestive only
	Chatterjee et al. (1981)	Yes	Yes	Health, interpersonal
	Bebbington et al. (1981)	Yes, men	Not reported	Events of severe and moderate threat
	Murphy (1982)	Yes	Suggestive	Health
	Billings et al. (1983)	Yes	Yes	Various negative events
	Faravelli and Ambonetti (1983)	Yes	Not reported	Undesirable, exit and severe
	Bidzinska (1984)	Yes	No	Marital and family conflicts, work overload, failures
	Roy et al. (1985)	Yes	No	Undesirable events
	Brugha and Conroy (1985)	Yes	Not reported	Undesirable, threatening; not independent, uncontrolled
	Ezquiaga et al. (1987)	Yes	Not reported	Threatening, independent

			Social factors
Medical patients			
Forrest et al. (1965)	Yes, weak	No	
Hudgens et al. (1967)	Yes, weak	No	Moves, interpersonal discord
Other psychiatric patients			
Schizophrenics			
Beck and Worthen (1972)	Yes	Suggestive	Events of higher rated hazard
Brown et al. (1973b)	Yes	Not reported	Events of moderate and marked threat over longer time
Jacobs et al. (1974)	Yes	Yes	Undesirable, health financial, interpersonal discord
Leff and Vaughn (1980)	Suggestive	Not reported	Not for undesirable events
Suicide attempters			
Paykel et al. (1975)	Fewer events in depressives	No	Fewer events in depressives, especially undesirable, unsetting
Slater and Depue (1981)	Fewer events in depressives	No; fewer exits	Fewer independent events
Cohen-Sandler et al. (1982)	Fewer events in depressives	Fewer deaths, separations	Case-note study in children
Mixed psychiatric patients			
Sethi (1964)	Yes	Yes	Not reported
Levi et al. (1966)	Yes	Yes	Not reported
Malmquist (1970)	No	No	No
Uhlenhuth and Paykel (1973)	No	No	No

Also common in the studies are arguments and discord with various key interpersonal figures. They may involve threat of separation. Blows to the self-esteem and failures have not usually been explicitly reported but are probably also common. As can be seen from the table, a wide variety of events is involved. In general the studies suggest only weak specificity. There is some relationship between depression and interpersonal losses, but these also precede other disorders, and many depressions are not preceded by them. The strongest relationship appears when events are categorised in rather broad terms such as threatening or undesirable. This extends well beyond interpersonal loss.

All studies in Table 1 were of patients with disorders sufficiently severe for them to present to psychiatrists. It has sometimes been argued that although life events may be important for milder disorders identified in community surveys, they are not implicated to any great degree in true major disorder. The findings in Table 1 do not sustain this view.

Psychotic and Endogenous Depression

A further issue involves the distinctions between psychotic or endogenous and neurotic depression. This is important in the present discussion, since we are dealing with the place of events in schizoaffective psychotic states. Terminology is confusing here since the terms "psychotic" and "endogenous" have been used as overlapping in the literature on depression.

A proportion of depressive episodes are not endogenous in the sense that they are not preceded by life events: perhaps about 20% in the controlled studies. However, as the term is usually employed, endogenous depressions are also regarded as showing a specific symptom pattern overlapping with psychotic depression including greater severity, psychomotor retardation or agitation, sometimes depressive delusions, early-morning wakening, and diurnal variation with morning worsening (Rosenthal and Klerman 1966).

A number of studies using careful life-event methods have shown that life events and symptom pattern are only weekly related. In our first New Haven study, symptoms were rated by one rater and life-event information was collected blind by another. Absence of life stress showed only a low correlation, although in the predicted direction, with an endogenous symptom factor (Paykel 1974). In a later study of outpatients (Paykel et al. 1984), again only a very weak relationship between the two aspects was found, reaching significance only when persisting problems at the time of presentation were examined, rather than life events at onset.

Several other studies have given similar findings (Brown et al. 1979; Benjaminsen 1981; Katschnig and Berner 1984; Monroe et al. 1985). Brugha and Conroy (1985) found greater patient-control life-event differences for CATEGO R (retarded or endogenous) depressives than for N (neurotic), rather than the reverse. Matussek and Neuner (1981) using a lengthy and probing interview, found differences between neurotic and endogenous depression only for separations from an important partner. In a small study, Bebbington et al. (1981) did find fewer life events in patients with an endogenous symptom pattern, but they found little evidence of this in a larger sample (Bebbington et al. 1988), although absence of social support more strongly predicted a poor outcome at 4 months in neurotic depressives (Brugha et al. 1987). However, Roy et al. (1985) found that the neurotic depressives had significantly more life events than endogenous depressives, and only they experienced more events than normal controls.

The ambiguities of terminology mean that in some of these studies patients showed the endogenous symptom pattern but were not psychotic in the sense of having delusions or hallucinations. Nevertheless, it would appear that life events bear only a weak relationship to symptom pattern, and that the latter is predominantly determined by some other mechanism.

Bipolar Manic Depressive Disorder

One aspect which is also important in the context of schizoaffective disorder and has not yet been adequately studied is that of elated affective disorder. Bipolar manic depressives have been in a small minority or absent in most studies. Three studies have explicitly examined mania. Ambelas (1979) studied a time period of 4 weeks preceding admission and found that manic patients had four times as many stressful life events as a surgical control group. Information on manic subjects was based mainly on case notes, but most of the events listed did appear to be independent. Ambelas found that the events experienced were mostly unpleasant ones. Whenever a pleasant event was found an element of threat or loss was also strongly suspected. Stresses were categorised into two types, losses and threats; losses were present twice as often as threats, and bereavement was found in five of 14 cases. In the second study, Kennedy et al. (1983) looked at the 4 months before onset in manic patients, using both a matched control group and patients as their own controls. They found a twofold increase in life events during the 4-month period. The within-patient control comparison was used to test whether or not these patients might have more life events in any 4-month period, for reasons such as personality traits, but this was not found to be the case. A third recent case-note study (Ambelas 1987), which may have overlapped to some extent in samples with Ambelas (1979), gave similar findings, with a much more marked effect for first attacks. This is consistent with the finding of another study in a lithium clinic that fluctuations in treated manic depressives were not stress related (Hall et al. 1977). A major life crisis may contribute to the onset of a disorder for which subsequent attacks are much more biologically determined. However, Aronson and Shukla (1987) found a sudden peak of relapses in bipolar disorder in a lithium clinic shortly after a hurricane, a clearly independent event. One study (Glassner and Haldipur 1983) found more evidence of stressful life events in bipolars with onset over the age of 20 than under, suggesting that constitutional factors might be more important in the latter.

Mania is a disorder producing increased activity and disinhibition and readily leading to new dependent events such as job changes, financial problems from overspending, arguments, and disruptions of old relationships and initiation of new ones. Particular care therefore needs to be taken to define independent events in such studies. Except for the study by Aronson and Shukla (1987), the existing studies have not fully ruled out such events.

Life Events and Outcome of Depression

In recent years, the relationship between life events and outcome of depression has come under investigation. Several studies have examined events at onset – really one aspect of endogenous and reactive depression. In relatively short term studies of 4–6 weeks' outcome in drug trials, Lloyd et al. (1981) found that presence of life events at onset did not influence outcome, while Rowan et al. (1982) found a weak trend for outcome to be worse where a major life event had occurred (unpublished analyses). In a community survey, Tennant et al. (1981) found better outcome where a threatening event had occurred in the 3 months before onset.

In longer follow-ups of 6–9 months, Parker et al. (1988) found in neurotic depressives that preceding breaks of intimate relationships, but not other events, were associated with good outcome. Monroe et al. (1983, 1985) found that more onset events predicted a better outcome, especially in patients with endogenous symptoms. In a 1-year follow-up of elderly depressives (Murphy 1983) life events at onset did not predict outcome.

In a somewhat different retrospective study, Billings and Moos (1984) compared depressives with either a recurrent or a nonrecurrent illness, for onset stressors. No differences were found between them.

Events concurrent with treatment might be expected to have greater effects. In the study cited earlier, Lloyd et al. (1981) found that patients with poor outcome were more likely to have experienced stressful events during the 4-week period. Rowan et al. (1982) found that events occurring during a 6-week treatment period had no significant effect on outcome, but few major independent events occurred. In a study of community cases, Tennant et al. (1981) found that remission was more likely over a 1-month period after a "neutralising" event, i.e. one which caused minimal threat but counteracted the effect of an earlier threatening event or chronic difficulty.

Three studies have examined concurrent events over follow-up periods of between 3 and 9 months. Surtees (1980) found that greater event stress was associated with worse outcome. Paykel and Tanner (1976) examined relapse in women in a continuation study of drugs and psychotherapy. Relapse was found to be associated with concurrent undesirable life events in the 3 months prior to relapse. These relapses appeared to be separate from those related to drug withdrawal. The third study (Monroe et al. 1983, 1985) failed to find outcome influenced by concurrent events.

Among longer term follow-up studies of patients, Murphy (1983) and Giel et al. (1978) both provided evidence supporting the hypothesis that outcome is worse if a threatening event has occurred. Among women in the community,

Brown et al. (1988) found recovery from chronic depression preceded by reduction in ongoing difficulties and occurrence of events implying a fresh start towards a better future. However, in a 12-month follow-up of a small sample of patients on maintenance therapy, Mendlewicz et al. (1986) found no overall effect of life events on relapse, although there was a nonsignificant association with bereavement.

The picture emerging from these studies is that life events at onset do not greatly effect outcome, but that there is a weak trend to better outcome in stress-related depressions. However, where events occur concurrently with treatment negative events lead to a worse outcome, and positive events to a better outcome.

Schizophrenia

In the aetiology of schizophrenia, twin and adoption studies provide evidence of a moderately strong genetic element. Concordance rates in monozygotic twins nevertheless leave considerable room for environmental influences, and there is strong evidence that social factors have important effects on the course.

Several studies have examined recent life events. Findings are shown in Tables 1 and 2. Brown and Birley (1968) found more independent events than in general population controls, but only in the 3 weeks before onset or relapse. The differences were considerably less than in Brown's later studies of depression. Most studies of depression also suggest an excess of events extending back for 6 months to a year. Using our methods, Jacobs and Myers (1976) found more life events in the year before first onset than in the general population, but here, too, differences were relatively weak, and for a small group of events categorised as likely to be independent of the subject's control they did not reach significance. The studies by Schwartz and Myers (1977a,b) involved schizophrenics in the

Table 2. Controlled studies of life events in schizophrenia

Controls	Author	Findings of excess events in schizophrenics
General population	Brown and Birley (1968)	3 weeks before onset
	Jacobs and Myers (1976)	Yes, relatively weak
	Schwartz and Myers (1977a,b)	Yes, minor symptoms in community
	Canton and Fraccon (1985)	Yes, especially undesirable, high objective negative impact
	Al Khani et al. (1986)	Yes. Saudi Arabia; only significant for married women
	Gureje and Adewunmi (1988)	No
Nonrelapsing schizophrenics	Leff et al. (1973)	Yes. Relapses on placebo
Neurotics	Hendrie et al. (1975)	No; more male schizophrenics in low stress category
	Harder et al. (1980)	No differences from neurotics and other psychiatric patients
Depressives	See Table 1	See Table 1

community not undergoing major relapse. Life events were more common in those showing minor symptoms, particularly of depression and anxiety, than in the general population. Canton and Fraccon (1985) found more life events in the 6 months before admission among Italian schizophrenics than controls, particularly for first onsets. Al Khani et al. (1986) compared Saudi Arabian schizophrenics and controls for the 6 months before onset. Differences were only significant for married women but were suggestive for other groups. In Nigerians with first episodes Gureje and Adewunmi (1988) found no excess of events.

Among studies using other kinds of control groups, Leff et al. (1973) found life events more common in schizophrenics who relapsed than in those who did not, but only in placebo rather than active drug groups from two maintenance drug trials. In extension of these findings Leff and Vaughn (1980) later found that life events tended to occur in relapsing schizophrenics whose families did not show high expressed emotionally. Hendrie et al. (1975) compared schizophrenics with neurotics and personality disorder patients using the Holmes-Rahe questionnaire. Among male but not female patients, schizophrenics were predominantly characterized by low stress, neurotics by high stress. Using similar stress scores for the year before first admission, Harder et al. (1980) found no differences between schizophrenics and other psychiatric patients, mainly neurotic, in the level of stress, although there were some differences in temporal pattern.

Comparisons with depressives have already been shown in Table 1. They tend to show fewer events, or fewer subjects having a major event, among the schizophrenics. Types of event have not been very critically examined in these studies, although in our own data exit events were more closely related to depression.

One other study used different methods. In an epidemiological study, Steinberg and Durell (1968) found the inception rate for schizophrenia significantly raised in the early months of military service. Overall life events do appear to contribute to schizophrenic onset and relapse, but to a much lesser extent than they do to depression, and possibly over a shorter time period.

Other Disorders

Studies of other disorders are beyond the scope of this chapter and are reviewed in detail elsewhere (Paykel and Dowlatshahi 1988). A number of studies of suicide attempters have shown a marked peak of events shortly before the attempt. Comparisons with depressives and other psychiatric patients confirm that the greatest frequency of events in any psychiatric disorder is among the suicide attempters in the period just before the attempt, suggesting, in the retrospective frame, the greatest causative effect.

Anxiety disorders have received less study than depressions. Event rates appear to be elevated before episodes, at rates comparable to, or a little lower than, those for depressions.

Magnitude of Causative Effect

The studies which have been reviewed suggest a ranking of magnitude of life-event occurrence, with suicide attempters experiencing most events, depressives next, and schizophrenics experiencing fewer events, although more than normal controls in a comparable time period. How are these differences to be interpreted? These are retrospective studies which select patients for a period just before the onset of the disorder. If the disorder is associated with recent life events, more events will be expected to occur in the time period under consideration. The more numerous the events, or the more common the occurrence of a major event, the greater will be the association.

The life events implicated in psychiatric disorder, although stressful and unpleasant, are not usually of catastrophic magnitude. Critics have pointed out that they are often experienced by the general population without any disorder following. It is therefore desirable to quantify the magnitude of effects.

An epidemiological measure which can be used in this context is the relative risk (Paykel 1978). This is the ratio of the rate of disease among those exposed to a causative factor to the rate among those not exposed. When this was applied to some of our own studies, it was found that the risk of developing depression in the 6 months after the most stressful classes of events was approximately 6:1, falling off rapidly with time after the event. Other studies have given similar findings. The relative risks for schizophrenia were much lower at only 2–3 over 6 months, but for suicide attempts they were higher.

Relative risks of this magnitude indicate an effect which is important, but not overwhelming (Paykel 1979). The findings suggest disorders with multifactorial causation, in which any single factor may account for only a relatively small proportion of the variance. Although events are important, a large part in determining whether an event is followed by disorder must be attributed to other modifying factors. There may be a whole host of these, both genetic and environmental, ranging from biochemical, through personality and coping mechanisms, to social support.

Schizoaffective Disorders

Findings on affective disorders and schizophrenia indicate differences between the disorders, and suggest that it might be profitable to seek parallel data on schizoaffective disorders. Much of the literature on schizoaffective disorders examines associated factors and the extent to which they suggest a closer relationship to affective or schizophrenic disorder. Affective episodes appear related to life events to a considerably greater extent than are schizophrenic episodes, both in terms of likely event occurrence and in magnitude of causative effect. There may also be possible differences with respect to the length of time over which the effect extends and the types of events involved, but these are not sufficiently consistent to provide reliable markers. It would be particularly interesting to know the magnitude of life events effects, and whether they occur, in schizoaffective disorders.

Care must be taken with the definition of the disorder in such studies. Some definitions of atypical psychoses derive from ideas of reactive psychosis, which include presence of a precipitant stress. In order to avoid circularity, it is important that studies of life events in schizoaffective disorders adopt a syndromal definition for the disorder.

Unfortunately, there are no studies of life events in schizoaffective disorders which conform fully to the methodological criteria laid out in the introductory section of this chapter. The plentiful studies contrasting schizoaffective, affective and schizophrenic disorders have concentrated on history, symptoms, family history, course and outcome, and response to treatment. There is still room for a careful study of life events in schizoaffectives and appropriate comparison groups.

A few studies do bear on the area. Chung et al. (1986) carried out a small study using Brown's methods to examine antecedent stress in 15 schizophrenics, 14 hypomanics, 9 subjects with schizophreniform disorder, and a mixed sample of normal and surgical controls, using DSM-III diagnoses. Patients with schizophreniform disorder were significantly more likely than controls or hypomanics to have experienced a life event in the preceding 6 months, and suggestively more than schizophrenics. In the preceding 1 month, rates were suggestively raised for hypomanics and schizophrenics but less so for schizophreniform patients. Unfortunately, there were no patients in the analysis who satisfied DSM-III criteria for schizoaffective rather than schizophreniform psychoses, which in DSM-III are psychoses satisfying schizophrenic criteria except for 6 months' duration, and the low numbers in all samples limit possible conclusions.

Using data from the NIMH Collaborative Study of the Psychobiology of Depression, van Eerdewegh et al. (1987) contrasted patients with different RDC diagnoses, on raters' and subjects' global judgements of preceding stress. For both ratings there were significant differences and a ranking from high stress to low, progressing from unipolar schizoaffectives and unipolar depressives, who were approximately equal, through bipolar schizoaffectives to bipolar affectives. Marneros et al. (1988a,b,c) examined course of schizoaffective disorders over a mean length of 25.6 years. Life-event information was obtained from case notes. Events at conset were not related to course but there were weak relationships of around 10% significance between occurrence of life events during the course and occurrence of more episodes, and a shorter cycle length, particularly for the first cycle. Seventy-six percent of the patients had at least one life event which could be considered a possible precipitating factor for an episode; 33% of the episodes were involved, with a peaking of reported events in the 4 weeks before the episode. First episodes were commonly preceded by life events. Events did not appear related to symptoms between the episodes or to age at onset. No individual event appeared preferentially involved, but episodes in male subjects more often than episodes in female subjects were preceded by an occupational change or an examination.

We have carried out a comparison of patients who had severe postpartum disorders with normal postpartum controls (Dowlatshahi and Paykel, in press).

About one-third were depressive and one-third schizoaffective, while one-third had other diagnoses. There was no excess of life events in patients compared with controls, or between diagnoses.

Clearly, these studies merely open up an area which would repay further detailed study.

Conclusions

Reliable and valid study of life events requires careful interview with attention to distortions of recall and elimination of events which may be secondary consequences of disorder. The relationship between life events and depression has received much study. There are elevated rates prior to onset and to relapse. The findings appear virtually the same for depressives of endogenous (and probably, pyschotic) symptom pattern as for neurotics. Rates are probably raised before episodes of depression and mania in bipolar disorder, but studies here have been fewer, and effects, at least in patients on lithium, may be less.

There have not been as many studies of schizophrenia, but the numbers are sufficient to permit reliable conclusions. Event rates tend to be elevated prior to schizophrenic onset and relapse compared with normal controls, but to a much less striking extent than for depression. Overall measures of causative effect show a less strong effect in schizophrenia than in depression.

Studies of preceding life events in schizoaffective disorders offer the possibility of an additional index of the relationship of these disorders to clinical pure affective and schizophrenic illnesses. Unfortunately, few such studies have been carried out. The available evidence suggests, but far from conclusively, that life events are involved in the first and subsequent attacks of schizoaffective disorders. Further studies are indicated.

References

Al Khani MAF, Bebbington PE, Watson JP, House F (1986) Life events and schizophrenia: a Saudi Arabian study, Br J Psychiatry 148:12–22

Ambelas A (1979) Psychologically stressful events in the precipitation of manic episodes. Br J Psychiatry 135:15–21

Ambelas A (1987) Life events and mania. A special relationship? Br J Psychiatry 150:235–240

Aronson TA, and Shukla S (1987) Life events and relapse in bipolar disorder: the impact of a catastrophic event. Acta Psychiatr Scand 75:571–576

Bebbington PE, Tennant C, Hurry J (1981) Adversity and the nature of psychiatric disorder in the community. J Affective Disord 3:345–366

Bebbington PE, MacCarthy B, Brugha T, Potter J, Sturt E, Wykes T, Katz R McGuffin P (1988) The Camberwell collaborative Depression Study. I. Depressed probands: adversity and the form of depression. Br J Psychiatry 152:754–765

Beck JC, Worthen K (1972) Precipitating stress, crisis theory and hospitalization in schizophrenia and depression. Arch Gen Psychiatry 26:123–129

Benjaminsen S (1981) Stressful life events preceding the onset of neurotic depression, Psychol Med 11:369–378

Bidzinska EJ (1984) Stress factors in affective diseases. Br J Psychiatry 144:161–166

Billings AG, Moos RH (1984) Chronic and nonchronic unipolar depression. The differential role of environment stressors and resources. J Nerv Ment Dis 172:65–75

Billings AG, Cronkite RC, Moos RH (1983) Social-environment factors in unipolar depression: comparisons of depressed patients and nondepressed controls. J Abnorm Psychol 92(2):119–133

Brown GW, Birley JLT (1968) Crises and life changes and the onset of schizophrenia. J Health Soc Behav 9:203–214

Brown GW, Harris T (1978) The social origins of depression: a study of psychiatric disorder in women. Tavistock, London

Brown GW, Sklair F, Harris TO, Birley JLT (1973a) Life-events and psychiatric disorders. I. Some methodological issues. Psychol Med 3:74–87

Brown GW, Harris TO, Peto J (1973b) Life events and psychiatric disorders. 2. Nature of causal link. Psychol Med 3:159–176

Brown GW, Bhrolchain NIM, Harris TO (1979) Psychotic and neurotic depression. 3. Aetiological and background factors. J Affective Disord 1:195–211

Brown GW, Adler Z, Bifulco A (1988) Life events, difficulties and recovery from chronic depression. Br J Psychiatry 152:487–498

Brugha TS, Conroy R (1985) Categories of depression: reported life events in a controlled design. Br J Psychiatry 147:641–646

Brugha TS, Bebbington B, MacCarthy B, Potter J, Sturt E, Wykes T (1987) Social networks, social support and the type of depressive illness. Acta Psychiatr Scand 76:664–673

Cadoret RJ, Winokur G, Dorzab J, Baker M (1972) Depressive disease: life events and onset of illness. Arch Gen Psychiatry 26:133–136

Canton G, Fraccon IG (1985) Life events and schizophrenia. A replication. Acta Psychiatr Scand 71:211–216

Chatterjee RN, Mukherjee SP, Nandi DN (1981) Life events and depression. Indian J Psychiatry 23:333–337

Chung RK, Langeluddecke P, Tennant C (1986) Threatening life events in the onset of schizophrenia, schizophreniform psychosis and hypomania. Br J Psychiatry 148:680–685

Cohen-Sandler R, Berman AL King RA (1982) Life stress and symptomatology: determinants of suicidal behavior in children. J Am Acad Child Psychiatry 21:178–186

Dowlatshahi D, Paykel ES (in press) Life events and social stress in puerperal psychoses: absence of effect psychol med

Eisler RM, Polak PR (1971) Social stress and psychiatric disorder. J Nerv Ment Dis 153:227–233

Ezquiaga E, Gutierrez JLA, Lopez AG (1987) Psychosocial factors and episode number in depression. J Affective Disord 12:135–138

Faravelli C, Ambonetti A (1983) Assessment of life events in depressive disorders. A comparison of three methods. Soc Psychiatry 18:51–56

Fava GA, Munari F, Pasvan L, Kellner R (1981) Life events and depression. A replication. J Affective Disord 3:159–165

Forrest AD, Fraser RH, Priest RG (1965) Environmental factors in depressive illness. Br J Psychiatry 111:243–253

Fowler RC, Liskow BI, Tanna VL (1980) Alcoholism, depression and life events. J Affective Disord 2:127–135

Giel R, Ten Horn GHMM, Ormel J, Schudel WJ, Wiersma O (1978) Mental illness, neuroticism and life events in a Dutch village sample: a follow-up. Psychol Med 8:235–243

Glassner B, Haldipur CVG (1983) Life events and early and late onset of bipolar disorder. Am J Psychiatry 140:215–217

Gureje O, Adewunmi A. (1988) Life events and schizophrenia in Nigerians. A controlled investigation. Br J Psychiatry 153:367–375

Hall KS, Dunner DL, Zeller G, Fieve RR (1977) Bipolar illness: a prospective study of life events. Compr Psychiatry 18:497–502

Harder DW, Strauss JS, Kokes RF, Ritzler BA, Gift TE (1980) Life events and psychopathology severity among first psychiatric admissions. J Abnorm Psychol 89:165–180

Hendrie HC, Lachar D, Lennox K (1975) Personality trait and symptom correlates of life change in a psychiatric population. J Psychosom Res 19:203–208

Holmes TH, Rahe RH (1967) The social readjustment rating scale. J Psychosom Res 11: 213–218

Hudgens RW, Morrison JR, Barchha R (1967) Life events and onset of primary affective disorders. A study of 40 hospitalised patients and 40 controls. Arch Gen Psychiatry 16:134–145

Jacobs S, Myers J (1976) Recent life events and acute schizophrenic psychosis: a controlled study. J Nerv Ment Dis 162:75–87

Jacobs SC, Prusoff BA, Paykel ES (1974) Recent life events in schizophrenia and depression. Psychol Med 4:444–453

Katschnig H, Berner P (1984) The poly-diagnostic approach in psychiatric research. In Proceedings of the International Conference on Diagnosis and Classification of Mental Disorder and Alcohol and Drug-Related Problems, Copenhagen, April 13–17, 1982. World Health Organization, Geneva

Kennedy S, Thompson R, Stancer HC, Roy A, Persad E (1983) Life events precipitating mania. Br J Psychiatry 142:398–403

Kosten TR, Rounsaville BJ, Kleber HD (1983) Relationship of depression to psychosocial stressors in heroin addicts. J Nerv Ment Dis 171:97–104

Lahniers CE, White K (1976) Changes in environmental life events and their relationship to psychiatric hospital admissions. J Nerv Ment Dis 163:154–158

Leff J, Vaughn C (1980) The interaction of life events and relatives' expressed emotion in schizophrenia and depressive neurosis. Br J Psychiatry 136:146–153

Leff J, Hirsch SR, Gaind R, Rohde PD, Stevens B (1973) Life events and maintenance therapy in schizophrenic relapse. Br J Psychiatry 123:659–660

Levi LD, Fales CH, Stein M, Sharp VH (1966) Separation and attempted suicide. Arch Gen Psychiatry 15:158–165

Lloyd C, Zisook S, Click M, Jaffe KE (1981) Life events and response to antidepressants. J Human Stress 7:2–15

Malmquist CP (1970) Depression and object loss in psychiatric admissions. Am J Psychiatry 126:1782–1787

Marneros A, Deister A, Rohde A, Junemann H, Fimmers R (1988a) Long-term course of schizoaffective disorders. I. Definitions, methods, frequency of esisodes and cycles. Eur Arch Psychiatry Neurol Sci 237:264–275

Marneros A, Rohde A, Deister A, Junemann H, Fimmers R (1988b) Long-term course of schizoaffective disorders. II. Length of cycles, episodes and intervals. Eur Arch Psychiatry Neurol Sci 237:276–282

Marneros A, Rohde A, Deister A, Fimmers R, Junemann H (1988c) Long-term course of schizoaffective disorders. III. Onset, type of episodes and syndrome shift, precipitating factors, suicidality, seasonality, inactivity of illness, and outcome. Eur Arch Psychiatry Neurol Sci 237:283–290

Matussek P, Neuner R (1981) Loss events preceding endogenous and neurotic depressions. Acta Psychiatr Scand 64:340–350

Mendlewicz J, Charon F, Linkowski P (1986) Life events and the dexamethasone suppression test in affective illness. J Affective Disord 10:203–206

Monroe SC, Bellack AS, Hersen M, Himmelhoch JM (1983) Life events, symptom course, and treatment outcome in unipolar depressed women. J Consult Clin Psychol 51:604–615

Monroe SC, Thase ME, Hersen M, Himmelhoch JM, Bellack AS (1985) Life events and the endogenous-nonendogenous distinction in the treatment and posttreatment course of depression. Comp Psychiatry 26:175–185

Murphy E (1982) Social origins of depression in old age. Br J Psychiatry 141:135–142

Murphy E (1983) The prognosis of depression in old age. Br J Psychiatry 142:111–119

Parker G, Blignault I, Manicavasagar V (1988) Neurotic depression: delineation of symptom profiles and their relation to outcome. Br J Psychiatry 152:15–23

Paykel ES (1974) Recent life events and clinical depression. In: Gunderson EK, Rahe RH (eds) Life stress and illness Thomas, Springfield, pp 134–163

Paykel ES (1978) Contribution of life events to causation of psychiatric illness. Psychol Med 18:245–253

Paykel ES (1979) Causal relationships between clinical depression and life events. In: Barrett JE (ed) Stress and mental disorder. Raven, New York, pp 71–86

Paykel ES (1982) Life events and early environment. In: Paykel ES (ed) Handbook of affective disorders Churchill Livingstone, Edinburgh, pp 146–161

Paykel ES (1983) Methodological aspects of life events research. J Psychosom Res 27:341–352

Paykel ES, Dowlatshahi D (1988) Life events and mental disorder, In: Fisher S, Reason J (eds) Handbook of life stress, cognition and health, chap 13. Wiley, Chichester, pp 241–263

Paykel ES, Tanner K (1976) Life events, depressive relapse and maintenance treatment. Psychol Med 6:481–485

Paykel ES, Myers JK, Dienelt MN, Klerman GL, Lindenthal JJ, Pepper MP (1969) Life events and depression: a controlled study. Arch Gen Psychiatry 21:753–760

Paykel ES, Prusoff BA, Myers JK (1975) Suicide attempts and recent life events: a controlled comparison. Arch Gen Psychiatry 32:327–333

Paykel ES, McGuiness B, Gomez J (1976) An Anglo-American comparison of the scaling of life events. Br J Med Psychol 49:237–247

Paykel ES, Rao BM, Taylor CM (1984) Life stress and symptom pattern in out-patient depression. Psychol Med 14:559–568

Prusoff B, Thompson WD, Sholomskas D, Riordan C (1977) Psychosocial stressors and depression among former heroin-dependent patients maintained on methadone. J Nerv Ment Dis 165:57–63

Rosenthal SH, Klerman GL (1966) Content and consistency in the endogenous depressive pattern. Br J Psychiatry 112:471–484

Rowan PR, Paykel ES, Parker RR (1982) Phenelzine and amitriptyline: effects on symptoms of neurotic depression. Br J Psychiatry 140:475–483

Roy A, Thompson R, Kennedy S (1983) Depression in chronic schizophrenia. Br J Psychiatry 142:465–470

Roy A, Breier A, Doran AR, Pickar D (1985) Life events in depression. Relationship to subtypes. J Affective Disord 9:143–148

Schwartz CC, Myers JK (1977a) Life events and schizophrenia. I. Comparison of schizophrenics with a community sample. Arch Gen Psychiatry 34:1238–1241

Schwartz CC, Myers JK (1977b) Life events and schizophrenia. II. Impact of life events on symptom configuration. Arch Gen Psychiatry 34:1242–1245

Sethi BB (1964) Relationship of separation to depression. Arch Gen Psychiatry 10:186–195

Slater J, Depue RA (1981) The contribution of environmental events and social support to serious suicide attempts in primary depressive disorder. J Abnorm Psychol 90:275–285

Steinberg HR, Durell J (1968) A stressful social situation as a precipitant of schizophrenia symptoms: an epidemiological study. Br J Psychiatry 114:1097–1105

Surtees PG (1980) Social support, residual adversity and depressive outcome. Soc Psychiatry 15:71–80

Tennant C, Bebbington P, Hurry J (1981) The short-term outcome of neurotic disorders in the community: the relation of remission to clinical factors and to "neutralizing" life events. Br J Psychiatry 139:213–220

Thomson KC, Hendrie HC (1972) Environmental stress in primary depressive illness. Arch Gen Psychiatry 26:130–132

Uhlenhuth EH, Paykel ES (1973) Symptom configuration and life events. Arch Gen Psychiatry 28:743–748

Vadher A, Ndetei DM (1981) Life events and depression in a Kenyan setting. Br J Psychiatry 139:134–149

Van Eerdewegh MM, Van Eerdewegh P, Croyell W, Clayton PJ, Endicott J, Koepke J, Rochberg N (1987) Schizo-affective disorders: bipolar-unipolar subtyping. Natural history variables: a discriminant analysis approach. J Affective Disord 12:223–232

Follow-Up Studies of Schizoaffective Disorders: A Comparison with Affective Disorders

M.T. Tsuang[1]

Introduction

Kasanin (1933) coined the term "schizoaffective psychoses" to characterize a group of patients who presented a mixture of both affective and schizophrenic features, and described the disorder as having a rapid onset, precipitated by either chronic or acutely stressful life events. Kasanin further noted that the psychosis typically lasted for a short period of time – a few weeks to a few months – and a complete recovery was the rule rather than the exception.

In this paper results will be presented on the long-term follow-up of a group of patients who were given a diagnosis of schizophrenia by clinicians but did not meet Washington University criteria (Feighner et al. 1972) for schizophrenia. These patients were atypical because of the presence of both affective and schizophrenic clinical features, acute onset with short duration of illness, and/or insufficient information at the time of diagnostic assessment. It is hoped that the results of follow-up studies of these atypical patients can shed light on the nature of these patients by comparing them with individuals who meet Feighner et al. (1972) criteria for either affective disorder or schizophrenia.

Material and Methods

All patients consecutively admitted to the University of Iowa Psychiatric Hospital during the period between 1934–1944 were screened for participation in a long-term follow-up study. Based on detailed case notes of these patients, 100 manics, 225 depressives, and 200 schizophrenics were selected. In addition, another group of 310 patients who did not meet the criteria for schizophrenia, even though their original chart diagnosis was schizophrenia, were selected. These 310 patients presented a mixture of affective and schizophrenic features and, for the purpose of this paper, were called "schizoaffectives." The schizoaffective group was followed in the same manner as the typical groups. Finally, a group of patients, admitted during a similar period of time, with no history of psychiatric illness were selected from the surgical department of the University of Iowa and were also followed over the same number of years in order to

---

[1] Harvard Schools of Medicine and Public Health, Brockton/West Roxbury VA Medical Center, 940 Belmont Street, Brockton, MA 02401, USA

Affective and Schizoaffective Disorders
Edited by A. Marneros and M.T. Tsuang
© Springer-Verlag Berlin Heidelberg 1990

provide a comparison with the affective, schizophrenic, and schizoaffective groups.

We were able to trace 97% of all study subjects 35–40 years after admission. This included locating subjects at their current address if alive, and obtaining a death certificate if deceased. Of the control group 31% had died at follow-up compared with 38% for schizoaffective disorder, 40% for schizophrenia, 59% for mania, and 73% for depression. Information to rate long-term outcome was obtained from personal interview, if the subject was alive, and from follow-up mental health records and other material if the subject was deceased. We were able to successfully rate the outcome status on 95% of all study cases. The details of the selection and field follow-up of these patients can be found in our previous publications (Tsuang et al. 1979; Tsuang and Fleming 1987).

Results

The long-term outcome of these subjects was measured on four dimensions and rated by researchers who were blind to the original diagnoses. The following criteria were used to evaluate outcome: for marital status, married or widowed was considered good, divorced or separated was considered fair, and being single was considered poor. For residental status, living at home or at a relatives' residence was seen as good, living at a nursing or county home was seen as fair, and confinement in a mental hospital was seen as poor. For occupational status, being employed or retired, a housewife or student was considered good, being unable to work due to physical incapacity was considered fair, and being unable to work due to mental illness was seen as poor. And finally, for psychiatric status, the absence of symptoms was seen as good, presence of some symptoms was considered fair, and the presence of incapacitating symptoms was considered poor.

Since our group of interest was the schizoaffectives they were compared with schizophrenia, mania, and depression based on the four outcome measures described above. For marital status the percentage of good outcome (42%) was significantly higher ($P < 0.01$) than that for schizophrenia (21%) but significantly lower than the manic (70%) and depressive (81%) groups. A very similar pattern was seen for residential status. For occupational status the percentage of good ratings (44%) was higher for schizoaffective disorder when compared with schizophrenia (35%). This difference, however, did not meet statistical significance. On the other hand, the percentage of good occupational status ratings for schizoaffective disorder was significantly ($P < 0.01$) lower than the percentage of good ratings for mania (67%) and depression (67%). Finally, for psychiatric status the percentage of good ratings in schizoaffective disorder (34%) was significantly higher ($P < 0.01$) than the percentage in schizophrenia (20%) but significantly lower than the percentages in mania (50%) and depression (61%). As can be seen here, the outcome results of the schizoaffective group consistently fell between those of the affective and schizophrenic groups in terms of marital, residential, occupational, and psychiatric status.

In order to test the hypothesis that these results were a reflection of the heterogeneous nature of the schizoaffective group, composed essentially of affective and schizophrenic subgroups, these patients were further subtyped and reanalyzed based on long-term outcome. Using previously published methods (Tsuang et al. 1986), we statistically generated three subgroups of schizoaffective disorder: affective, schizophrenic, and undifferentiated. The first step in the analysis was to determine which admission variables most significantly separated our sample of 310 schizoaffective patients into definable subgroups. Based on our previous research (Tsuang 1979), we hypothesized that two of the subtypes would be one that was affective-like and one which was schizophrenic-like, and therefore, the admission variables selected for the analysis needed to distinguish affective disorder from schizophrenia at the 0.05 level of significance. In addition, the variables chosen had a lower percentage of missing values and an adequate distribution of values in order to best discriminate between the detect subtypes of schizoaffective disorder. Eleven variables that met the above criteria were chosen for the analysis: age at admission, sex, marital status, education, precipitating factors, self-reproach, poor premorbid adjustment, persecutory delusions, auditory hallucinations, motor symptoms, and short-term outcome.

Since we were interested in subdividing schizoaffective disorder into affective and schizophrenic subtypes, our schizophrenic ($n = 200$) and affective disorder ($n = 325$) groups were used in conjunction with the 11 variables to generate a multivariate system of classifying each schizoaffective patient into the appropriate subtype. Using all follow-up information, including personal interviews and mental health records, we rediagnosed those psychiatric patients (schizophrenic and affective disorder) based on DSM-III criteria. This diagnostic exercise resulted in 160 schizophrenics and 177 affective disorder cases. Subjects with inadequate follow-up information were not rediagnosed.

The statistical technique used to classify schizoaffective disorder by subtype was logistic regression (Feinberg 1981; Engelman 1981). This method is a form of regression analysis which generates a prediction equation using a binary dependent variable and independent variables which may be either categorical or continuous. For our purposes the dependent variable was "diagnostic group" as defined by two categories (160 schizophrenics and 177 affectives) and was coded 1 for "schizophrenic" and 0 for "not schizophrenic" (i.e., affective disorder). The independent variables were the 11 discussed above. They were all categorical variables coded as 0 or 1, except age at admission which was continuous. The resulting regression equation predicts the probability of a subject being schizophrenic (P(S)).

Some of the 310 schizoaffectives had missing data on one or more of the 11 predictor variables. These subjects were omitted from the analysis, leaving 271 cases with complete data. The calculated probability values for these cases were ordered from smallest (0.2) to largest (0.97). The distribution of probabilities is shown in Fig. 1. The working hypothesis was that there were three distinct subtypes, and, by examination of Fig. 1 and by statistically comparing various subdivisions of the distribution, we determined that adequate breaks occurred at probabilities of 0.5 and 0.75. We propose that these groups, defined

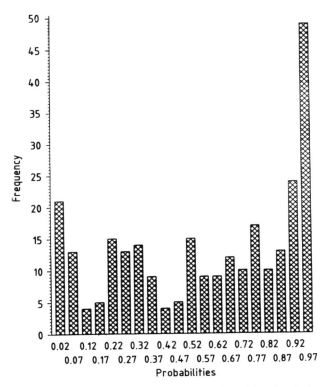

Fig. 1. Distribution of probabilities for being schizophrenic ($n = 271$ schizoaffectives)

by the above cut-off points, represent three subtypes of schizoaffective disorder: (a) schizophrenic ($n = 111$, P(S) > 0.75), (b) undifferentiated ($n = 57$, P(S) = (0.5 − 0.75)), and (c) affective ($n = 103$, P(S) < 0.5).

In order to substantiate these groupings of schizoaffective disorder, we compared all 11 predictor variables across the three subtypes. Only two variables did not statistically discriminate between subtypes at the 0.05 level – "sex" and "persecutory delusions." The results on the remaining nine variables generally place the undifferentiated subtype between the schizophrenic and affective subtypes. So for marital status (single), poor premorbid adjustment, and motor symptoms, the schizophrenic subtype had the highest percentages, the affective subtype had the lowest percentages, and the undifferentiated group fell in the middle. For age at admission, members of the schizophrenic subtype averaged 24 years, the undifferentiated subtype averaged 29 years, and the affective subtype averaged 30 years old. For education beyond high school, precipitating factor(s), and short-term outcome (recovered), the affective group had the highest percentage, the schizophrenic group had the lowest percentage, and the undifferentiated subtype was in the middle.

Examining the long-term outcome results in these three subtypes, independent of the above 11 variables, we clearly see that there are statistically significant differences in all four long-term outcome measures between those of the schizophrenic and affective subtypes as shown in Table 1. Although the undifferentiated subtype falls between the schizophrenic and affective subtype, statistically it seems to be closer to the schizophrenia subtype. For marital status the undifferentiated subtype is significantly different from both schizophrenia and affective disorder. For the other three outcomes there was no difference between the undifferentiated and schizophrenic subtypes.

We also compared the three subtypes with our original schizophrenic and affective disorder groups in terms of long-term outcome. The schizophrenic subtype was similar to the schizophrenic group and significantly different from the affective group based on all four outcome measures. Conversely, the affective subtype was similar to the affective disorder group but different from the schizophrenic group.

Table 2 presents comparisons between the undifferentiated subtype and the typical groups of affective disorder and schizophrenia. For marital status, the undifferentiated subtype is significantly different from both schizophrenia and affective disorder. For residential status, the undifferentiated subtype is similar to affective disorder and different from schizophrenia. For occupational status and psychiatric status, the undifferentiated subtype is similar to schizophrenia but is significantly different from affective disorder. Hence, as can be seen from Table 2, the undifferentiated subtype falls between the affective and schizophrenic groups in terms of long-term outcome.

Table 1. Long-term outcome comparisons among three subtypes of schizoaffective disorder

Outcome variable	Subtypes			Statistical comparison		
	S (n = 111)	U (n = 57)	A (n = 103)			
Marital status (%)						
Good	25 (22.5)	25 (43.9)	64 (62.1)	S:U**	S:A**	U:A*
Fair	10 (9.0)	16 (28.1)	18 (17.5)			
Poor	76 (68.5)	16 (28.1)	21 (20.4)			
Occupational status (%)						
Good	41 (36.9)	24 (42.1)	56 (54.4)	S:U	S:A*	U:A
Fair	4 (3.6)	5 (8.8)	11 (10.7)			
Poor	66 (59.5)	28 (49.1)	36 (35.0)			
Psychiatric status (%)						
Good	28 (25.2)	15 (26.3)	50 (48.5)	S:U	S:A**	U:A**
Fair	29 (26.1)	17 (29.8)	22 (21.4)			
Poor	54 (48.6)	25 (43.9)	31 (30.1)			
Residential status (%)						
Good	46 (41.4)	32 (56.1)	69 (67.0)	S:U	S:A**	U:A
Fair	53 (47.7)	20 (35.1)	27 (26.2)			
Poor	12 (10.8)	5 (8.8)	7 (6.8)			

*, $P < 0.05$; **, $P < 0.01$ (pairwise comparisons of good outcome).
S, schizophrenic subtype; U, undifferentiated subtype; A, affective subtype.

Table 2. Long-term outcome in the "undifferentiated" subtype of schizoaffective disorder (SA) compared with schizophrenia and affective disorder

Outcome variable	Study group SA		
	Schizophrenia ($n = 186$)	Undifferentiated subtype ($n = 57$)	Affective disorder ($n = 298$)
Marital (%)			
Good	39 (21.0)**	25 (43.9)	232 (77.9)**
Fair	22 (11.8)	16 (28.1)	27 (9.1)
Poor	125 (67.2)	16 (28.1)	39 (13.1)
Residential (%)			
Good	64 (34.4)**	32 (56.1)	207 (69.5)
Fair	89 (47.8)	20 (35.1)	54 (18.1)
Poor	33 (17.7)	5 (8.8)	37 (12.4)
Occupational (%)			
Good	65 (34.9)	24 (42.1)	200 (67.1)**
Fair	14 (7.5)	5 (8.8)	40 (13.4)
Poor	107 (57.5)	28 (49.1)	58 (19.5)
Psychiatric (%)			
Good	38 (20.4)	15 (26.3)	172 (57.7)**
Fair	48 (25.8)	17 (29.8)	55 (18.5)
Poor	100 (53.8)	25 (43.9)	71 (23.8)

**, $P < 0.01$ (comparison of good outcome with the undifferentiated subtype).

Discussion

The results of this long-term outcome study tend to support our hypothesis that the atypical schizophrenic group or schizoaffective group is a heterogeneous group consisting of affective and schizophrenic subgroups, and probably a third group of undifferentiated patients. The tripartite nature of the schizoaffective group can be seen in the trimodal distribution of subtypes based on the 11 selection variables and long-term outcome results, with the undifferentiated subgroup falling between the schizophrenic and affective disorder subgroups. Clearly researchers and clinicians must attempt, at the outset, to classify atypical patients as either affectively disordered or schizophrenic, leaving only those patients with a mixture of both affective and schizophrenic features in a more circumscribed schizoaffective group; otherwise the term "schizoaffective," as a diagnostic category, will become meaningless both from the clinical and research points of view.

We are currently analyzing each patient who remains in the undifferentiated group using both a cross-sectional and longitudinal prognostic perspective to better understand the symptomatology and outcomes of these patients. It is hoped that more narrowly defined boundaries for schizoaffective disorder can be developed so that future research will be based on rigorous, demonstrable criteria. This will allow for much needed study of these atypical patients from clinical, descriptive, therapeutic, pathophysiological, genetic, and other etiological perspectives.

References

Engelman L (1981) Stepwise logistic regression. In: Dixon W (ed) BMDP statistical software. University of California Press, Berkeley, pp 330–344

Feighner JP, Robins E, Guze SB, Woodruff RA, Winokur G, Munoz R (1972) Diagnostic criteria for use in psychiatric research. Arch Gen Psychiatry 26:57–63

Feinberg SE (1981)The analysis of cross-classified categorical data. 2nd edn. MIT Press, Cambridge, pp 102–116

Kasanin J (1933) The acute schizo-affective psychoses. Am J Psychiatry 13:97–126

Tsuang MT (1979) Schizoaffective disorder: dead or alive? Arch Gen Psychiatry 36:633–634

Tsuang MT, Fleming JA (1987) Long-term outcome of schizophrenia and other psychoses. In: Häfner H, Gattaz WF, Jan Zarik W (eds) Search for the causes of schizophrenia. Springer, Berlin Heidelberg New York

Tsuang MT, Woolson RF, Fleming JA (1979) Long-term outcome of major psychoses: schizophrenia and affective disorders compared with psychiatrically symptom-free surgical conditions. Arch Gen Psychiatry 36:1295–1301

Tsuang MT, Simpson JC, Fleming JA (1986) Diagnostic criteria for subtyping schizoaffective disorder. In: Marneros A, Tsuang MT (eds) The schizoaffective psychoses. Springer, Berlin Heidelberg New York

Sociodemographic and Premorbid Features
of Schizophrenic, Schizoaffective, and Affective Psychoses

A. MARNEROS, A. DEISTER, and A. ROHDE[1]

Introduction

Sociodemographic and premorbid features could be among the validating criteria for distinguishing between diagnostic groups of mental disorders. Schizoaffective disorders were assumed as belonging to the group of schizophrenias (Bleuler 1972; Huber et al. 1979; WHO 1979). Modern research, however, has shown that there are some interesting differences regarding course and outcome between schizophrenic and schizoaffective disorders (Marneros et al. 1986a–c, 1987, 1989a–d, 1990). Conversely, similarities between affective and schizoaffective disorders have also been reported (Angst 1986).

In this contribution we compare some sociodemographic, premorbid, and general data of affective, schizoaffective, and schizophrenic disorders with the aim of distinguishing between these diagnostic groups.

Subjects, Definitions, and Methods

Subjects

This study is part of the Cologne study on the long-term course of schizophrenic, schizoaffective, and schizophrenic disorders (Marneros et al. 1986a–c, 1988a–d, 1989a–e).

This contribution is based on the follow-up investigations of 291 inpatients fulfilling the diagnostic criteria of schizophrenic, schizoaffective, and affective disorders, as they are defined below (see Definitions). We compared 97 patients with schizophrenic disorders (mean follow-up period, 19.6 years), 88 patients with schizoaffective disorders (mean follow-up period, 25.8 years), and 106 patients with unipolar and bipolar affective disorders (mean follow-up period, 27.9 years).

Definitions

The definitions applied distinguish between "episode" (defined cross-sectionally) and "disorder" or "illness" (defined longitudinally). The diagnostic criteria for

[1] Psychiatrische Universitätsklinik, Sigmund-Freud-Straße 25, 5300 Bonn 1, FRG

Affective and Schizoaffective Disorders
Edited by A. Marneros and M.T. Tsuang
© Springer-Verlag Berlin Heidelberg 1990

episodes are based on the criteria and definitions of DSM-III and DSM-III-R respectively, only slightly modified. Eight different types of episodes are defined (see Appendix).

The diagnosis "schizoaffective disorder" according to the criteria used (see Appendix) requires concurrent or sequential schizophrenic *and* manic or melancholic symptomatology at least once during the course. The diagnosis "schizophrenic disorder" can only be made if only schizophrenic symptomatology occurred during the course, and there was never any melancholic or manic symptomatology. The diagnosis "affective disorder," according to the criteria used, can only be made if only manic or melancholic symptomatology occurred during the course, and there was never any schizophrenic or schizoaffective symptomatology.

Instruments of Evaluation

All patients were interviewed by one of us at follow-up. The exploratory framework used was the German translation of the Present State Examination (PSE; Wing et al. 1974, 1982) and a pool of items based on some instruments measuring psychological and social outcome, i.e., the Disability Assessment Schedule (WHO/DAS; WHO 1986), the Psychological Impairment Rating Schedule (WHO/PIRS; Schubart et al. 1986), and the Global Assessment Scale (GAS; Spitzer et al. 1976) – for details see Deister et al., this volume.

In addition to the interview, all available case records on hospitalizations of the patient were evaluated using a standardized protocol containing sections on general information, history, social factors, family history, life events, psychopathological symptoms, somatic findings, and treatment. The symptom list of this protocol was AMDP-oriented.

Results

Sociodemographic Data

Sex Distribution

The sex distribution differs between schizophrenic disorders and the other two diagnostic groups (Table 1). We found a female to male ratio of 3:1 in affective disorders. In schizoaffective disorders there were almost twice as many women as men, while in schizophrenic disorders we found more male than female patients (1:0.8).

Age at Onset

In schizophrenic disorders more than one-half of the patients became ill before the age of 26 years. In contrast about one-half of the patients with affective

Table 1. Sociodemographic features

	Schizophrenic (n = 97)	p1	Schizoaffective (n = 88)	p2	Affective (n = 106)	p3
Sex		0.003**		0.103		0.000** (1)
Famale	43%		65%		76%	
Male	57%		35%		24%	
Sex distribution (f:m)	0.8:1		1.9:1		3.0:1	
Age at onset (years)		0.012*		0.012*		0.000** (1)
15–25	54%		34%		16%	
26–35	15%		31%		35%	
>35	31%		35%		49%	
Arithmetic mean	29.9	0.411	31.2	0.002**	36.1	0.000** (2)
Median	25.0	0.219	29.5	0.003**	35.0	0.000** (3)
Season of birth		0.402		0.355		0.235 (1)
Spring (March-May)	35%		26%		23%	
Summer (June to August)	22%		18%		29%	
Autumn (September to November)	20%		26%		24%	
Winter (December to February)	24%		30%		25%	
Marital status at onset (all patients)		0.000**		0.013*		0.000** (1)
Single	65%		33%		19%	
Married	27%		61%		78%	
Widowed	7%		2%		2%	
Divorced/separated	1%		2%		1%	
Marital status at onset (patients between 26 and 65 years at onset)	(n = 45)	0.003**	(n = 58)	0.461	(n = 89)	0.000** (1)
Single	31%		10%		14%	
Married	51%		81%		82%	
Widowed	16%		3%		2%	
Divorced/separated	2%		5%		1%	

	Schizophrenic	p1	Schizoaffective	p2	Affective	p3
Mental illness in the family	43%	0.003**	65%	0.529	60%	0.015* (1)
Patients with mentally ill						
Female relatives	24%	0.000**	50%	1.000	50%	0.000** (1)
Male relatives	34%	0.514	39%	0.690	36%	0.785 (1)
Patients with relatives with						
Schizophrenia	14%	0.262	9%	0.697	8%	0.115 (1)
Schizoaffective disorder	—	0.009**	7%	0.189	3%	0.095 (1)
Affective disorder	1%	0.000**	31%	0.119	42%	0.000** (1)
Not identified psychoses	7%	0.151	14%	0.776	12%	0.228 (1)
Other mental disorders	19%	0.008**	6%	0.158	2%	0.000** (1)
Broken Home	27%	0.361	33%	0.252	26%	0.829 (1)

p1, Significance of schizophrenic vs schizoaffective disorder; p2, Significance of schizoaffective vs affective disorder; p3, Significance of affective vs schizophrenic disorder.

*, $P < 0.05$; **, $P < 0.01$, using (1) chi-square test, (2) t-test, and (3) Mann-Whitney "U"-test.

disorders became ill after the age of 35 years. Schizoaffective patients occupy a position between the two other groups (Table 1).

Season of Birth

There were no significant differences among the investigated groups regarding the season of birth (Table 1).

Marital Status at Onset

In affective disorders 78% of the patients were married at the time of first manifestation, as opposed to only 27% in schizophrenic patients. The differences between the groups are significant.

Investigating only patients who had an age at first manifestation greater than 25 years and younger than 65 years we also found significant differences between schizophrenic psychoses on the one hand and schizoaffective and affective psychoses on the other, but there was no longer a significant difference between schizoaffective and affective patients. That means that the differences are independent of age and sex.

Mental Illness in the Family

Significantly more schizoaffective (65%) and affective patients (60%) than schizophrenic patients (43%) were found to have at least one relative with a mental illness (Table 1). It is a very interesting finding that this difference relates only to patients with mentally ill female relatives. In regard to patients with mentally ill male relatives there are no differences among the investigated groups.

Upon investigating what kind of mental disorder the relatives have, we found significant differences in regard to patients who have relatives with affective disorders. In the affective group 42% of the patients have at least one relative with an affective psychosis as opposed to only one patient in the schizophrenic group.

In the schizoaffective group 31% of the patients had relatives with affective psychosis, but this difference in comparison with the affective group is not significant. We found a family history of schizoaffective disorders in 7% of the schizoaffective patients and in only 3% of the affective patients, but in none of the schizophrenics.

Broken Home

In all of the three investigated groups, the majority of the patients did not come from broken homes. A broken home – mainly the loss of one or both of the parents, or their separation before the patient reached the age of 16 – was found in only 26% of patients with affective disorders and in 33% of patients with schizoaffective disorders. The differences among the diagnostic groups were not significant (Table 1).

Premorbid Features

Premorbid Personality

Because of the mainly retrospective estimation of the premorbid personality structure we did not use standardized evaluation instruments, relying instead on interviewers' opinions and case records. We used three global categories: (a) obsessoid personality (typus melancholicus of Tellenbach 1976, similar to "obsessive compulsive personality" of DSM-III-R), (b) asthenic/low self-confident personality (similar to the "dependent personality" of DSM-III-R), and its opposite (c) sthenic/high self-confident personality (see criteria in Marneros et al. 1989d).

Of the patients with affective disorders about one-half (51%) fulfilled the criteria of obsessoid personality (typus melancholicus), but only 25% did so in the schizoaffective group, as did only one of the schizophrenic patients (1%).

We were unable to allocate the premorbid personality to one of these three categories in 54% of the patients with schizophrenic disorders; most of the residual patients in this group showed an asthenic/low self-confident premorbid personality structure (Table 2).

Premorbid Social Interaction Patterns

Information about the premorbid social interactions of the patients was gathered in the same way as that on personality structure. The premorbid social contacts of schizoaffective and affective patients were found in general to be good (Table 2). In contrast, almost one-half of the purely schizophrenic patients had a tendency towards isolation and only 41% had good premorbid social contacts.

Stable Heterosexual Partnership Before Onset

Significantly more affective and schizoaffective than schizophrenic patients had a stable heterosexual partnership before onset (married, engaged or with steady girlfriend/boyfriend for at least 6 months before onset, Table 2). This finding has proved to be independent of age and sex (Marneros et al. 1987).

Premorbid Social Class

Social class was first judged according to the criteria of Kleining and Moore (Kleining 1975a,b; Kleining and Moore 1968; Moore and Kleining 1960) and then transferred to the categorization of Hollingshead and Redlich (1958). According to German sociological investigations, there are no significant differences in social structure among Western industrial countries, especially between the USA and the Federal Republic of Germany (Kleining 1975a,b; Kleining and Moore 1968; Moore and Kleining 1960), so the two classifications are compatible. The findings regarding original (parents') social class, social class at onset, and social mobility were as follows (Table 3):

1. There were significant differences between schizophrenic patients and the two other groups regarding both original social class and social class at onset.

Table 2. Premorbid features

	Schizophrenic (n = 97)	p1	Schizoaffective (n = 88)	p2	Affective (n = 106)	p3
Premorbid personality (global categories)		0.000**		0.001**		0.000**
Obsessoid	1%		25%		51%	
Sthenic/high self-confidence	6%		28%		24%	
Asthenic/low self-confidence	42%		38%		25%	
Not classifiable	54%		2%		—	
Premorbid social interactions		0.000**		0.152		0.000**
Tendency to isolation	49%		24%		37%	
No tendency to isolation	41%		75%		62%	
Other	10%		1%		1%	
Stable heterosexual partnership before onset (>6 months)	33%	0.000**	67%	0.055	79%	0.000*
Educational level		0.019*		0.299		0.000*
Very low level	24%		8%		3%	
Low level	45%		51%		54%	
Intermediate level	17%		16%		12%	
High level	14%		25%		31%	
Broken off education	37%	0.000**	13%	0.093	6%	0.000**
Occupational status at onset		0.000**		0.106		0.000**
Unemployed	14%		1%		1%	
Housewife	14%		32%		45%	
No vocational training	47%		26%		16%	
Skilled laborer	7%		8%		6%	
White-collar worker	11%		23%		22%	
Senior white-collar worker	2%		10%		6%	
Self-employed	2%		—		5%	
Retired	1%		—		—	
Life event before onset	24%	0.000**	51%	0.979	51%	0.000**

p1, significance of schizophrenic vs schizoaffective disorder (chi-square test); p2, significance of schizoaffective vs affective disorder (chi-square test); p3, significance of affective vs schizophrenic disorder (chi-square test).
*, $P < 0.05$; **, $P < 0.01$.

Table 3. Social class. (According to Kleining and Moore 1968; transferred into social classes according Hollingshead and Redlich 1958)

	Federal Republic of Germany	Schizophrenic (n = 97)	p1	Schizoaffective (n = 88)	p2	Affective (n = 106)	p3
Parent's social class	To 1960[a]		0.000**		0.256		0.035
I + II	21%	21%		29%		22%	
III	30%	14%		30%		26%	
IV	28%	36%		38%		36%	
V	21%	29%		7%		16%	
Patient's social class at onset	1960–1974[b]		0.000**		0.946		0.000*
I + II	19%	18%		30%		29%	
III	35%	11%		26%		29%	
IV	30%	22%		38%		34%	
V	16%	50%		7%		8%	
Patient's social mobility (parents' class to patient's social class at onset)			0.007**		0.184		0.000*
Downward		33%		17%		12%	
Upward		7%		22%		33%	
Same level		58%		61%		55%	

[a] Moore and Kleining 1960; Kleining and Moore 1968.
[b] Kleining 1975a,b.
p1, significance of schizophrenic vs schizoaffective (chi-square test); p2, significance of schizoaffective vs affective (chi-square test); p3, significance of affective vs schizophrenic (chi-square test).
*, P < 0.05; **, P < 0.01.
I + II, Upper classes, higher middle class, middle middle class; III, Lower middle class; IV, Higher low class; V, Lower low class.

2. These differences were found mainly in the lowest social classes, with schizophrenic patients significantly more frequent than schizoaffective and affective
   disorders in the lower low class (V).
3. Schizophrenic patients had often (33%) already "drifted downward" before
   onset. Patients for whom social mobility was impossible because their original
   social class was already the lowest (V) (downward drift) or the highest (I)
   (upward drift) one were excluded.
4. There were no significant differences between schizoaffective and affective
   patients regarding social class and social mobility up to first manifestation.
5. A comparison with the general population of the Federal Republic of Germany showed a closer relationship between this distribution and the schizoaffective and affective patients than to the schizophrenic patients. Schizophrenic patients are overrepresented in the lower classes.

Education

In evaluating educational level we used four categories: (a) school for the
retarded/children with learning difficulties or elementary school not completed
(very low level); (b) completed elementary school or intermediate school/
vocational school not completed (low level); (c) completed intermediate
school/vocational school or high school not completed (intermediate level); (d)
completed high school or university (high level) (Table 2).

   Affective and schizoaffective patients had on average a higher level of
education than schizophrenic patients. On the schizophrenic patients 24% had
only a very low educational level in contrast to 3% of affective patients.

   An interesting finding was the high proportion of schizophrenic patients who
ended their education without completing the course or without passing the
exams (37%, as opposed to 13% in schizoaffective and 6% in affective patients).
This was independent of the level of institution (from elementary school up to
university).

Occupational Status at Onset

Between schizophrenic and schizoaffective patients as well as between schizophrenic and affective patients we found significant differences regarding occupational status at first manifestation. Of the schizophrenic patients 47% had no
vocational training. In the affective group most patients were housewives at
onset (Table 2).

Life Event Before Onset

About one-half of the affective and schizoaffective patients (51%) had a life
event-situation in the last 12 months before first manifestation. In schizophrenic
patients only 24% showed such a situation (Table 2).

Conclusions and Discussion

The present study shows relevant differences in both sociodemographic and premorbid features among schizophrenic, schizoaffective, and affective disorders, whereby the most relevant differences were found between schizophrenic disorders on the one side and schizoaffective and affective disorders on the other.

In both affective and schizoaffective disorders females were found to be more frequently represented than males, in contrast to schizophrenia. This is in agreement with other investigations (Angst 1980, 1987; Berner and Lenz 1986; Schubart et al. 1986; Möller and von Zerssen 1986; Omata 1985; Tsuang et al. 1986).

Schizophrenic patients became ill at a significantly younger age than patients with affective disorders; the age at onset in schizoaffective disorders was found to be intermediate between affective and schizophrenic disorders. Affective and schizoaffective patients significantly more frequently had a stable heterosexual partnership before onset than schizophrenic patients. This finding was proved to be independent of age and sex (Achte and Tuulio-Henriksson 1983; Roy 1981).

Although no special premorbid personality for any of the investigated groups was found, patients with obsessoid personality were found more frequently in the group of affective disorders but patients with low self-confident personality were more frequently in the schizoaffective and schizophrenic groups. It seems that significantly more schizophrenic patients have premorbidly a tendency towards social isolation than schizoaffective and affective patients (Achte and Tuulio-Henriksson 1983).

Patients with schizophrenic disorders were found more frequently in a lower social class, having a lower educational and occupational level than schizoaffective and affective patients, which again is in agreement with other investigations (Achte and Tuulio-Henriksson 1983; Dahl 1983; Maj 1985; Roy 1981; Rzewuska and Angst 1982). The lower educational and occupational levels of schizophrenic patients prove to be independent of age at onset. It is interesting that almost one-half of the schizophrenic patients had drifted to a lower social class before onset.

No significant differences were found between schizoaffective and affective patients regarding social class and social mobility. With regard to a broken home situation, no differences were found among the investigated groups.

All together the present study does not support earlier assumptions that schizoaffective disorders belong to the group of schizophrenias, but it does show some interesting similarities between affective and schizoaffective disorders.

Appendix: Definit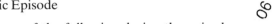

1. Diagnostic Criteria of Episodes

Schizophrenic Episode

A. At least one of the following during the episode:
   1. Delusions of being controlled, thought broadcasting, thou₅
      thought withdrawal
   2. Delusions of persecution or jealousy, somatic, grandiose, religiou
      istic, or other delusions, if accompanied by at least one of the following:
      (a) hallucinations; (b) blunted, flat, or inappropriate affect; (c) catatonic
      or other grossly disorganized behavior
   3. Auditory hallucinations in which either a voice keeps up a running
      commentary on the individual's behavior or thoughts, or two or more
      voices converse with each other, or the patient hears his own thoughts
      spoken aloud
   4. Auditory hallucinations on several occasions with content of more than
      one or two words, having no apparent relation to depression or elation
   5. Incoherence, marked loosening of associations, markedly illogical think-
      ing, or marked poverty of speech if associated with at least one of the
      following: (a) blunted, flat, or inappropriate affect; (b) delusions or hal-
      lucinations; (c) catatonic or other grossly disorganized behavior
B. Duration: at least 1 week
C. Absence of a melancholic, manic, or manic-depressive mixed episode – as
   defined in this paper – during, immediately before, or immediately after
   (without free interval) the presence of the symptoms of (A)
D. Not due to any organic mental disorder

Paranoid Episode

A. Persistent persecutory delusions or delusional jealousy or grandiose, relig-
   ious, nihilistic, or other delusions, but no delusions of (A1) of schizophrenia
   (i.e., no delusions of being controlled, thought broadcasting, thought inser-
   tion, or thought withdrawal)
B. Emotion and behavior appropriate to the content of the delusional system
C. Duration: at least 1 week
D. None of the symptoms of criterion (A) of schizophrenia
E. No prominent hallucinations
F. Absence of a melancholic or manic or manic-depressive mixed episode – as
   defined in this paper – during, immediately before, or immediatelly after
   (without free interval) the presence of the symptoms of (A)
G. Not due to any organic mental disorder

Melancholic Episode

A. Loss of pleasure in all or almost all activities
B. Lack of reactivity to usually pleasurable stimuli

C. At least three of the following:
   1. Distinct quality of depressed mood, i.e., the depressed mood is perceived as distinctly different from the kind of feeling experienced following the death of a loved one
   2. The depression is regularly worse in the morning
   3. Early morning awakening (significantly earlier than usual)
   4. Marked psychomotor retardation or agitation
   5. Significant anorexia or weight loss
   6. Excessive or inappropriate guilt, or excessive or inappropriate feelings of insufficiency
D. Duration: at least 1 week
E. Absence of the criteria of the schizophrenic, paranoid, manic, or manic-depressive mixed episode, during, immediately before, or immediately after (without free interval) the melancholic episode
F. Not due to any organic mental disorder

Manic Episode

A. One or more distinct periods with a predominantly elevated, expansive, or irritable mood
B. Duration of at least 1 week (or any duration if hospitalization is necessary), during which, for most of the time, at least three of the following symptoms have persisted (four if the mood is only irritable) and have been present to a significant degree:
   1. Increase in activity (either socially, at work, or sexually) or physical restlessness
   2. More talkative that usual or pressure to keep talking
   3. Flight of ideas or subjective experience that thoughts are racing
   4. Inflated self-esteem (grandiosity, which may be delusional)
   5. Decreased need for sleep
   6. Distractibility, i.e., attention is too easily drawn to unimportant or irrelevant external stimuli
   7. Excessive involvement in activities that have a high potential for painful consequences which is not recognized, e.g., buying sprees, sexual indiscretions, foolish business investments, reckless driving
C. Absence of the symptomatological features of the schizophrenic, paranoid, melancholic, or manic-depressive mixed episode, during, immediately before, or immediately after (without free interval) the manic episode
D. Not due to any organic mental disorder

Manic-Depressive Mixed Episode

A. The episode involves the symptomatic picture of both melancholic and manic episode intermixed or alternating without free interval
B. Not due to any organic mental disorder

Schizodepressive Episode

A. The episode involves the symptomatic picture of both schizophrenic or paranoid *and* melancholic episodes intermixed or alternating without free interval
B. If the symptomatology is a mixture of the symptoms of a paranoid and a melancholic episode the delusions have to be mood-incongruent (i.e., no nihilistic delusions or delusions of guilt or insuffiency or other melancholic delusions)
C. Not due to any organic mental disorder

Schizomanic Episode

A. The episodes involves the symptomatic picture of both schizophrenic or paranoid and manic episode intermixed or alternating without free interval
B. If the symptomatology is a mixture of the symptoms of a paranoid and a manic episode the delusions have to be mood-incongruent (i.e., no grandiose or other manic delusions)
C. Not due to any organic mental disorder

Schizomanic-Depressive Mixed Episode

A. The episode involves the symptomatic picture of both schizophrenic or paranoid *and* manic-depressive mixed episodes intermixed or alternating without free interval
B. If the symptomatology is a mixture of a paranoid and a manic-depressive mixed episode the delusions have to be mood-incongruent (as in schizodepressive and schizomanic episode)
C. Not due to any organic mental disorder

Noncharacteristic Episodes

Episodes not fullfilling the criteria of the episodes mentioned above have been defined as noncharacteristic.

2. Diagnostic Criteria of Disorder

Schizoaffective Disorder

During the whole course:
A. Presence of at least one schizoaffective episode, i.e., schizodepressive, schizomanic, or schizomanic-depressive mixed episode, as defined in this paper
or
B. If schizophrenic (or paranoid) episodes and affective episodes change from one to another independently of their number, sequence, or proportional representation
C. If (A) or (B) positive, noncharacteristic episodes can occur within the course; their presence does not have any influence on the diagnosis

Pure Schizophrenia

During the whole course:
A. Presence of schizophrenic episodes
B. Absence of schizoaffective or affective episodes, as defined in this paper
C. If (A) and (B) are positive during the whole course, the presence of paranoid or noncharacteristic episodes does not have any influence on the diagnosis

Pure Affective Disorder

During the whole course:
A. Presence of affective episodes
B. Absence of schizoaffective, schizophrenic, or paranoid episodes, as defined in this paper
C. If (A) and (B) positive, the occurrence of noncharacteristic episodes does not have any influence on the diagnosis

Pure Paranoid Disorder

During the whole course:
A. Presence of paranoid episodes, as defined in this paper
B. Absence of schizophrenic, affective, or schizoaffective episodes, as defined in this paper
C. If (A) and (B) positive, the occurrence of noncharacteristic episodes makes the diagnosis uncertain.

References

Achte K, Tuulio-Henriksson A (1983) Schizophrenia and schizoaffective psychosis. Psychiatr Clin (Basel) 16:126–140
AMDP (Arbeitsgemeinschaft für Methodik und Dokumentation in der Psychiatrie (ed) (1979) Das AMDP-System – Manual zur Dokumentation psychiatrischer Befunde, 3rd edn. Springer, Berlin Heidelberg New York
American Psychiatry Association (1980) Diagnostic and statistical manual of mental disorders, 3rd edn. APA, Washington
American Psychiatric Association (1987) Diagnostic and statistical manual of mental disorders. 3rd revised edn. APA, Washington
Angst J (1980) Verlauf schizoaffektiver Psychosen. In: Schimmelpenning GW (ed) Psychiatrische Verlaufsforschung Huber, Bern
Angst J (1986) The course of schizoaffective disorders. In: Marneros A, Tsuang MT (eds) Schizoaffective psychoses. Springer, Berlin Heidelberg New York
Angst J (1987) Epidemiologie der affektiven Psychosen. In: Kisker KP, Lauter H, Meyer JE, Müller C, Strömgren E (eds) Psychiatrie der Gegenwart, vol 5, 3rd edn. Springer, Berlin Heidelberg New York
Berner P, Lenz G (1986) Definitions of schizoaffective psychosis: mutual concordance and relationship to schizophrenia and affective disorder. In: Marneros A, Tsuang MT (eds) Schizoaffective psychoses. Springer, Berlin Heidelberg New York
Bleuler M (1972) Die schizophrenen Geistesstörungen im Lichte langjähriger Kranken- und Familiengeschichten. Thieme, Stuttgart
Dahl A (1983) Ego function assessment of schizoaffective patients as compared to schizophrenic and affective psychotic patients. Psychiatr Clin (Basel) 16:275–285
Hollingshead AB, Redlich FC (1958) Social class and mental illness. Wiley, New York

Huber G, Gross G, Schüttler R (1979) Schizophrenie. Springer, Berlin Heidelberg New York

Kleining G (1975a) Soziale Mobilität in der Bundesrepublik Deutschland. I. Klassenmobilität. Koeln Z Soziol Sozialpsychol 27:97–121

Kleining G (1975b) Soziale Mobilität in der Bundesrepublik Deutschland. II. Status- oder Prestige-Mobilität. Koeln Z Soziol Sozialpsychol 27:273–292

Kleining G, Moore H (1968) Soziale Selbsteinstufung (SSE) – Ein Instrument zur Messung sozialer Schichten. Koeln Z Soziol Sozialpsychol 20:502–552

Maj M (1985) Clinical course and outcome of schizoaffective disorders. Acta Psychiatr Scand 72:542–550

Marneros A, Tsuang MT (eds) (1986) Schizoaffective psychoses. Springer, Berlin Heidelberg New York

Marneros A, Deister A, Rohde A (1986a) The Cologne study on schizoaffective disorders and schizophrenia suspecta. In: Marneros A, Tsuang MT (eds) Schizoaffective psychoses. Springer, Berlin Heidelberg New York

Marneros A, Rohde A, Deister A, RisseA (1986b) Features of schizoaffective disorders. In: Marneros A, Tsuang MT (eds) Schizoaffective psychoses. Springer, Berlin Heidelberg New York

Marneros A, Rohde A, Deister A, Risse A (1986c) Features of schizoaffective disorders: the "cases-in-between." In: Marneros A, Tsuang MT (eds) Schizoaffective psychoses. Springer, Berlin Heidelberg New York

Marneros A, Deister A, Rohde A (1987) Schizophrene und schizoaffektive Psychosen. Die Langzeitprognose. In: Huber G (ed) Fortschritte in der Psychosenforschung. Schattauer, Stuttgart

Marneros A, Deister A, Rohde A, Jünemann H, Fimmers R (1988a) Long-term course of schizoaffective disorders. I. Definitions, methods, frequency of episodes and cycles. Eur Arch Psychiatry Neurol Sci 237:264–275

Marneros A, Rohde A, Deister A, Jünemann H, Fimmers F (1988b) Long-term course of schizoaffective disorders. II. Length of cycles, episodes and intervals. Eur Arch Psychiatry Neuro Sci 237:276–282

Marneros A, Rohde A, Deister A, Fimmers R, Jünemann H (1988c) Long-term course of schizoaffective disorders. III. Onset, type of episodes and syndrome shift, precipitating factors, suicidality, seasonality, inactivity of illness and outcome. Eur Arch Psychiatry Neurol Sci 237:283–290

Marneros A, Deister A, Rohde A (1988d) Syndrome shift in long-term course of schizo-affective disorders. Eur Arch Psychiatry Neurol Sci 238:97–104

Marneros A, Deister A, Rohde A, Steinmeyer EM, Jünemann H (1989a) Long-term outcome of schizoaffective and schizophrenic disorders: a comparative study. I. Definitions, methods, psychopathological and social outcome. Eur Arch Psychiatry Neurol Sci 238: 118–125

Marneros A, Steinmeyer EM, Deister A, Rohde A, Jünemann H (1989b) Long-term outcome of schizoaffective and schizophrenic disorders: a comparative study. III. Social consequences. Eur Arch Psychiatry Neurol Sci 238:135–139

Marneros A, Deister A, Rohde A (1989c) Quality of affective symptomatology and its importance for the definition of schizoaffective disorders. Psychopathology 22:152–160

Marneros A, Deister A, Rohde A (1989d) Unipolar and bipolar schizoaffective disorders: a comparative study. I. Premorbid and sociodemographic features. Eur Arch Psychiatry Neurol Sci 239:158–163

Marneros A, Rohde A, Deister A, Steinmeyer EM (1990) Behinderung und Residuum bei schizoaffektiven Psychosen: Daten, methodische Probleme und Hinweise für zukünftige Forschung. Fortschr Neurol Psychiatr 58:66–75

Möller HJ, von Zerssen D (1986) Der Verlauf schizophrener Psychosen unter den gegenwärtigen Behandlungsbedingungen. Springer, Berlin Heidelberg New York

Möller HJ, von Zerssen D (1987) Prämorbide Persönlichkeit von Patienten mit affektiven Psychosen. In: Kisker KP, Lauter H, Meyer JE, Müller C, Strömgren E (eds) Psychiatric der Gegenwart, vol 5, 3rd edn. Springer, Berlin Heidelberg New York

Moore H, Kleining G (1960) Das soziale Selbstbild der Gesellschaftsschichten in Deutschland. Koeln Z Soziol Sozialpsychol 12:86–119

Omata W (1985) Schizoaffektive Psychosen in Deutschland und Japan – eine transkulturell-psychiatrische Studie. Fortschr Neurol Psychiatr 53:168–176

Roy A (1981) Acute schizo-affective disorder. Can J Psychiatry 26:468–469

Rzewuska M, Angst J (1982) Aspects of the course of bipolar manic-depressive, schizoaffective, and paranoid schizophrenic psychoses. Arch Psychiatry Nervenkr 231:487–501

Schubart C, Schwarz R, Krumm B, Biehl H (1986) Schizophrenie und soziale Anpassung. Springer, Berlin Heidelberg New York

Spitzer RL, Gibbon M, Endicott J (1976) The global assessment scale. Arch Gen Psychiatry 33:768

Tellenbach H (1976) Melancholie. Springer, Berlin Heidelberg New York

Tsuang MT, Simpson JC, Fleming JA (1986) Diagnostic criteria for subtyping schizoaffective disorder. In: Marneros A, Tsuang MT (eds) Schizoaffective psychoses. Springer, Berlin Heidelberg New York

Wing JK, Cooper JE, Sartorius N (1974) Measurement and classification of psychiatric symptoms. Cambridge University Press, Cambridge

Wing JK, Cooper JE, Sartorius N (1982) Die Erfassung und Klassifikation psychiatrischer Symptome: Beschreibung und Glossar des PSE (present state examination). Beltz, Weinheim

World Health Organization (WHO) (1979) Schizophrenia. An international follow-up study. Wiley, Chichester

World Health Organization (WHO) (1986) WHO psychiatric disability assessment schedule (WHO/DAS). WHO, Geneva

Course of Affective and Schizoaffective Disorders

A. ROHDE, A. MARNEROS, A. DEISTER, H. JÜNEMANN, and B. STAAB[1]

Introduction

In the discussion on the question of how to classify schizoaffective disorders –
i.e., as a subgroup of one of the major functional psychoses or as a separate
nosological entity – a position often taken in recent years is that schizoaffective
disorders appear at least partially to be subtypes of affective disorders (Levinson
and Levitt 1987; Sovner and McHugh 1976; Winokur 1984; Winokur et al., this
volume). One of the reasons for this point of view is that several studies have
shown similarities in course between affective and schizoaffective disorders, for
instance, the well-known Zurich studies of Angst and coworkers (Angst 1980;
Angst et al. 1973, 1980) or the Cologne Study of Marneros and coworkers
(Marneros et al. 1988a–d). Regarding affective disorders, there has been
general agreement in recent years that the unipolar and bipolar forms should be
investigated separately because of several relevant differences (Angst 1966,
1987). Recent work shows that the subgrouping of schizoaffective disorders –
similarly to affective disorders – into unipolar and bipolar forms is also indicated
(Angst 1989, Marneros et al. 1989a–c). The differentiation between unipolar
and bipolar forms of affective and schizoaffective disorders is necessary not only
because of relevant differences in premorbid, sociodemographic, and therapeutic aspects, but also considering the longitudinal approach. Conversely, the
division of schizoaffective disorders into schizodepression and schizomania
(Brockington et al. 1980; Maj 1985) has the disadvantage of taking only the
cross-sectional aspect into consideration (Marneros et al. 1986a–c, 1989b). The
division of affective and schizoaffective disorders into unipolar and bipolar
forms also solves the problem of syndrome shift and polymorphism of the course
(Marneros et al. 1988d).

In this paper the course of affective and schizoaffective disorders will be
compared. In addition, several course variables for unipolar and bipolar subgroups will be compared.

---

[1] Psychiatrische Universitätsklinik, Sigmund-Freud-Straße 25, 5300 Bonn 1, FRG

Affective and Schizoaffective Disorders
Edited by A. Marneros and M.T. Tsuang
© Springer-Verlag Berlin Heidelberg 1990

Subjects and Methods

Subjects

The present contribution is part of the Cologne study on the long-term course and outcome of affective, schizoaffective, and schizophrenic disorders. For this contribution we compared various elements of course of 106 patients with affective and 88 with schizoaffective disorder. Table 1 shows some features of the sample, like sex, age at onset, age at follow-up, and duration of follow-up. The methods, instruments of evaluation, and diagnostic criteria are described in Marneros et al. (this volume).

The *subgrouping into unipolar and bipolar foms* of affective and schizoaffective disorders depends on the presence or absence of manic symptomatology. Disorders with manic symptomatology (similar to the manic episode of DSM-III) at least once during the course were classified as "bipolar," and disorders without any manic symptoms as "unipolar" forms (1989a–c). Seventy-six of the patients with affective and 40 with schizoaffective disorder were unipolar, and 30 affective patients and 48 schizoaffective patients had a bipolar course.

Elements of Course

Course was defined according to Angst (1986), as "the signs and symptoms over the whole lifetime following the first manifestation of a psychiatric disorder. Its criterial elements are onset, episodes or cycles, intervals, and outcome, which normally designates the present state at the last follow-up." In this paper we are going to compare the following cours variables: (a) type of episodes, (b) annual frequency of episodes (AFE), (c) annual frequency of cycles (AFC), (d) length of cycles, and (e) inactivity of the illness. Definitions of these elements of course will be given in the appropriate sections below (see also Marneros et al. 1988a).

Statistical Evaluation

As already demonstrated by Angst, there is considerable individual variation in the number and length of episodes and cycles, so that it is uncertain whether or not parametric methods, especially those based on the assumption of a normal distribution, could be used for analysis. For some variables, the information available from earlier studies (Angst 1980; Angst and Weis 1967; Angst et al. 1973) suggests a log-normal distribution. The findings of Angst could be confirmed by Marneros et al. (1988a) and were found to be valid for affective disorders as well as for schizoaffective disorders. Figure 1 gives an example, taking the mean length of cycles for schizoaffective disorders. Unlike the raw data, the logarithmically transformed values give an approximately normal distribution (checked graphically and using the Kolmogorov-Smirnov test). Checking the same variable for affective disorders the picture is almost identical. Thus, for the cases in question, the empirical distribution functions were checked (graphically and using the Kolmogorov-Smirnov test) and if necessary a logar-

Table 1. Characteristics of study population

	Affective ($n = 106$)	Schizoaffective ($n = 88$)
Sex		
Female	76%	65%
Male	24%	35%
Age at onset (mean no. of years)	36.1	31.2
Duration of follow-up period (mean no. of years)	27.9	25.8
Age at end of follow-up period (mean no. of years)	64.0	57.0

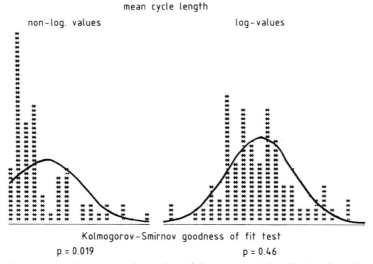

Fig. 1. Logarithmic transformation of the mean lengths of cycles for schizoaffective disorders

ithmic transformation was applied. After that, comparison of goups was done using the Mann-Whitney "U"-test (nonparametric) or the t-test (parametric).

Results

Frequency of Episodes

The 105 affective patients had 3.8 episodes on average (geometric mean) during the course and the 86 schizoaffective patients had an average of 4.6 episodes (one affective patient and two schizoaffective patients who were permanently hospitalized were excluded). A *monophasic course* (only one episode during

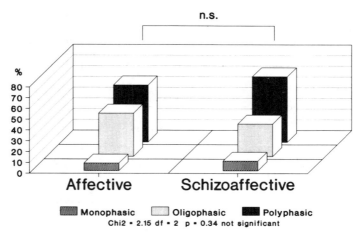

Fig. 2. Type of course of affective and schizoaffective disorders

course) was found in 7% of the affective and 9% of the schizoaffective group (Fig. 2). The course was oligophasic (up to three episodes) in 40% of the affective and 30% of the schizoaffective patients. The majority of both groups had a *polyphasic* course (four or more episodes): 53% and 61% respectively (Fig. 2). The differences between affective and schizoaffective disorders regarding the monophasic, oligophasic, and polyphasic courses and the number of episodes were not significant (χ^2, $P = 0.34$, t-test (log values) $P = 0.07$).

Annual Frequency of Episodes

To achieve better comparability among the various individual cases with follow-up periods varying from 10 to 61 years, the AFE was introduced (Marneros et al. 1988a). The AFE is calculated by dividing the number of episodes by the duration of illness in years. The AFE is individually calculated. It was found to be 0.14 episodes for the affective and 0.19 for the schizoaffective group (geometric mean), showing a significant difference (t-test (log-values), $P = 0.006$; Table 2).

Annual Frequency of Cycles

Different results were found regarding the AFC, defined as the number of episodes divided by the activity period of illness in years, that is the time up to the last relapse-free period. The AFC is relatively independent from the not accurately definable beginning and ending of episodes, and it is also independent from the inactivity period of the disorders (last relapse-free period), as well as from the monophasic cases. Affectives ($n = 97$) had 0.26 cycles per year (geometric mean), the 78 schizoaffectives with at least two episodes had 0.318 cycles per year (no significant difference; Table 2).

Table 2. Elements of course: schizoaffective vs affective disorder

	Affective	Schizoaffective	Significance
Annual frequency of episodes	($n = 105$)	($n = 86$)	
Geometric mean	0.144	0.194	$P = 0.006^{**}$ (1)
Median	0.136	0.203	$P = 0.003^{**}$ (2)
Annual frequency of cycles	($n = 97$)	($n = 78$)	
Geometric mean	0.264	0.318	$P = 0.164$ (1)
Median	0.232	0.332	$P = 0.075$ (2)
Inactivity of the illness	($n = 63$)	($n = 82$)	
Arithmetic mean (years)	14.85	13.86	$P = 0.444$ (3)
Median (years)	17	11	$P = 0.215$ (2)

**, $P < 0.01$; (1) t-test (log values); (2) Mann-Whitney test; (3) t-test (nonlog values).

Cycle Length

A cycle was defined by Angst as the period of time between the beginning of one episode and the beginning of the next (Angst 1980). The average length of cycles 1 to 7 (geometric mean) is shown in Fig. 3. We decided to compare only the first seven cycles because the number of patients with a higher number of cycles is limited. Similar patterns occur for both groups. The first cycle is longer than the succeeding ones in both groups. For the affective group this is 37.96 months, for the schizoaffective 37.20 months. Comparing cycle 1 to cycle 7 no significant difference was found between affective and schizoaffective disorders.

Inactivity of the Illness

"Inactivity of the illness" was defined in a former paper by Marneros and coworkers as a period of at least 3 years since the end of the last episode, independently of the presence or absence of residual symptoms (Marneros et al. 1988c). The 3-year period was arbitrary and a compromise, but nevertheless based on empirical data (for details see Marneros et al. 1988c).

A last relapse-free period of more than 3 years was noted in 73% of the schizoaffective and 78% of the affective patients. The average inactive period (median) was 11 years for schizoaffective and 17 years for affective patients, showing no significant differences between the two groups (Table 2).

Unipolar and Bipolar Forms of Affective and Schizoaffective Disorders

Frequency of Episodes in Unipolar and Bipolar Disorders

Comparing monophasic, oligophasic, and polyphasic types of course between unipolar and bipolar affective and schizoaffective patients, significant differences were found between the unipolar and bipolar affective as well as between the unipolar and bipolar schizoaffective patients (Fig. 4).

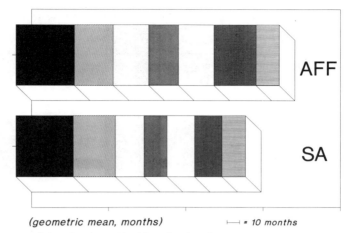

(geometric mean, months)   ⊢——⊣ = 10 months

Fig. 3. Cycle length (cycles 1–7) in affective and schizoaffective disorders

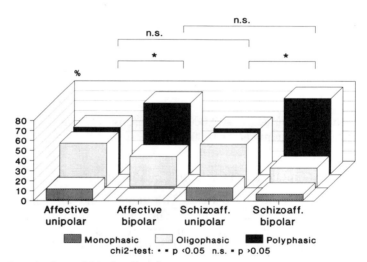

Fig. 4. Type of course in unipolar and bipolar disorders

Annual Frequency of Episodes in Unipolar and Bipolar Disorders

Comparing the AFE for unipolar and bipolar forms of illness, nearly identical values were found. Unipolar affective patients show an AFE of 0.12, and unipolar schizoaffective patients 0.13 (Table 3). For the bipolar affective patients the AFE is 0.23, and for the bipolar schizoaffectives patients it is 0.26 (geometric mean). The difference between the unipolar affective and schizoaffective patients is not statistically significant ($P = 0.316$) which is also the case between the bipolar affective and schizoaffective patients ($P = 0.488$). But on testing unipolar versus bipolar affective patients there is a highly significant difference

Table 3. Elements of course: unipolar vs bipolar affective and schizoaffective disorders

	Affective		Schizoaffective
Annual frequency of episodes (geometric mean)			
Unipolar	0.12	ns	0.14
| **	| **		| **
Bipolar	0.23	ns	0.26
Annual frequency of cycles (geometric mean)			
Unipolar	0.22	ns	0.24
	| **		| *
Bipolar	0.41	ns	0.39
Inactivity of the illness (median no. of years)			
Unipolar	19.0	ns	19.0
	| ns		| *
Bipolar	10.0	ns	10.0

*, $P < 0.05$; **, $P < 0.01$; ns, $P > 0.05$.

(t-test (log values $P = 0.000$), as there is between unipolar and bipolar schizo-affective patients ($P = 0.000$).

Annual Frequency of Cycles in Unipolar and Bipolar Disorders

The AFC results for patients with unipolar and bipolar disorders are similar to those for the AFE (Table 3). Unipolar forms of affective and schizoaffective disorders do not differ significantly from one another (0.22 and 0.24 respectively; geometric mean, $P = 0.596$), neither do bipolar forms (0.41 and 0.39 respectively; $P = 0.793$). On the other hand, there is a highly significant difference between unipolar and bipolar affective patients (0.22 and 0.41 respectively; $P = 0.002$) and a significant difference between unipolar and bipolar schizoaffective disorders (0.24 and 0.39 respectively; $P = 0.011$).

Cycle Length in Unipolar and Bipolar Disorders

In Fig. 5, which shows the mean length of cycles 1 to 7 (geometric mean), the first cycle is of special interest. The shortest average first cycle was found in the bipolar affectives of our group (19.4 months), followed by the bipolar schizo-affectives (27.4 months) and unipolar affectives (50.6 months). The unipolar schizoaffectives had the longest average first cycle (56.4 months).

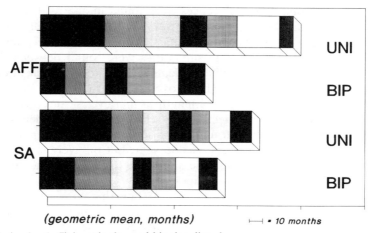

(geometric mean, months)   ⊢──⊣ = 10 months

Fig. 5. Cycle length (cycles 1–7) in unipolar and bipolar disorders

Inactivity of the Illness in Unipolar and Bipolar Disorders

At the time of follow-up, the period of inactivity of the illness in the unipolar patients of our sample was nearly twice as high as that in bipolars, in affective disorders as well as schizoaffective disorders (Table 3; $P = 0.03$ for schizoaffective patients, $P = 0.09$ for affective patients).

Conclusions and Discussion

The course of schizoaffective disorders has considerable similarities with that of affective disorders (Angst 1980; Angst et al. 1980; Rzewuska and Angst 1982). Both disorders are polyphasic, they have nearly identical annual frequency of episodes and cycles, both of them relapse according to similar patterns (Angst 1980, 1986; Marneros et al. 1988a–c). Studies on the course of affective disorders show that there are relevant differences between uni- and bipolar affective disorders (Angst 1986). Similar differences were found in the course of unipolar and bipolar schizoaffective disorders (Marneros et al. 1989a–c).

The global comparison of affective and schizoaffective disorders showed interesting similarities, supporting the suggestion that schizoaffective disorders should be subgrouped within the affective disorders. But similarities and differences in the course of affective and schizoaffective disorders should not be globally estimated, because they might be sample-dependent, i.e., dependent on the proportion of the unipolar and bipolar forms in the respective groups. The comparison of affective and schizoaffective disorders is much more reliable if it is limited to a comparison of a unipolar affective sample with a unipolar schizoaffective sample and of a bipolar affective with a bipolar schizoaffective sample. Doing this, differences were found in nearly all investigated variables between unipolar and bipolar forms, for affective as well as for schizoaffective disorders, with the exception of inactivity of illness between unipolar and bipolar affective patients. Striking similarities were found between unipolar affective and unipolar schizoaffective patients and between bipolar affective and bipolar schizoaffective patients. This proved to be true for all the selected variables: type of course, AFE, AFC, length of first cycles, and inactivity of the illness. Patients with bipolar affective and schizoaffective disorders relapse much more often than patients with unipolar disorders. The bipolar patients of this study had a relapse nearly every second year, but on average patients with unipolar disorders had only one relapse in 4 years. In particular the first cycle was shorter in the bipolar than in the unipolar forms.

The findings of the present study show that unipolar disorders – affective as well as schizoaffective – have a significantly more favorable course than do bipolar disorders regarding probability of relapse. This contradicts Welner et al. (1977), who found no differences between unipolar and bipolar schizoaffective patients with regard to course of illness.

All in all, the courses of affective and schizoaffective disorders show important similarities, especially if we differentiate between unipolar and bipolar forms. The distinction into unipolar and bipolar forms of affective and schizoaffective disorders is not only relevant but is also of interest for clinical practice, for instance, in deciding when a prophylactic treatment should begin. There is evidence that as is the case with bipolar affective disorders, which respond better to lithium prophylaxis than do unipolar forms (Mendlewicz et al. 1973; Zvolsky et al. 1974; Bunney et al. 1970), also schizoaffective bipolar disorders respond better to lithium propylaxis than do unipolars (Bastianello et al. 1985; Küfferle and Lenz 1983).

The prognosis of unipolar disorders with regard to course is more favorable than that of bipolar disorders. But the prognosis also includes the outcome of a disorder. As Marneros et al. (1989a–c) have shown, no significant differences between unipolar and bipolar forms of affective and schizoaffective disorders were found regarding the social and psychopathological outcome.

In conclusion, it can be said that the findings on the course of affective and schizoaffective disorders support the assumption of the existence of two groups of disorders, (a) unipolar disorders and (b) bipolar disorders, each of them having an affective and a schizoaffective subgroup.

References

Angst J (1966) Zur Ätiologie und Nosologie endogener depressiver Psychosen. Eine genetische, soziologische und klinische Studie. Springer, Berlin Heidelberg New York
Angst J (1980) Verlauf unipolar depressiver, bipolar manisch-depressiver and schizo-affektiver Erkrankungen und Psychosen. Fortschr Neurol Psychiatr 48:3–30
Angst J (1986) The course of schizoaffective disorders. In: Marneros A, Tsuang MT (eds) Schizoaffective psychoses. Springer, Berlin Heidelberg New York

Angst J (1987) Verlauf der affektiven Psychosen. In: Kisker KP, Lauter H, Meyer J-E, Müller
    C, Strömgren E (eds) Psychiatrie der Gegenwart, vol 5, 3rd edn. Springer, Berlin Heidel-
    berg New York
Angst J (1989) Der Verlauf schizoaffektiver Psychosen. In: Marneros A (ed) Schizoaffektive
    Psychosen. Therapie und Prophylaxe. Springer, Berlin Heidelberg New York
Angst J, Weis P (1967) Periodicity of depressive psychoses. In: Brill H, Cole JO, Deniker P,
    Hippius H, Bradley BP (eds) Neuro-psychopharmacology. Proceedings of the fifth inter-
    national congress of the Collegium Internationale Neuro-Psychopharmacologicum,
    Washington DC 1966. Excerpta Medica, Amsterdam
Angst J, Baastrup P, Grof P, Hippius H, Pöldinger W, Weis P (1973) The course of monopolar
    depression and bipolar psychoses. Psychiatr Neurol Neurochir 76:489–500
Angst J, Felder W, Lohmeyer B (1980) Course of schizoaffective psychoses: results of a
    follow-up study. Schizophr Bull 6:579–585
Bastianello RR, Janiri L, Mauro P, Pirrongelli C (1985) Slow-release lithium in treatment of
    schizoaffective syndromes. Int J Clin Pharmacol Res 5:205–211
Brockington I, Wainwright S, Kenell R (1980) Depressed patients with schizophrenic or
    paranoid symptoms. Psychol Med 10:665–675
Bunney WE, Brodie KH, Murphy DL, Goodwin FK (1970) Psychopharmacological differ-
    entiation between two subgroups of depressed patients. Proceedings of the 78th Annual
    Convention of the APA
Küfferle B, Lenz G (1983) Classification and course of schizo-affective psychoses. Psychiatr
    Clin (Basel) 16:169–177
Levinson DF, Levitt MEM (1987) Schizoaffective mania reconsidered. Am J Psychiatry
    144:415–425
Maj M (1985) Clinical course and outcome of schizoaffective disorders. Acta Psychiatr Scand
    72:542–550
Marneros A, Deister A, Rohde A (1986a) The Cologne study on schizoaffective disorders and
    schizophrenia suspecta. In: Marneros A, Tsuang MT (eds) Schizoaffective psychoses.
    Springer, Berlin Heidelberg New York
Marneros A, Rohde A, Deister A, RisseA (1986b) Features of schizoaffective disorders. In:
    Marneros A, Tsuang MT (eds) Schizoaffective psychoses. Springer, Berlin Heidelberg
    New York
Marneros A, Rohde A, Deister A, Risse A (1986c) Schizoaffective disorders: the prognostic
    value of the affective component. In: Marneros A, Tsuang MT (eds) Schizoaffective
    psychoses. Springer, Berlin Heidelberg New York
Marneros A, Deister A, Rohde A, Jünemann H, Fimmers R (1988a) Long-term course of
    schizoaffective disorders. I. Definitions, methods, frequency of episodes and cycles. Eur
    Arch Psychiatry Neurol Sci 237:264–275
Marneros A, Rohde A, Deister A, Jünemann H, Fimmers R (1988b) Long-term course of
    schizoaffective disorders. II. Length of cycles, episodes, and intervals. Eur Arch Psy-
    chiatry Neurol Sci 237:276–282
Marneros A, Rohde A, Deister A, Fimmers R, Jünemann H (1988c) Long-term course of
    schizoaffective disorders. III. Onset, type of episodes and syndrome shift, precipitating
    factors, suicidality, seasonality, inactivity of illness, and outcome. Eur Arch Psychiatry
    Neurol Sci 237:283–290
Marneros A, Rohde A, Deister A, Jünemann H (1988d) Syndrome shift in long-term course
    of schizoaffective disorders. Eur Arch Psychiatry Neurol Sci 238:97–104
Marneros A, Deister A, Rohde A (1989a) Unipolar and bipolar schizoaffective disorders: a
    comparative study. I. Premorbid and sociodemographic features. Eur Arch Psychiatry
    Neurol Sci 239:158–163
Marneros A, Rohde A, Deister A (1989b) Unipolar and bipolar schizoaffective disorders: a
    comparative study. II. Long-term course. Eur Arch Psychiatry Neurol Sci 239:164–170
Marneros A, Deister A, Rohde A, Jünemann H (1989c) Unipolar and bipolar schizoaffective
    disorders: a comparative study. III. Long-term outcome. Eur Arch Psychiatry Neurol
    239:171–176
Marneros A, Rohde A, Deister A, Steinmeyer A (1990) Behinderung und Residuum bei
    schizoaffektiven Psychosen: Daten, methodische Probleme und Hinweise für zukünftige
    Forschung. Fortschr Neurol Psychiatr 58:66–75

Mendlewicz J, Fieve RR, Stallone F (1973) Relationship between effectiveness of lithium therapy and family history. Am J Psychiatry 130:1011–1013
Rzewuska M, Angst J (1982) Prognosis of periodic bipolar manic-depressive and schizoaffective psychoses. Arch Psychiatr Nervenkr 231:471–486
Sovner RD, McHugh PR (1976) Bipolar course in schizo-affective illness. Biol Psychiatry 11:195–204
Welner A, Croughan J, Fishman R, Robins E (1977) The group of schizoaffective and related psychoses: a follow-up study. Compr Psychiatry 18:413–422
Winokur G (1984) Psychosis in bipolar and unipolar affective illness with special reference to schizoaffective disorder. Br J Psychiatr 145:236–242
Zvolsky P, Vinarova E, Dostal T, Soucek K (1974) Family history of manic-depressive and endogenous patients and clinical effect of treatment with lithium. Act Nerv Super (Praha) 16:194–195

Long-Term Outcome of Affective, Schizoaffective, and Schizophrenic Disorders: A Comparison

A. Deister, A. Marneros, A. Rohde, B. Staab, and H. Jünemann[1]

Introduction

In the past decade most empirical studies investigating schizoaffective psychoses have confirmed that regarding outcome these psychoses occupy an intermediate position between schizophrenic and affective disorders (Angst 1980a,b, 1986; Brockington et al. 1980a,b; Harrow and Grossman 1984; Pope et al. 1980; Rzewuska and Angst 1982). In the Cologne study (using narrow definitions based on the longitudinal approach and employing standardized instruments of evaluation) we found that the long-term outcome of schizoaffective disorders is much more favorable than that of schizophrenia (Marneros et al. 1986c, 1989a,b).

More than 20 years ago Angst stated that affective disorders had been considerably less intensively investigated than schizophrenic disorders (Angst 1966). Despite methodological shortcomings (Angst 1987; Marneros et al. 1990), since that statement some follow-up studies have shown that the prognosis and outcome of affective disorders seem to be less favorable than originally described by Kraepelin in 1909 (e.g., Angst 1987; Bratfos nd Haug 1968; Lee and Murray 1988; Rao et al. 1977). It must not be forgotten, however, that the outcome of a mental disorder has many aspects: social disability, psychopathological residuum, psychological deficit, or social consequences (Angst 1986; Marneros et al. 1990). Each of these aspects can be differently influenced by the illness, and therefore they have to be investigated separately. The aim of this paper is to compare the various aspects of the outcome of schizophrenic, schizoaffective, and affective disorders.

Subjects, Methods, and Instruments

Subjects and Methods

This paper is part of the Cologne study (Marneros et al. 1986a–c, 1988a–d). The subjects and methods of the follow-up investigation have already been described by Marneros et al. (this volume). In addition to the population compared regarding long-term course (88 patients with schizoaffective disorders and 106 patients with affective disorders) we report here on the long-term outcome of 97

---

[1] Psychiatrische Universitätsklinik, Sigmund-Freud-Straße 25, 5300 Bonn 1, FRG

Affective and Schizoaffective Disorders
Edited by A. Marneros and M.T. Tsuang
© Springer-Verlag Berlin Heidelberg 1990

patients diagnosed as having schizophrenia (mean follow-up period, 19.6 years; mean age at follow-up, 49.5 years).

Instruments of Evaluation

The evaluation of long-term outcome is based on personal follow-up investigation using the standardized instruments (Marneros et al. 1989a) as described below.

Global Assessment Scale (GAS)

The GAS, developed by Spitzer et al. (1976; Endicott et al. 1976) is a rating scale for evaluating the overall functioning of a subject during a specified period on a continuum from psychological or psychiatric illness to health.

Disability Assessment Schedule (WHO/DAS)

This instrument was developed by the WHO (1979, 1988) for the assessment of social behavior and disability during or after mental illness. "Disability," in this instrument, is defined as a disturbance or loss of the ability to perform specific social functions and roles in the family, at work, and/or in social groups, according to the normal expectations of the community (Schubart et al. 1986a). We used the German version of the WHO/DAS, developed by the Central Institute of Mental Health in Mannheim (Schubart et al. 1986b).

We decided, on the grounds of sample-dependent specificities, to omit some items of section 2 of the WHO/DAS (social role performance). The main reason for this decision was the permanent hospitalization of some patients in the schizophrenic group or the absence of required conditions for performance of the social roles rated by these items, especially parental or occupational role (Marneros et al. 1989a). For every item the interviewer had to rate both intensity and duration. The scores finally assigned were the sums of the scores for intensity and duration.

Psychological Impairment Rating Schedule (WHO/PIRS)

The WHO/PIRS was developed by the WHO (1979) for the assessment of psychological impairment after mental illness. It reflects the opinion of the observing expert. The WHO/PIRS is strongly related to the Present State Examination (Biehl et al. 1986, 1989; Schubart et al. 1986b).

Evaluation of Social Consequences

From the group of all evaluated factors reflecting social consequences of the illnesses (Marneros et al. 1989b) we selected as most representative and, at the same time, reliable the following: (a) occupational mobility (only downward drift), (b) social mobility, (c) premature retirement, and (d) achievement of the expected social development. (For definitions of the variables see the respective subsections of the Results section.)

Results

Global Assessment Scale

The findings according to the GAS are shown in Table 1 and Fig. 1. Only 12.4% of the schizophrenic but 50.0% of the schizoaffective and 64.2% of the affective patients had no difficulties at the time of follow-up. The differences between both affective and schizoaffective patients and schizophrenic patients are highly significant, but there is no significant difference between the schizoaffective and affective groups regarding the parameter "no difficulties in global functioning."

Grouping the findings into the categories: (a) no difficulties (score 91–100), (b) moderate difficulties (score 51–90), (c) severe difficulties (score 31–50), and (d) extreme difficulties (score 0–30), see Table 1, we found highly significant differences between schizoaffective and affective disorders. In affective disorders only 3.8% had a score lower than 51, and no patient showed extreme difficulties.

Differences between schizoaffective and affective patients were also found in comparing the arithmetic means (Table 2). The affective group seems to be more homogeneous than the schizoaffective and schizophrenic patients. As shown in Fig. 1, the median score of the schizoaffective group (90.5) is very similar to that of the affective group (95), while the minimum value in the schizoaffective group is the same as that in the schizophrenic group (10 in both groups).

Disability Assessment Schedule

Global Evaluation

In section 5 of the WHO/DAS the investigator's overall assessment of the patients social adjustment is given, considering all information recorded and

Table 1. Global Assessment Scale (GAS)

	Schizophrenic ($n = 97$)	Schizoaffective ($n = 88$)	Affective ($n = 106$)
No difficulties (Score, 91–100)	12 (12.4%)	44 (50.0%)	68 (64.2%)
Moderate difficulties (Score, 51–90)	13 (13.4%)	24 (27.3%)	34 (32.1%)
Severe difficulties (Score, 31–50)	22 (22.7%)	15 (17.0%)	4 (3.8%)
Extreme difficulties (Score, 0–30)	50 (51.5%)	5 (5.7%)	0

Schizophrenic vs schizoaffective disorder: $\chi^2 = 59.4$, $df = 3$; $P = 0.000$,**; schizophrenic vs affective disorder: $\chi^2 = 110.9$, $df = 3$; $P = 0.000$,**; schizoaffective vs affective disorder: $\chi^2 = 16.7$, $df = 3$; $P = 0.001$.**
**, $P < 0.01$.

GAS-Score

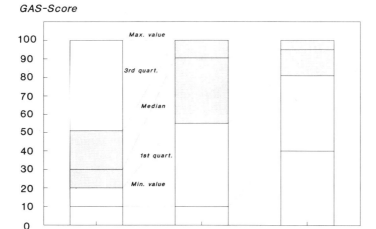

Fig. 1. Global Assessment Scale (GAS). Minimum value, first quartile, median, third quartile, maximum value

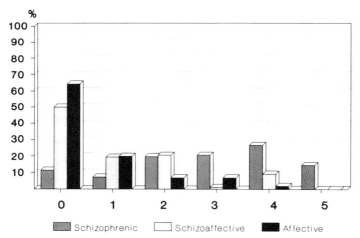

Fig. 2. Disability Assessment Schedule (WHO/DAS). Global evaluation: 0, excellent adjustment; 1, good adjustment; 2, fair adjustment; 3, poor adjustment; 4, very poor adjustment; 5, severe maladjustment. Significance: schizophrenic vs schizoaffective disorder, $P = 0.000$ ($df = 5$); schizophrenic vs affective disorder, $P = 0.000$ ($df = 5$); schizoaffective vs affective disorder, $P = 0.003$ ($df = 4$)

rated in the schedule (see Fig. 2). In the schizophrenic group a good adjustment after a long-term course of the illness is very rare (11%). Schizoaffective (50%) and affective patients (64.2%) show a significantly more favorable adjustment than schizophrenic patients. The schizoaffective patients occupy a position between the other two groups.

Table 2. Global Assessment Scale (GAS)

	Schizophrenic ($n = 97$)	Schizoaffective ($n = 88$)	Affective ($n = 106$)
Arithmetic mean	41.97	75.18	87.43
Standard deviation	26.77	27.65	15.64

t-test: schizophrenic vs schizoaffective disorder, $P = 0.000$,**; schizophrenic vs affective disorder, $P = 0.000$,**; schizoaffective vs affective disorder, $P = 0.000$.**
**, $P < 0.01$.

Table 3. Disability Assessment Schedule (WHO/DAS): patient's average score

	Schizophrenic ($n = 97$)	Schizoaffective ($n = 88$)	Affective ($n = 106$)
0	7%	48%	54%
0.01–0.50	6%	11%	18%
0.51–1.00	7%	16%	12%
1.01–1.50	8%	4%	5%
1.51–2.00	7%	6%	4%
2.01–2.50	10%	7%	3%
2.51–3.00	9%	6%	2%
3.01–3.50	14%	1%	1%
3.51–4.00	10%	1%	—
4.01–4.50	12%	—	—
4.51–5.00	7%	—	—
Arithmetic mean[a]	2.583	0.731	0.487
Median[b]	2.833	0.333	0.000

[a] t-Test: schizophrenic vs schizoaffective disorder, $P = 0.000$,**; schizophrenic vs affective disorder, $P = 0.000$,**; schizoaffective vs affective disorder, $P = 0.072$.
[b] Mann-Whitney u-test: schizophrenic vs schizoaffective disorder, $P = 0.000$,**; schizophrenic vs affective disorder $P = 0.000$,**; schizoaffective vs affective disorder, $P = 0.166$.
**, $P < 0.01$.

Patient's Average Score (PAS)

The PAS is the arithmetic mean of all equally weighted item scores for each individual patient. The results are shown in Table 3. Again the schizoaffective patients had a position in between the two other groups. About one-half of schizoaffective and of the affective patients had no disturbances in all six evaluated items (PAS = 0), the differences between these groups are not significant.

Item's Average Score (IAS)

The IAS is the arithmetic mean of an item score rated in a group of patients. Figure 3 shows the profile of the six evaluated items for the three diagnostic groups. Between schizoaffective and affective patients there are significant differences only in regard to the items "self-care" and "emergency behavior,"

Score-Mean

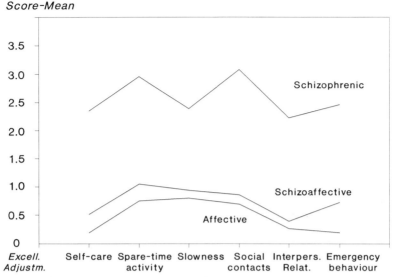

Fig. 3. Disability Assessment Schedule (WHO/DAS): profile of Item's Average Score (IAS)

while in schizophrenic patients the disturbances are more severe in all the investigated items.

Psychological Impairment Rating Schedule (WHO/PIRS)

For each section of the WHO/PIRS an "overall impression" was evaluated. The profile of these ten sections (Fig. 4) shows highly significant differences between schizophrenic patients and the other two groups investigated, while schizoaffective and affective patients show nearly the same profile.

Social Consequences

Downward Occupational Drift

Occupational drift is defined as the difference in occupational status between the beginning of occupational life and the time of the follow-up investigation or, for retired patients, the time of retirement. We considered only those patients for whom downward occupational drift was possible, i.e., those classified as housewives, because of marriage or birth of a child, were excluded.

In the schizophrenic patients downward occupational drift was significantly more frequent (Table 4) than in the other groups; affective patients had the lowest frequency (29%).

Social Drift

The social drift was estimated by comparing the patient's original social class (parent's social class) with the patient's social class at the end of the observation

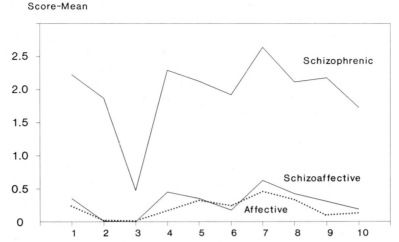

Fig. 4. Psychological Impairment Rating Schedule (PIRS): profile of Item's Average Score (IAS). Global evaluation: *1*, slowness; *2*, attention withdrawal; *3*, fatiguability; *4*, initiative; *5*, facial expression; *6*, body language; *7*, affect display; *8*, conversation skills; *9*, self presentation; *10*, cooperation

Table 4. Social consequences

	Schizo-phrenic	p1	Schizo-affective	p2	Affective	p3
Downward occupational drift	($n = 81$) 65%	0.015*	($n = 58$) 45%	0.086	($n = 55$) 29%	0.000**
Downward social drift	($n = 59$)		($n = 55$)		($n = 45$)	
Total	58%	0.000**	18%	0.808	24%	0.000**
Female patients	65%	0.000**	12%	0.047*	36%	0.053
Male patients	54%	0.011*	23%	0.229	10%	0.001**
Upward social drift	($n = 73$)		($n = 57$)		($n = 48$)	
Total	7%	0.058	18%	0.006**	42%	0.000**
Female patients	8%	0.291	19%	0.106	39%	0.010*
Male patients	6%	0.132	17%	0.026*	44%	0.000**
Premature retirement	($n = 81$) 44%	0.025*	($n = 58$) 26%	0.960	($n = 55$) 26%	0.024*
Achievement of the expected social development	($n = 97$) 43%	0.000**	($n = 88$) 72%	0.083	($n = 106$) 82%	0.000

Chi^2-test: p1, significance of schizophrenic vs schizoaffective disorders; p2, significance of schizoaffective vs affective disorders; p3, significance of schizophrenic vs affective disorders.
*, $P < 0.05$; **, $P < 0.01$.

time. The social class was estimated according to the criteria of Kleining and Moore (1968) transferred to the classification of Hollingshead and Redlich (1958). We excluded all patients for whom social drift was impossible because their original social class was already the lowest (downward drift) or the highest one (upward drift), and housewives because of marriage or birth of a child.

Significantly more schizophrenics (58%) than schizoaffective (18%) and affective (24%) patients experienced a downward social drift. An upward social drift was found to be most frequent in affective patients (42%).

Premature Retirement

Regarding premature retirement we found no significant differences between affective and schizoaffective patients (Table 4). Schizophrenic patients had the highest frequency of premature retirement. Housewives were excluded.

Achievement of the Expected Social Development

The factor achievement of the expected social development reflects the opinion of the interviewer as to whether the patient is fulfilling his or her expected social role and whether he or she has achieved the social status which would be expected on the basis of the status of the family, education, possibilities of upward social drift, and so on.

Evaluating this parameter, we found more patients fulfilling this definition in the affective group (82%) than in the schizoaffective (72%) and the schizophrenic groups (43%).

Conclusions and Discussion

Schizophrenic patients had a more unfavorable long-term outcome than patients with schizoaffective and affective disorders. They were significantly more frequently disabled, showed more severe psychological impairment, and a significantly higher proportion of patients experienced negative social consequences. The disturbances are not only more frequent but also more intense than in affective and schizoaffective disorders (Marneros et al. 1989a,b). This result has been repeatedly confirmed (Angst 1986; Harrow and Grossman 1984; Opjordsmoen 1989). Investigations finding no differences between schizophrenic and schizoaffective disorders and between schizophrenic and affective disorders are exceptions, being due to different diagnostic criteria or sample-dependent differences (Marneros et al. 1990).

In evaluating long-term outcome it is important to consider that "outcome" is not a monolithic term. Outcome is only a compromise, characterizing the present psychopathological, psychological, and social state of the patient usually some months or years after onset of the illness (Angst 1980b, 1986; Marneros et al. 1989a,c, 1990). Each of the aspects of outcome mentioned can be differently affected.

Investigating the course of schizoaffective and affective disorders we were able to show that the course of these illnesses is dependent on their polarity

(Rohde et al., this volume). In contrast to course (Angst 1989; Marneros et al. 1989c,d; Rohde et al., this volume), we did not find any significant differences in outcome between unipolar and bipolar forms both in schizoaffective (Marneros et al. 1989e) and affective disorders. This allows a comparison of the outcome of affective and schizoaffective disorders regardless of their polarity.

We were able to show that it is insufficient to evaluate and compare only proportions of patients who did not have disturbances at the time of follow-up. Evaluating the overall functioning using the GAS (Spitzer et al. 1976; Endicott et al. 1976) we did not find significant differences in the number of patients with no difficulties between the two groups. But comparing the distributions there are significant differences: the group of affective patients seems to be more homogeneous regarding long-term outcome, while the group of schizoaffective patients shows similarities in this respect with the group of schizophrenic patients.

Angst (1989) reported GAS scores for both schizoaffective and affective patients. The patients in his study had about 20 score points less (median) at the end of the observation time than in our study. One possible explanation for the differences between the two studies may be the different point in time at which global functioning was evaluated. In the Cologne study the GAS was estimated on average more than 10 years after the last episode, while in Angst's study the GAS score was estimated significantly earlier. Although the two studies exhibit discrepancies in the level of the GAS scores in each group in both studies, the relationships between the groups and the distribution within each group seem to be similar.

Kettering et al. (1987) reported mean GAS scores of 63 in unipolar non-psychotic depression and of 56.5 in unipolar psychotic depression after a follow-up period of only 14 months on average. Opjordsmoen (1989) investigated three groups of functional psychosis diagnosed according to the RDC and DSM-III after an observation period of between 3 and 39 years. He found mean GAS scores of 73 for unipolar affective, 67 for schizodepressive, and 47 for schizo-phrenic patients. A total of 66% of the patients were judged to be healthy at the end of the observation time.

Disability according to the WHO (Schubart et al. 1986a) means a disturbance or loss of the ability to perform specific social functions and roles in the family, at work, and/or in social groups in line with the normal expectations of the community. In the schizoaffective group about every second patient had impaired social adjustment. Of the patients with affective disorders more than one-third also experienced social impairment or negative social consequences.

Angst (1987) estimated that about one-half to two-thirds of the affective patients remitted socially. Similarly to our results, Lehmann et al. (1988) found that 32% of depressed patients are moderately or severely impaired regarding social functioning. Follow-up studies of affective disorders are less comparable (Angst 1987; Lee and Murray 1988; Opjordsmoen 1989). However, it can be assumed that there is a group of one-third to one-half of the patients who are not fully remitted, which is a result similar to ours.

In conclusion, it can be said that the great majority of the schizophrenic patients were found to be unable to function in several areas, or their behavior was considerably influenced by psychotic symptomatology, or they showed serious impairment in communication or judgement. On the other hand, patients with affective disorders do not have such a favorable outcome as the Kraepelinian dichotomy suggests, either psychopathologically or socially.

Schizoaffective disorders occupy a position between these two groups: although the differences between schizophrenic and schizoaffective patients seem to be more marked, there are also important differences between schizoaffective and affective disorders, especially if other than only global instruments have been used for assessing the long-term outcome.

References

Angst J (1966) Zur Ätiologie und Nosologie endogener depressiver Psychosen. Springer, Berlin Heidelberg New York
Angst J (1980a) Clinical typology of bipolar illness. In: Belmaker RH, van Praag HM (eds) Mania. An evolving concept. Spectrum, Jamaica
Angst J (1980b) Verlauf unipolar depressiver, bipolar manisch-depressiver und schizo-affektiver Erkrankungen und Psychosen. Fortschr Neurol Psychiatr 48:3–30
Angst J (1986) The course of schizoaffective disorders. In: Marneros A, Tsuang MT (eds) Schizoaffective psychoses. Springer, Berlin Heidelberg New York
Angst J (1987) Verlauf der affektiven Psychosen. In: Kisker KP, Lauter H, Meyer J-E, Müller C, Strömgren E (eds) Psychiatrie der Gegenwart, vol 5, 3rd edn. Springer, Berlin Heidelberg New York
Angst J (1989) Der Verlauf schizoaffektiver Psychosen. In: Marneros A (ed) Therapie und Prophylaxe schizoaffektiver Psychosen. Springer, Berlin Heidelberg New York
Biehl H, Maurer K, Schubart C, Krumm B, Jung E (1986) Prediction of outcome and utilization of medical services in a prospective study of first onset schizophrenics – results of a prospective 5-year follow-up study. Eur Arch Psychiatry Neurol Sci 236:139–147
Biehl H, Maurer K, Jablensky A, Cooper JE, Tomov T (1989) The WHO/PIRS. I. Introducing a new instrument for rating observed behaviour and the rationale of the psychological impairment concept. Br J Psychiatry 155 (suppl. 7):68–70
Bratfos O, Haug JO (1968) The course of manic-depressive psychosis. Acta Psychiatr Scand 44:89–112
Brockington I, Wainwright S, Kendell R (1980a) Manic patients with schizophrenic or paranoid symptoms. Psychol Med 10:73–83
Brockington I, Wainwright S, Kendell R (1980b) Depressed patients with schizophrenic or paranoid symptoms. Psychol Med 10:665–675
Endicott J, Spitzer RL, Fleiss JL, Cohen J (1976) The global assessment scale. A procedure for measuring overall severity of psychiatric disturbance. Arch Gen Psychiatry 33:766–771
Harrow M, Grossman LS (1984) Outcome in schizoaffective disorders: a critical review and reevaluation of the literature. Schizophr Bull 10:87–108
Hollingshaed AB, Redlich FC (1958) Social class and mental illness. Wiley, New York
Kettering RL, Harrow M, Grossman L, Meltzer HY (1987) The prognostic relevance of delusions in depression: follow-up study. Am J Psychiatry 144:1154–1160
Kleining G, Moore H (1968) Soziale Selbsteinstufung (SSE) – Ein Instrument zur Messung sozialer Schichten. Köln Z Soziol Sozialpsychol 20:502–552
Kraepelin E (1909) Psychiatrie. Ein Lehrbuch für Studierende und Ärzte, vol 1, 8th edn. Barth, Leipzig
Lee AS, Murray RM (1988) The long-term outcome of Maudsley depressives. Br J Psychiatry 153:741–751
Lehmann HE, Tenton FR, Deutsch M, Feldman S, Engelsman F (1988) An 11-year follow-up study of 110 depressed patients. Acta Psychiatr Scand 78:57–65
Marneros A, Deister A, Rohde A (1986a) The Cologne study on schizoaffective disorders and schizophrenia suspecta. In: Marneros A, Tsuang MT (eds) Schizoaffective psychoses. Springer, Berlin Heidelberg New York

Marneros A, Rohde A, Deister A (1986b) Features of schizoaffective disorders: the "cases-in-between." In: Marneros A, Tsuang MT (eds) Schizoaffective psychoses. Springer, Berlin Heidelberg New York

Marneros A, Rohde A, Deister A, Risse A (1986c) Schizoaffective disorders: the prognostic value of the affective component. In: Marneros A, Tsuang MT (eds) Schizoaffective psychoses. Springer, Berlin Heidelberg New York

Marneros A, Deister A, Rohde A, Jünemann H, Fimmers R (1988a) Long-term course of schizoaffective disorders. Definitions, methods, frequency of episodes and cycles. Eur Arch Psychiatry Neurol Sci 237:264–275

Marneros A, Rohde A, Deister A, Jünemann H, Fimmers R (1988b) Long-term course of schizoaffective disorders. Length of cycles, episodes and intervals. Eur Arch Psychiatry Neurol Sci 237:276–282

Marneros A, Rohde A, Deister A, Fimmers R, Jünemann H (1988c) Long-term course of schizoaffective disorders. Onset, type of episodes and syndrome shift, precipitating factors, suicidality, seasonality, inactivity of illness and outcome. Eur Arch Psychiatry Neurol Sci 237:283–290

Marneros A, Deister A, Rohde A (1988d) Syndrome shift in long-term course of Schizoaffective disorders. Eur Arch Psychiatry Neurol Sci 238:97–104

Marneros A, Deister A, Rohde A, Steinmeyer EM, Jünemann H (1989a) Long-term outcome of schizoaffective and schizophrenic disorders: a comparative study. I. Definitions, methods, psychopathological and social outcome. Eur Arch Psychiatry Neurol Sci 238: 118–125

Marneros A, Steinmeyer EM, Deister A, Rohde A, Jünemann H (1989b) Long-term outcome of schizoaffective and schizophrenic disorders: a comparative study. III. The social consequences. Eur Arch Psychiatry Neurol Sci 238:135–139

Marneros A, Deister A, Rohde A (1989c) Unipolar and bipolar schizoaffective disorders: a comparative study. I. Premorbid and sociodemographic features. Eur Arch Psychiatry Neurol Sci 239:158–163

Marneros A, Rohde A, Deister A (1989d) Unipolar and bipolar schizoaffective disorders: a comparative study. II. Long-term course. Eur Arch Psychiatry Neurol Sci 239:164–170

Marneros A, Deister A, Rohde A, Staab B, Jünemann H (1989e) Unipolar and bipolar schizoaffective disorders: a comparative study. III. Long-term outcome. Eur Arch Psychiatry Neurol Sci 239:171–176

Marneros A, Rohde A, Deister A, Steinmeyer EM (1990) Behinderung und Residuum bei schizoaffektiven Psychosen: Daten, methodische Probleme und Hinweise für zukunftige Forschung. Fortschr Neurol Psychiatr 58:51–86

Opjordsmoen S (1989) Long-term course and outcome in unipolar affective and schizoaffective psychoses. Acta Psychiatr Scand 79:317–326

Pope H, Lipinski J, Cohen B, Axelrod D (1980) "Schizoaffective disorder": an invalid diagnosis? A comparison of schizoaffective disorder, schizophrenia, and affective disorder. Am J Psychiatry 137:91–97

Rao VA, Nammalvar N (1977) The course and outcome in depressive illness. BJ Psychiatry 130:392–396

Rzewuska M, Angst J (1982) Aspects of the course of bipolar manic-depressive, schizoaffective, and paranoid schizophrenic psychoses. Arch Psychiatr Nervenkr 231:487–501

Schubart C, Krumm B, Biehl H, Schwarz R (1986a) Measurement of social disability in a schizophrenic patient group. Soc Psychiatry 21:1–9

Schubart C, Schwarz R, Krumm B, Biehl H (1986b) Schizophrenie und soziale Anpassung. Springer, Berlin Heidelberg New York

Spitzer RL, Gibbon M, Endicott J (1976) The global assessment scale. Arch Gen Psychiatry 33:768

World Health Organization (WHO) (1979) Schizophrenia. An international follow-up study. Wiley, Chichester

World Health Organization (WHO) (1988) WHO psychiatric disability assessment schedule (WHO/DAS). WHO, Geneva

Suicide in Affective and Schizoaffective Disorders

J. Angst, H.H. Stassen, G. Gross, G. Huber, and M.H. Stone[1]

Introduction

Suicide is a neglected but frequent outcome of the spontaneous course of affective disorders. Lifetime suicide rates for depression were reported in 1970 by Guze and Robins to be between 12% and 19%. Fifty to sixty percent of all suicides in the normal population are due to affective disorders. Barraclough et al. (1974) found a depression in 64% of the suicides they studied, Hagnell et al. (1982) in more than 50% of subjects in the Lundby Study. Robins et al. (1959) found an affective disorder in 45% of cases. Rich et al. (1986) investigated 286 cases in the San Diego Suicide Study: in the younger age-group, less than 30 years old, 38% were depressives, in the older group 56%. Hagnell et al. (1982) found that especially men commit suicide very early after onset of the first depressive episode and after a relatively short ambulatory treatment. The high suicide rate for affective disorders is frequently not noticed; particularly short-term observations and treatments usually neglect the problem totally. In a small group treated over a short period, suicide is a rare event. Therefore, most reports on such treatments as psychotherapy or drugs do not mention suicide at all, and one might believe that the majority of depressives feel just fine after a treatment. In fact, as far as we know, modern psychiatric interventions have not yet been proven capable of reducing the suicide rate of depressives. On the contrary, in many Western countries the suicide rates of hospitalized psychiatric patients have increased more than the population growth and also more than the suicide rates for the total population (Ernst et al. 1980).

Modern antidepressant treatments can reduce the symptoms and suffering of depression considerably, but in the majority of cases some minor residual symptoms persist as long as the episode lasts. In cases of premature cessation of the medication, a relapse is observed. The median length of a depressive episode is about 5.5 months. This figure does not deviate from data collected almost 100 years ago. Ziehen (1896), Pilcz (1901), and Wertham (1929a,b) described a median episode length of 4–6 months. We have to conclude that in the majority of cases, treatment does not shorten the length of episodes.

Long-term medication of patients at high risk for suicide may be successful. Montgomery et al. (1979, 1983, 1988) treated patients who had a previous

---

[1] Psychiatric University Hospital Zürich, Research Department, P.O. Box 68, 8029 Zürich, Switzerland

Affective and Schizoaffective Disorders
Edited by A. Marneros and M.T. Tsuang
© Springer-Verlag Berlin Heidelberg 1990

history of at least three suicide attempts over 1 year with flupenthixol and were able to reduce the rates of suicide attempts by active medication. Another three studies also indicate that long-term lithium medication can decrease the frequency of suicide attempts (Poole et al. 1978; Hanus and Zapletalek 1984; Causemann and Müller-Oerlinghausen 1988). These observations are encouraging if there is an association between frequency of suicide attempts and suicides. But long-term medication can have this effect only if the suicide risk does not diminish with time. Tsuang and Woolson (1978) reported that the risk of suicide was highest in depressive men during the first 10 years of illness and then decreased. On the other hand, we know that suicide rates in the normal population increase with age, a fact which is not easily compatible with the former observation. A basic problem is therefore whether the risk of suicide is constant or diminishes, or even increases with age. The second question is whether suicide due to depression is linked with diagnosis or personality characteristics, such as aggression, impulsiveness, or being capable of making difficult decisions.

The study of Angst and Clayton (1986) showed that male subjects who committed suicide were clearly more aggressive than controls, measured with the Freiburger Personality Inventory of Fahrenberg and Selg (1970). Their study indicates that the subgroup of depressives characterized by aggression may be especially at risk for committing suicide. If that is correct, this finding may be unspecific and may also be true for other diagnostic groups such as schizoaffectives, schizophrenics, or the borderline personalities. At present, we do not have any empirical data to answer this question. Except for aggression, which is also very common among subjects who do not commit suicide, it has up to now been impossible to predict which subjects will commit suicide based on such general characteristics as sex, age, marital status, or social class.

This paper deals especially with the question of whether the suicide risk of psychiatric patients varies during their lifetime or remains constant. This question will be answered by comparing four diagnostic groups of patients: those with affective disorders, those with schizoaffective disorders, those with schizophrenia, and those with borderline personality disorders. The data consist of three different samples collected by different methods, from Bonn (Huber et al. 1979), New York (Stone et al. 1987), and Zurich (Angst et al. 1980). Special emphasis will be given to the Zurich sample.

Study Samples

Between 1959 and 1963 we started a prospective longitudinal study on the course of affective disorders of patients admitted to the Psychiatric University Hospital, Zurich. The patients were followed up every 5 years until 1985. Of 406 cases, 18 were excluded from the sample because they did not meet DSM-III criteria for major depression or bipolar disorder. The remaining sample consisted of 133 unipolar depressive, 110 bipolar depressive, and 145 schizoaffective patients. These diagnoses were based on the total information collected up to the end of

Table 1. Zurich sample, suicides

	UP n (%)	BP n (%)	SA n (%)	Total n (%)
Patients	133	110	145	388
Deaths	85 (64)	59 (54)	68 (47)	212 (55)
Suicides	17 (20)	7 (12)	13 (19)	37 (17)

UP, Unipolar depressive; BP, bipolar depressive; SA, schizoaffective.

observation. A substantial number of patients (n = 212) died during this period (see Table 1; the respective suicide rates are given in parentheses): 64% (20% suicides) of the unipolar depressives, 54% (12% suicides) of the bipolar depressives, and 47% (19% suicides) of the schizoaffectives. From another study on reactive depressive patients (Rosner 1988), involving records of selected patients at the psychiatric University Hospital, Zurich, between 1959 and 1962, we have included 65 additional cases (14 suicides and 51 patients who died of other causes).

A follow-up study on the psychopathological and social courses of development of 758 schizophrenic patients hospitalized between 1945 and 1959 was carried out at the Psychiatric University Clinic of Bonn (Huber et al. 1979). Follow-ups were done from 1967 to 1973 on 502 of these patients, 67% of whom had become probands on the occasion of their first psychiatric hospitalization. A total of 142 persons died, 30 of them by suicide (suicide rate 21.1%). For present purposes, we have combined this subgroup of 142 persons who died with the data material of Zurich. All patients have been rediagnosed by G. Gross on the basis of clinical records and according to the Zurich criteria in order to identify schizoaffective cases.

For comparisons only, we have also included the data of 49 suicides collected by Stone et al. (1987) in New York. This latter sample comprises 42 cases with "borderline" diagnoses.

Statistics

Survival analysis models the time to some particular event in terms of risk functions. Several well-established approaches to the problem of modeling longitudinal course and outcome exist. The most popular model in this context is the proportional hazards model, which was introduced by Cox in 1972, whereas the Kaplan-Meier (Kaplan and Meier 1958) estimate of the population cumulative distribution of times and its generalization (Turnbull 1976) are widely used as the fundamental summary of a given data set. Our analyses are based on the nonparametric Kaplan-Meier approach, although, as we will see later, some results of our investigation suggest a parametric solution, in particular, a linear approach as well. The nonparametric Kaplan-Meier maximum likelihood estimator $\hat{S}_{KM}(t)$ at failure time t_i is given by

$$\hat{S}_{KM}(t_i) = \prod_{j \in \{j|t_j < t_i\}} \left(1 - \frac{d_j}{r_j}\right)$$

where d_j is the number of failures at t_j, and r_j is the number at risk, that is, the number of objects which have neither failed nor been censored, immediately prior to t_j. For present purposes, one has solely to replace "failure" by "onset", "death", or "duration of illness" in order to apply the above model to our data.

The Lifelong Course of Affective and Schizoaffective Psychoses

In the Zurich sample of endogenous affective psychoses meeting the DSM-III diagnostic criteria for major mood disorders, 212 patients died during the follow-up period up to 1985. In a second step we will subgroup these patients into those with suicidal and nonsuicidal deaths.

Table 2 describes similarities and differences in course and outcome in affective and schizoaffective patients, both consisting of uni- and bipolar sub-groups. The two groups do not differ in average length of episodes, length of cycles, episodes per year, and total time spent in illness from onset to last observation. This means that both affective and schizoaffective patients have the same periodicity of their disorder. There are two differences; one is explained by the earlier onset of schizoaffective disorder, which is linked with a higher length of illness and a higher number of episodes observed during a lifetime. The second difference consists of a lower final Global Assessment Scale (GAS) score (Endicott et al. 1976) which was computed during the last interval prior to death or prior to the development of an organic brain syndrome. Therefore, this score reflects impairment due to the affective or schizoaffective psychosis. The impairment is definitely more severe in the schizoaffective group than in the affective group. Most of the patients suffer from depressive neurasthenic and hypochondriacal symptoms.

Table 2. Data from Zurich study, 1985: all deaths, affective versus schizoaffective psychoses

No.	Affective 144	Schizoaffective 68	P
Age at onset	48	31	0.0000
Age at death	73	66	0.009
Length of episodes (months)	5.33	5.15	ns
Length of cycles (years)	3.5	3.1	ns
Episodes per year	0.42	0.37	ns
Total no. of episodes	6	8	0.0003
Length of illness (years)	17.5	29.1	0.0000
% time ill	0.26	0.2	ns
Final GAS score	60.5	51	0.003

All figures are medians.

The results would not disprove the hypothesis that schizoaffective psychoses are a more severe form of the same disorder as affective psychoses; the earlier onset and higher disability would certainly be compatible with the hypothesis. The hypothesis is further supported by the same periodicity of the two subforms. This conclusion is not totally justified, of course, because there is a major difference in the course between uni- and bipolar subgroups in both affective and schizoaffective psychoses.

The two diagnostic groups – affective and schizoaffective – can now be broken down according to nonsuicidal and suicidal deaths. Unfortunately, the groups are too small to be broken down further by polarity of the illness into uni- and bipolar subgroups. The statistical comparisons are made for:

1. Suicides versus other deaths
2. Affective versus schizoaffective suicides
3. Other deaths: affective versus schizoaffective psychoses

Suicides Versus Other Deaths

In the affective group, subjects who committed suicide had a significantly earlier onset and died earlier, but also showed a shorter length of the episodes and more episodes per year than the subjects who died for other reasons (Table 3). The finding that the residual symptomatology and social impairment (GAS score) during the last interval was less severe in the group of those who committed suicide may be explained by the much younger age at death of this group.

Schizoaffective patients who died by suicide and those who died of other causes do not differ remarkably from each other, but the group of those who committed suicide is rather small for statistical comparisons. Therefore, the results may not yet be conclusive.

Affective Versus Schizoaffective Suicides

For this analysis the 24 suicides as a consequence of affective disorders are compared with the 13 due to a schizoaffective disorder (Table 4). These two groups do not differ very much, but here again, the differences is perhaps obscured by the smallness of the schizoaffective group. For instance, schizo-affective patients experienced almost twice as many episodes as affective patients before they committed suicide. It should be mentioned in this context that the suicide event was counted as a final episode. The final GAS indicates again a higher impairment during the interval for schizoaffective patients com-pared with affective patients.

Other Deaths After Affective or Schizoaffective Psychoses

In contrast to the groups who committed suicide, in which the subjects are rather similar, the remaining groups of patients who died for other reasons differ remarkably, and these findings are much more compatible with findings drawn from total samples of patients with affective and schizoaffective psychoses

Table 3. Course of suicides and other deaths

	Affective			Schizoaffective		
	Suicides	Other deaths	P	Suicides	Other deaths	P
No.	24	120		13	55	
Age at onset	30.5	49	0.0003	32	31	ns
Age at death	56.5	74.5	0.0000	62	68	0.02
Length of episode	3.2	5.6	0.006	7.1	4.8	ns
Length of cycles	2.5	3.6	0.08	2.8	3.3	ns
Episodes/year	0.49	0.27	0.02	0.35	0.30	ns
Total no. of episodes	4.5	6	ns	8	8	ns
Length of illness	16.5	17.5	ns	22.7	31.6	ns
% time ill	18.7	17.2	ns	20.3	12.7	ns
Final GAS score	70	60	0.04	55	51	ns

All figures are medians.

Table 4. Course of affective versus schizoaffective psychoses

	Suicides			Other deaths		
	Aff.	Schizoaff.	P	Aff.	Schizoaff.	P
No.	24	13		120	55	
Age at onset	30.5	32	ns	49	31	0.001
Age at death	56.5	62	ns	74.5	68	0.01
Length of episodes (months)	3.2	7.1	ns	5.6	4.8	ns
Length of cycles (years)	2.5	2.8	ns	3.6	3.3	ns
Episodes per year	0.49	0.35	ns	0.27	0.30	ns
Total no. of episodes	4.5	8	ns	6	8	0.01
Length of illness	16.5	22.7	ns	17.5	31.6	0.001
% time ill	18.7	20.3	ns	17.2	12.7	ns
Final GAS score	70	55	0.01	60	51	0.05

All figures are medians.

(Table 4). Schizoaffective patients show a significantly earlier onset (31 versus 49 years), a lower age at death (68 versus 74.5), a larger number of episodes (8 versus 6), a greater length of illness (31.6 versus 17.5 years), and, again, a poorer remission during the interval (GAS score 51 versus 60). These results are about the same as those in Table 2. The main finding is that the suicidal patients with affective and those with schizoaffective disorders show some similarity, in contrast to the other deaths with the same diagnosis.

Subjects who committed suicide are characterized by a higher occurrence of previous suicide attempts, shown in Table 5. On the other hand, suicides among

first-degree relatives do not differ remarkably between the subgroups of probands (alive, dead, dead by suicide), as shown in Table 6.

The finding that affective and schizoaffective patients who committed
suicide were very similar in onset and course of their illness, except for the final
outcome, is of great interest and suggests the hypothesis that subjects who
commit suicide may have something in common across diagnostic groups. In
order to check this hypothesis, we will now analyze the three samples from
Bonn, Zurich, and New York with varying diagnoses (depression, schizophrenia, schizoaffective disorder, borderline personality disorder).

Table 7 describes sex and diagnosis of the patients from the three sites –
Zurich, Bonn, and New York – who committed suicide and of those subjects
who died for other reasons. In the Zurich sample the reactive depressives
admitted to the hospital from 1959 to 1962 are now included, too. Therefore, the
depressive group consists of endogenous and reactive depressives.

It is of interest to note that there is no marked sex difference in the suicide
samples of the three sites. Sixty men and 70 women committed suicide, 28% and
26% of the total male and female deaths respectively. The figures from New
York refer to a very young group which is at lower risk of dying for other reasons
than suicide. In the Zurich sample 18% and in the Bonn sample 21% of all
deaths were due to suicide. These figures are slightly higher than those reported
in the literature, but they are based on much longer follow-ups than are usually
carried out. Furthermore, they reflect the fact that the group studied consisted of
hospitalized patients with severe endogenous psychoses.

Table 8 describes some further characteristics, such as age at death, length
of observation until death (time after onset), and age at onset, of the total
material collected in Zurich, Bonn, and New York. These data show clearly that

Table 5. Number of suicide attempts (lifetime)

No. of suicide attempts	Percentage attempting suicide		
	Suicides ($n = 37$)	Other deaths ($n = 175$)	Patients alive ($n = 176$)
0	62	85	70
1	19	9	18
2	11	5	3
3 or more	8	1	9

Table 6. Suicides among relatives

	Patients		
	Suicides	Other deaths	Alive
No. of first-degree relatives	223	1267	1252
No. of suicides	10	33	43
%	4.5	2.6	3.4

Table 7. Description of the three samples

	Zurich	Bonn	New York
Suicides			
No.	51	30	49
Men	19	17	24
Women	32	13	25
Unipolar	29	—	—
Bipolar	9	—	4
Schizophrenic	—	21	3
Schizoaffective	13	9	—
Borderline	—	—	42
Other deaths			
No.	226	112	13
Men	94	48	10
Women	132	64	3
Unipolar	115	—	—
Bipolar	56	—	—
Schizophrenic	—	78	1
Schizoaffective	55	34	—
Borderline	—	—	12

the New York group consists mainly of borderline patients who are definitely younger, as shown by their earlier age of onset. But the patients from Bonn, not including bipolar and unipolar affective disorders, also have an earlier age of onset characteristic for schizoaffectives and schizophrenics.

The subjects who committed suicide differ from those who died other deaths clearly in their age distribution at death, as illustrated by Figs. 1 and 2. The nonsuicidal deaths show increasing probabilities with age, whereas the distribution of the suicides is almost normal. In the next step we give the results of the survival analyses in order to compare the mortality of the diagnostic groups taken together from all three sites.

Mortality of Affective, Schizoaffective, and Schizophrenic Patients

In a first step we have determined the mortality, separately for each diagnosis, from the nonsuicidal deaths among the unipolar, bipolar, schizoaffective, and schizophrenic patients of our samples. For this purpose, survival analysis has been applied in order to model the distribution of deaths as a function of age or duration of illness.

Figure 3 displays the survival of unipolar depressive patients as compared with bipolar depressive patients. The two curves are almost identical, indicating that there are no differences in mortality between the two populations. The survival curve shows a typical arctan characteristic: with increasing age, the curve drops off more and more steeply; in other words, the death risk increases substantially only at the most advanced ages. However, this finding is due to the fact that the distribution of "age at death" is right-skewed at a mean of 69.3

Table 8. Age, age at onset, and length of observation (time after onset) of the three samples (Zurich, Bonn, and New York)

| | Suicides | | | | | | | | | Other deaths | | | | | |
| | Zurich | | | Bonn | | | New York | | | Zurich | | | Bonn | | |
	Age at death	Time after onset	Age at onset	Age at death	Time after onset	Age at onset	Age at death	Time after onset	Age at onset	Age at death	Time after onset	Age at onset	Age at death	Time after onset	Age at onset
Mean	51.8	19.5	33.3	39.0	10.3	28.7	27.0	4.8	22.3	69.4	26.2	44.3	50.9	17.8	32.8
SD	14.3	13.0	13.8	11.5	8.0	12.0	7.1	5.3	5.4	12.1	14.3	15.8	14.5	11.3	11.7
Median	54.0	21.0	32.0	38.0	9.0	25.0	26.0	2.0	21.0	72.0	24.0	45.5	51.0	17.0	32.0
Q25	41.0	6.0	20.0	30.5	4.0	19.8	21.5	1.0	18.5	62.7	15.8	31.8	40.3	10.0	24.0

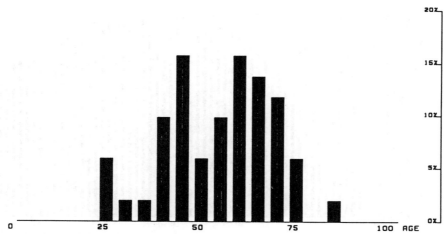

Fig. 1. Frequency distribution of "age at death" derived from the 51 suicides of the Zurich sample

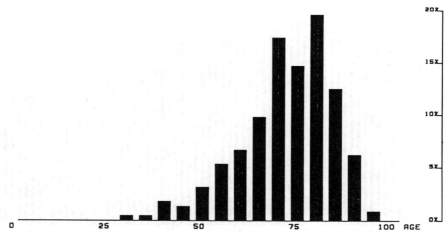

Fig. 2. Frequency distribution of "age at death" derived from the 226 nonsuicidal deaths of the Zurich sample

years (Fig. 1). Here, as in all subsequent mortality analyses, unipolar and bipolar depressive patients are combined in the "affective" subgroup (since they have identical mortalities).

The schizoaffective nonsuicidal deaths have a slightly increased mortality as compared with the affective subgroup (Fig. 4), whereas the schizophrenic subgroup displays a completely different survival curve (Fig. 5), indicating that the nonsuicidal schizophrenic patients die significantly earlier than all other nonsuicidal patients.

These findings are in contrast to the distribution of deaths among the suicide cases. As Figs. 6, 7, and 8 illustrate, their survival function is approximately

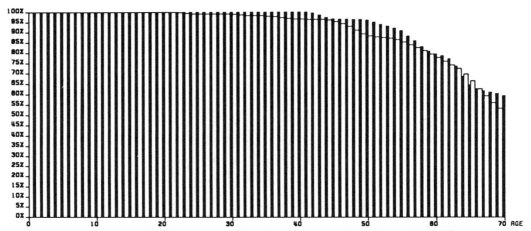

Fig. 3. Survival of nonsuicidal patients as a function of age: unipolar subgroup (*n* = 55) versus bipolar subgroup (*n* = 115). *Light bars* represent unipolars, *dark bars* represent bipolars

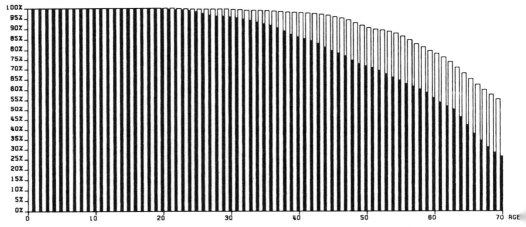

Fig. 4. Survival of nonsuicidal patients as a function of age: unipolar and bipolar subgroup (*n* = 170) versus schizoaffective subgroup (*n* = 97). *Light bars* represent affectives, *dark bars* represent schizoaffectives

linear, and the risk of committing suicide is practically constant over a lifetime. This holds true for depressive, schizoaffective, and schizophrenic, as well as for borderline patients (Fig. 9). In particular, we find a constant suicide risk in affectives for patients between 30 and 70 years (together with a 10% risk for male patients between 17 and 30 years), in schizoaffectives for patients between 34 and 72 years, in schizophrenics for patients between 20 and 54 years (together with a slightly decreased risk for patients over 50 years), in borderline patients between 17 and 35 years (together with a slightly decreased risk for those over 30 years) (Fig. 10). The steepness of the risk function is almost identical for

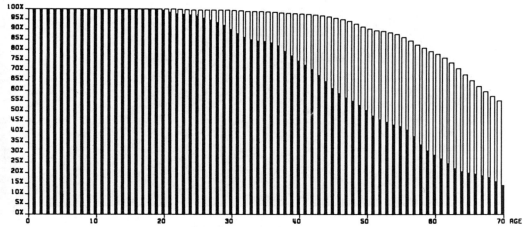

Fig. 5. Survival of nonsuicidal patients as a function of age: unipolar and bipolar subgroup ($n = 170$) versus schizophrenic subgroup ($n = 76$). *Light bars* represent affectives, *dark bars* represent schizophrenics

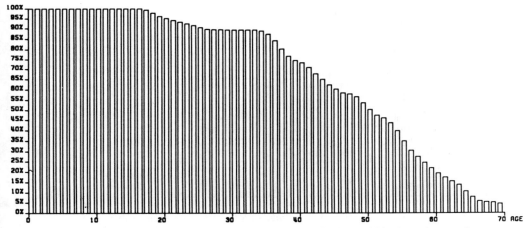

Fig. 6. Survival of suicidal patients as a function of age: unipolar and bipolar subgroup ($n = 38$)

affectives, schizoaffectives and schizophrenics, whereas for borderlines the respective risk function is twice as steep, indicating that the suicide risk is twice as high in these cases. No significant sex differences were revealed, except for the finding that men, as a group, start to commit suicide earlier. Their risk is already present at age 20, whereas for women this becomes true only after age 35 (significant at the 5% level). For both sexes, however, the risk remains constant over a lifetime, and, as mentioned above, there is no sex difference in the lifetime prevalence of suicide between men and women.

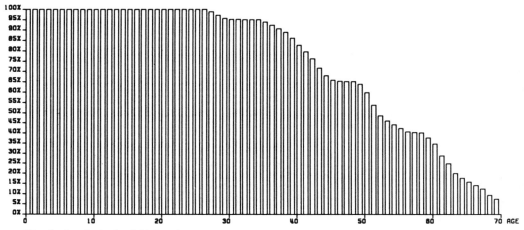

Fig. 7. Survival of suicidal patients as a function of age: schizoaffective subgroup (*n* = 20)

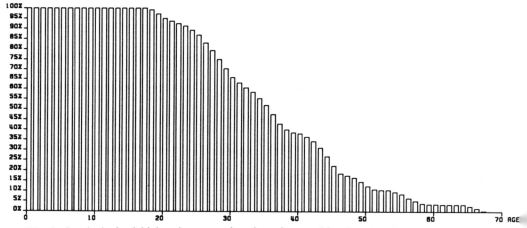

Fig. 8. Survival of suicidal patients as a function of age: schizophrenic subgroup (*n* = 29)

   With regard to the *age of onset*, our study revealed several interesting findings. Even though unipolar, bipolar, schizoaffective, and schizophrenic patients who died of other, nonsuicidal causes differ considerably in the age of onset distribution (depending on diagnosis), almost no such differences showed up in the suicides. Their age of onset distribution seems to be independent of diagnosis (Figs. 11 and 12), suggesting that suicides form a specific subgroup or psychiatric entity.

Discussion of Results

The results of this study are based on data from three groups of investigators with similar, but not identical diagnostic concepts. They are based on patients

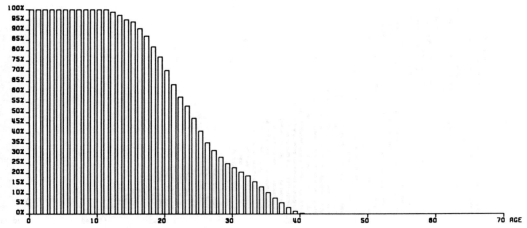

Fig. 9. Survival of suicidal patients as a function of age: borderline subgroup ($n = 42$)

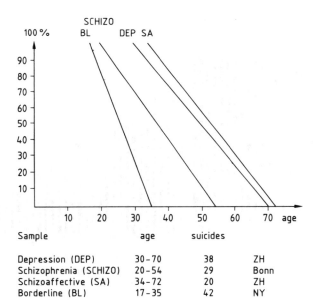

Fig. 10. Survival of suicidal patients as a function of age

Sample	age	suicides	
Depression (DEP)	30–70	38	ZH
Schizophrenia (SCHIZO)	20–54	29	Bonn
Schizoaffective (SA)	34–72	20	ZH
Borderline (BL)	17–35	42	NY

coming from three different countries, which could be an argument against unifying the material for data analysis. On the other hand, we are dealing with hard facts in dating the deaths of patients; the error in the assessment of age at onset is certainly very similar in all three sites. Differences in diagnoses between the sites do not matter to a great extent, because the schizophrenics were recruited in Bonn, the borderlines in New York, the affectives in Zurich, and only the group of schizoaffectives comes from Zurich and Bonn. The results therefore reflect reliable mortality data, collected from official registers of four different diagnostic classes of patients.

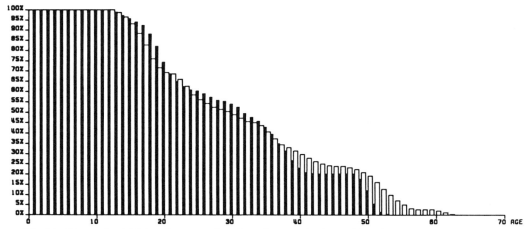

Fig. 11. Onset of suicidal patients as a function of age: unipolar and bipolar subgroup (*n* = 38) versus schizoaffective subgroup (*n* = 20). *Light bars* represent affectives, *dark bars* represent schizoaffectives

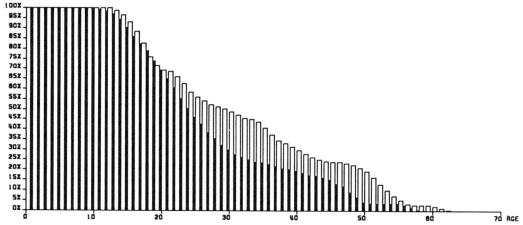

Fig. 12. Onset of suicidal patients as a function of age: unipolar and bipolar subgroup (*n* = 38) versus schizophrenic subgroup (*n* = 30). *Light bars* represent affectives, *dark bars* represent schizophrenics

Previous analyses of the data from Zurich (Angst and Stassen 1987) are confirmed. In this paper, age at onset, course, and outcome of affective and schizoaffective patients from Zurich were compared. The schizoaffective group is clearly a more severely ill group with an earlier age at onset, a longer course of illness, and a poorer outcome. Splitting patients who committed suicide from those who died for other reasons results in the disappearance of the differences within the two suicide groups. Whereas affective and schizoaffective nonsuicidal deaths differ in course from each other, this is not true for subjects who committed suicide. They do not differ to a significant extent in characteristics of their course except in terms of a poorer outcome, again for the schizoaffective group. It is remarkable that the two groups are otherwise very similar. This finding raised the hypothesis that the subgroup of those who committed suicide may be a very special one and may have common features across diagnostic classes. This hypothesis could be tested by studying the four diagnostic groups coming from the three centers. Applying survival analysis, several main findings stand out. First of all, uni- and bipolar affective disorders do not differ in their survival course. This material comes exclusively from Zurich and was therefore unified for further analysis into one group. As a function of age at death, subjects who committed suicide showed – independent of the diagnosis – linear risk functions. This is true for patients with affective or schizoaffective disorders, for schizophrenics, and for borderlines. In contrast to this major finding, survival curves of those with nonsuicidal deaths follow the typical arctan characteristic that is always found in analyses of the normal population. The linear distribution of suicides means that the risk of suicide for the whole group of patients is constant over a lifetime and does not decrease or increase with age. This finding does not confirm the results of Tsuang and Woolson (1978), who reported that the risk of suicide was highest in depressed men during the first 10 years of illness. The constant risk of suicide is remarkable in our study, because it is independent of sex and diagnosis. The four diagnostically different groups of subjects who committed suicide differ only in age at onset of the disorders and in their suicide risk. Men and women differ only in earliest age at suicide. In this respect, men, as a group, start about 15 years earlier than women to commit suicide. The risk for men is already present at age 20, whereas for women it begins at about age 35. However, after the onset, the risk remains constant for both sexes.

The constant group risk for committing suicide is remarkable from a clinical point of view. It means that patients never escape from their risk. In an individual case, of course, this risk may vary to a great extent and be completely dependent on the presence or absence of episodes and symptoms. In cases of recurrence, the risk of suicide comes up again and again to a great extent.

The remarkable finding that suicide groups show a linear risk function independent of diagnosis suggests that an additional factor across all diagnoses plays a major role in subjects who commit suicide. This factor must be independent of the diagnosis. About its nature we can only speculate. It could be a common biological feature, such as a brain deficit in certain transmitter systems, for instance, in the serotonin system. On the clinical level, it could be linked with certain personality features. Angst and Clayton (1986) compared personality measures of patients who later committed suicide with those of controls and found a clearly elevated aggression score in the former group. Aggression, or closely related other personality features such as impulsiveness, may be a basic predisposition of subjects who later commit suicide. This hypothesis can be tested by analyzing premorbid personality measures of different diagnostic groups and studying their outcome until death. Unfortunately, such studies have not yet been done.

For prevention and treatment, our results have some implications. On the one hand, it should be kept in mind that the suicide risk does not decrease with age and length of illness, and that, therefore, all possible measures should be taken to suppress symptoms or to prevent relapses or future episodes. A second consequence is that we should look more carefully for common features of all subjects who commit suicide and study their personality in more detail. The reports of positive results in suppressing suicide attempts by long-term medication are encouraging. These studies should be continued because, at the moment, this seems to be the only promising way to reduce suicide risk substantially in view of the correlation between suicide attempts and suicide.

References

Angst J, Clayton PJ (1986) Premorbid personality of depressive, bipolar, and schizophrenic patients with special reference to suicidal issues. Compr Psychiatry 27:511–532

Angst J, Stassen HH (1987) Verlaufsaspekte affektiver Psychosen: Suizide, Rückfallrisiko im Alter. In: Huber G (ed) Fortschritte in der Psychosenforschung? 7."Weissenauer" Schizophrenie-Symposion, Bonn 1986. Schattauer, Stuttgart, pp 145–164

Angst J, Frey R, Lohmeyer B, Zerbin-Rüdin E (1980) Bipolar manic-depressive psychoses: results of a genetic investigation. Hum Genet 55:237–254

Barraclough B, Bunch J, Nelson B, et al. (1974) A hundred cases of suicide: clinical aspects. Br J Psychiatry 125:355–373

Causemann B, Müller-Oerlinghausen B (1988) Does lithium prevent suicides or suicide attempts? In: Birch NJ (ed) Lithium: inorganic pharmacology and psychiatric use. IRL, Oxford

Cox DR (1972) Regression models and life tables. J R Stat Soc 34B:187–220

Endicott J, Spitzer RL, Fleiss, JL, Cohen J (1976) The Global Assessment Scale. A procedure for measuring overall severity of psychiatric disturbance. Arch Gen Psychiatry 33: 766–771

Ernst K, Moser U, Ernst C (1980) Zunehmende Suizide psychiatrischer Klinikpatienten: Realität oder Artefakt? Arch Psychiatr Nervenkr 228:351–363

Fahrenberg J, Selg H (1970) Das Freiburger Persönlichkeits Inventar (FPI), Handanweisung für die Durchführung und Auswertung. Hogrefe, Göttingen

Guze SB, Robins E (1970) Suicide and primary affective disorders. Br J Psychiatry 117: 437–438

Hagnell O, Lanke J, Rorsman B (1982) Suicide and depression in the male part of the Lundby study. Changes over time during a 25-year observation period. Neuropsychobiology 8:182–187

Hanus H, Zapletalek M (1984) Suicidal behavior during lithium prophylaxis in patients with affective disorders (in Czech). Czech Psychiatr 80:97–100

Huber G, Gross G, Schüttler R (1979) Schizophrenie. Verlaufs- und sozialpsychiatrische Langzeituntersuchungen an den 1945–1959 in Bonn hospitalisierten schizophrenen Kranken. Springer, Berlin Heidelberg New York

Kaplan EL, Meier P (1958) Nonparametric estimation from incomplete observations. J Am Stat Assoc 53:457–481

Montgomery SA, Montgomery D, McAuley R et al.(1979) Maintenance therapy in repeat suicidal behavior: a placebo-controlled trial. In: Proc. 10th International Congress for Suicide Prevention and Crisis Intervention, Ottawa, pp 227–229

Montgomery SA, Roy D, McAuley R, et al. (1983) The prevention of recurrent suicidal acts. Br J Clin Pharmacol 15:183S–188S

Montgomery SA, Green M, Baldwin D, Montgomery D (1988) Placebo-controlled studies of brief mood disturbances. Meeting of the British Association for Psychopharmacology, Galway, 15–17 Sept 1988

Pilcz A (1901) Die periodischen Geistesstörungen. Eine klinische Studie. Fischer, Jena

Poole AJ, James HD, Hughes WC (1978) Treatment experiences in the Lithium Clinic at St. Thomas' Hospital. J R Soc Med 71:890–894

Rich CL, Young D, Fowler RC (1986) San Diego Study. I. Young vs old subjects. Arch Gen Psychiatry 43:577–582

Robins E, Gassner S, Kayes J, et al. (1959) The communication of suicidal attempt: a study of 135 consecutive cases of successful (completed) suicide. Am J Psychiatry 115:724–733

Rosner H (1988) Reaktive Depression. Statistische Untersuchungen mit besonderer Berücksichtigung der katamnestisch Suizidierten. Med. Dissertation, University of Zurich

Stone MH, Hurt SW, Stone DK (1987) The PI 500: long-term follow-up of borderline inpatients meeting DSM-III criteria. J Pers Dis 1:291–298

Tsuang MT, Woolson RF (1978) Excess mortality in schizophrenia and affective disorders. Do suicides and accidental deaths solely account for this excess? Arch Gen Psychiatry 35:1181–1185

Turnbull BW (1976) The empirical distribution function with arbitrarily grouped, censored, and truncated data. J R Stat Soc 38B:290–295

Wertham FI (1929a) A group of benign chronic psychoses: prolonged manic excitements. With a statistical study of age, duration and frequency in 2000 manic attacks. Am J Psychiatry 9:17–78

Wertham FI (1929b) Die klinische Kerngruppe der chronischen Manie. Z Gesamte Neurol Psychiatr 121:770–779

Ziehen T (1896) Die Erkennung und Behandlung der Melancholie in der Praxis. Marhold, Halle

Schizoaffective Disorders: Interrelationships Between Familial Psychopathology, Neuroendocrine Assessments, and Outcome

W. Coryell[1]

Introduction

Among competing hypotheses concerning the nature of schizoaffective disorder, perhaps the most broadly supported holds that most individuals with schizoaffective disorders have in fact either schizophrenia or an affective disorder (Brockington and Meltzer 1983). According to this view, the diagnosis of schizoaffective disorder is equivalent to "undiagnosed" with a limited differential. Patients grouped under this label are therefore diagnostically heterogeneous; some have affective disorder, some have schizophrenia, and some may have other, as yet unspecified disorders.

Among the approaches used to dissect presumably heterogeneous groups, family and outcome studies are the most prominent. Indeed, these methods have yielded surprisingly consistent patterns across studies, despite wide differences in methodology and in the boundaries used to define schizoaffective disorder. Probands with this label have consistently higher familial loadings for affective disorder than do probands with schizophrenia (Coryell 1988), and with similar consistency, schizoaffective probands have higher familial loadings for schizophrenia than do probands with affective disorder. Together with the fact that outcome for schizoaffective disorder is regularly worse than that for affective disorder but better than that for schizophrenia (Coryell 1988), these patterns speak strongly both for the heterogeneity hypothesis and for the validity of these approaches to its study.

More recently, neuroendocrine assessments have joined follow-up and family studies as a frequently used approach to heterogeneity. Because a blunted TSH response to TRH and an abnormal cortisol escape from dexamethasone suppression were at one point both widely alleged to be specific to primary or endogenous depression, these two tests have appeared in many studies concerned with affective disorders masquerading as other illnesses.

Despite the widespread use of all these approaches, very few studies have quantified relationships between them. Such relationships are of interest, particularly in regard to the study of schizoaffective disorder. If all three measures – patterns of familial psychopathology, outcome, and neuroendocrine assessments – can usefully separate schizophrenia from affective disorder, then they should

---

[1] University of Iowa College of Medicine, Department of Psychiatry, Psychiatric Hospital, 500 Newton Road, Iowa City, IA 52242, USA

Affective and Schizoaffective Disorders
Edited by A. Marneros and M.T. Tsuang
© Springer-Verlag Berlin Heidelberg 1990

correlate within a group containing a mixture of those disorders, provided the component disorders are sufficiently represented. Moreover, two congruent test results should correspond more strongly to a third test result than either alone. Such combinations could then be used to more definitively separate schizo-affective patients who have an affective disorder from those who have other illnesses.

The data described below are particularly suited to these issues. First, all patients had schizoaffective disorder according to the Research Diagnostic Criteria (RDC; Spitzer et al. 1978), among the most inclusive and therefore heterogeneous definitions of schizoaffective disorder in wide use. Second, these patients underwent a prospective, semi-annual follow-up to 1 year and partici-pated in a family in which all willing first-degree relatives were interviewed by raters blind to proband diagnosis and to outcome. Finally, they underwent testing with both the dexamethasone suppression test (DST) and the thyroid releasing hormone-stimulation test (TRH-ST).

Methods

Subjects

Subject selection and assessment are described in detail elsewhere (Coryell and Zimmerman 1986; 1988). Consecutively admitted patients with nonorganic, nonmanic psychoses were invited to participate if they were not transients, knew their biological parents, and fulfilled medical and pharmacological conditions for valid DST and TRH-ST procedures. This last requirement was suspended during the intake of the final 30 patients; consequently, some patients (mostly those taking lithium) underwent a DST but not a TRH-ST.

These inclusion criteria produced a sample made up almost entirely of patients with RDC major depression, psychotic type; schizoaffective disorder, depressed type; or schizophrenia. Only those with schizoaffective disorder, depressed type are considered here. These patients were generally young (Table 1), had a slight female predominance,and were mostly unmarried and severely ill according to global measures. One third were bipolar, two fifths had the RDC subtype of chronic schizoaffective disorder, and nearly one half were "mainly schizophrenic."

Procedures

Within 1 week of admission, the author used an unstructured interview to diag-nose each patient. Another rater independently interviewed each subject using the full Schedule for Affective Disorders and Schizophrenia (SADS) and like-wise reached a diagnosis. The two raters then met and derived a consensus diagnosis. This diagnosis was used to define the group described here.

One year later, each diagnosis was reviewed by a senior diagnostician who was blind to neuroendocrine and family study results but not to 1-year outcome data. Some patients with an intake diagnosis of major depression or schizo-

Table 1. Baseline characteristics of 42 patients with RDC schizoaffective disorder, depressed type

Age, mean (SD)	34.6	(10.7)
No. (%) female	25	(59.5)
Marital status		
No. (%) single	19	(45.2)
No. (%) married	11	(26.2)
No. (%) separated/divorced	12	(28.6)
Episode duration at intake, weeks mean (SD)	272.4	(313.0)
GAS score at intake, mean (SD)	28.6	(6.0)
No. (%) bipolar (any history of mania or schizoaffective mania)	14	(33.3)
Schizoaffective subtypes		
No. (%) nonchronic	24	(57.1)
No. (%) chronic	18	(42.9)
No. (%) mainly affective	18	(42.9)
No. (%) mainly schizophrenic	20	(47.6)
No. (%) other	4	(9.5)

phrenia were rediagnosed at 1 year as having a schizoaffective disorder, but no patient considered schizoaffective at intake was given a different diagnosis at follow-up (Coryell et al. 1988).

Two patients did not know their biological parents and another three refused to allow the direct interview of their relatives. These three patients themselves provided a family history interview, however. The remaining 37 probands entered the family study and all living first-degree relatives over 17 years were contacted. Raters blind to proband diagnosis then administered a Diagnostic Interview Schedule (DIS) (Robins et al. 1981) for axis I diagnoses as well as a Structured Interview for DSM-III Personality Disorders (SIDP) (Pfohl et al. 1982).

Each patient also underwent a DST within 1 week of admission. Patients took 1 mg dexamethasone at 11 p.m., orally and in tablet form; post-dexamethasone samples were then drawn at 8 a.m., 4 p.m., and 11 p.m. and were assessed using RIA techniques.

Recommended post-dexamethasone thresholds for nonsuppression have most often varied between 4 µg/dl and 6 µg/dl, inclusive. Because of this lack of consensus, we (Coryell and Zimmerman 1989) and others at this center (Winokur et al. 1987) have designated an ambiguous range rather than a single, discrete cut-off value. Patients with post-dexamethasone values less of than 4 are here considered definite suppressors, while those with values over 6 are definite nonsuppressors.

The TRH-ST also took place within a week of admisson, 48 h or more before or after the DST. After an overnight fast, patients received 500 µg of TRH intravenously over a 1-min period, and samples for TSH were drawn through an indwelling catheter at -15, 0, 15, 30, 60, 90, and 120 min. As with post-dexamethasone cortisol values, Δ-maximum TSH values were assigned to one of three ranges. Since most previous studies have used either 5 or 7 μU/ml as the upper limit of a blunted or abnormal response, we identified this range as ambiguous. Those values below 4 μU/ml thus indicate definitely blunted responses.

Mark Zimmerman conducted follow-up interviews 6 months and 1 year later using an instrument patterned after the longitudinal interval follow-up evaluation (LIFE; Keller et al. 1987). The number and intensity of schizoaffective symptoms were rated on a weekly basis by identifying change points and by then characterizing the intervening time periods. LIFE conventions designated as recovered patients who had had 8 or more weeks with no more than one or two criteria symptoms to no more than a mild degree. In the present study we also determined recovery from psychosis – 8 or more weeks free of delusions or hallucinations and insight into those psychotic features demonstrable at follow-up. Finally, Global Assessment Scale (GAS) scores (Endicott et al. 1976) were used to quantify overall severity at intake and at the 1-year follow-up. This 100-point scale reflected both symptom intensity and social functioning. Lower scores indicated greater overall severity.

Results

Neuroendocrine Results and Outcome

Definite nonsuppressors were twice as likely to recover from their psychosis as were definite suppressors (Table 2), while patients with an intermediate post-dexamethasone cortisol value had an intermediate likelihood of recovery. Other definitions of recovery yielded similar patterns, and the GAS score at 1 year correlated negatively and significantly with the post-dexamethasone cortisol at intake ($n = 42$, $r = 0.35$, $P = 0.02$).

Table 2. Baseline DST results and 1-year outcome in RDC schizoaffective depression

	Baseline maximum Post-dexamethasone cortisol, μg/dl		
	<4	4–6	>6
Number (row %)	20 (47.6)	10 (23.8)	12 (28.6)
No. (%) recovered from psychotic features[a]	6 (30.0)	5 (50.0)	8 (66.7)
No. (%) recovered from episode	8 (40.0)	6 (60.0)	8 (66.7)
No. (%) recovered to "normal self"	11 (55.0)	7 (70.0)	10 (83.3)
GAS score, mean (SD)	49.5 (16.5)	58.8 (22.3)	61.6 (18.9)
Mean (SD) no. of weeks with full depressive syndrome[b]	17.0 (17.3)	7.1 (12.7)	7.0 (9.3)
Mean (SD) no. of weeks psychotic	27.5 (21.8)	22.6 (23.0)	14.2 (16.1)

[a] <4 μg/dl or >6 μg/dl, $\chi^2 = 4.1$, df = 1, $P = 0.04$.
[b] <4 μg/dl vs >6 μg/dl, $t = 2.1$, df = 29.8, $P = 0.04$.

Table 3. TRH-ST results and 1-year outcome in RDC schizoaffective disorder

	Baseline Δ-maximum TSH (μU/ml)		
	<5	5–7	>7
Number (row %)	6 (18.8)	7 (21.9)	19 (59.4)
No. (%) recovered from psychotic features	4 (66.7)	4 (57.1)	5 (26.3)
No. (%) recovered from episode	4 (66.7)	5 (71.4)	6 (31.6)
No. (%) recovered to "normal self"	4 (66.7)	3 (42.9)	12 (63.2)
GAS score, mean (SD)	63.2 (16.8)	57.7 (19.7)	47.7 (16.7)
Mean (SD) no. of weeks with full depressive syndrome	5.8 (10.9)	13.7 (14.9)	14.3 (17.2)
Mean (SD) no. of weeks psychotic	17.2 (18.1)	19.4 (21.0)	28.7 (23.0)

The results of the TRH-ST also yielded expected patterns in recovery rates (Table 3) – patients with definitely blunted responses were twice as likely to recover from their psychosis as were patients who had definitely nonblunted responses; the remaining patients again had an intermediate likelihood of recovery. However, Δ-maximum TSH values did not correlate significantly with 1-year GAS scores ($n = 32$, $r = -0.12$, $P = 0.51$).

Combinations of DST and TRH-ST results were not more strongly related to outcome. Of those 21 subjects with definite results from both tests, most (14, or 66.7%) exhibited both definite dexamethasone suppression and a definite normal response to TRH-ST; four (28.6%) of these patients recovered from psychosis. Only three had definite abnormal responses to both tests, and two (66.7%) of these patients recovered.

Family History and Outcome

Contrary to expectations, patients with family histories of affective disorder were generally (though not significantly) overrepresented among patients who failed to recover (Table 4). Patients with family histories positive for schizophrenia spectrum disorders were likewise overrepresented, however. Accordingly, the relatives of patients who recovered had somewhat lower morbid risks for affective disorder and for schizophrenia spectrum disorders than did patients who failed to recover, though none of these comparisons reached statistical significance.

Neuroendocrine Results and Family History

Suppressor status showed no perceptible relationship to familial loading for affective disorder (Table 5), but only probands with post-dexamethasone cortisol values less than 4 μg/dl had relatives with schizophrenia. Morbid risk figures for schizophrenia spectrum disorder did not vary by proband suppressor status, however. Patients with definitely blunted TRH responses had somewhat

Table 4. Familial psychopathology and recovery from psychotic features

	Status at 1 year			
	Recovered		Not recovered	
Number (row %)	19	(47.5)	21	(52.5)
Number (%) of probands FS/FH positive for				
– any major depression	9	(47.4)	13	(61.9)
– any mania	3	(15.8)	4	(19.0)
– either mania or major depression	9	(47.4)	13	(61.9)
– any schizophrenia	1	(5.3)	2	(9.5)
– any schizophrenia spectrum disorder	4	(21.1)	5	(23.8)
– any schizophrenia spectrum disorder and no major depression	1	(5.3)	0	
– any mania or major depression and no schizophrenia spectrum disorder	6	(31.6)	8	(38.1)
Number of relatives evaluated	141		123	
Age-corrected number of relatives at risk for				
– major depression	110.3		97.4	
– mania	115.4		102.2	
– schizophrenia spectrum disorder	126.9		112.6	
– schizophrenia	126.4		112.1	
Number of affected relatives (morbid risk)				
– major depression	18	(16.3)	21	(21.6)
– mania	3	(2.6)	5	(4.9)
– schizophrenia spectrum disorder	4	(3.2)	8	(7.1)
– schizophrenia	1	(0.8)	3	(2.7)

lower familial loadings for major depression and schizophrenia spectrum disorders, but the intermediate group did not have intermediate morbid risks.

Discussion

Among these three measures – family history, neuroendocrine, and outcome – several of the expected interactions emerged and several did not. Schizoaffective patients with neuroendocrine responses indicative of endogenous or psychotic depression were more likely to recover than were other schizoaffective patients. However, patients who recovered had neither higher morbid risks for affective disorder nor a lower morbid risk for schizophrenia spectrum disorders. Neither were patients with abnormal neuroendocrine results distinguished by higher familial loadings for affective disorder, though morbid risk figures for schizophrenia did assume the expected pattern.

Contrary to expectations based on presumed heterogeneity of schizoaffective disorder, probands who failed to recover from psychosis actually had a somewhat greater familial loading for affective disorder. Heavy familial loading for affective disorder has elsewhere been associated with chronicity among primary depressives (Akiskal 1982). This effect may well have overwhelmed the

Table 5. Neuroendocrine test results and familial psychopathology

	Baseline maximum post-dexamethasone cortisol (μg/dl)			Baseline Δ-maximum TSH (μU/ml)		
	<4	4–6	>6	<5	5–7	>7
Number (row%)	20.0 (50.0)	9.0 (22.5)	11.0 (27.5)	6.0 (19.4)	7.0 (22.6)	18.0 (58.1)
Number (%) of probands FS/FH positive for						
– any major depression	11.0 (55.0)	4.0 (44.4)	7.0 (63.6)	3.0 (50.0)	4.0 (57.1)	9.0 (50.0)
– any mania	3.0 (15.0)	2.0 (22.2)	2.0 (18.2)	0	1.0 (14.3)	2.0 (11.1)
– either mania or major depression	11.0 (55.0)	4.0 (44.4)	7.0 (63.6)	3.0 (50.0)	4.0 (57.1)	9.0 (50.0)
– schizophrenia	3.0 (15.0)	0	0	1.0 (16.7)	0	2.0 (11.1)
– any schizophrenia spectrum disorder	4.0 (20.0)	2.0 (22.2)	3.0 (27.3)	2.0 (33.3)	1.0 (14.3)	4.0 (22.2)
– any schizophrenia spectrum disorder and no major depression	1.0 (5.0)	0	0	1.0 (16.7)	0	0
– any mania or major depression and no schizophrenia spectrum	8.0 (40.0)	2.0 (22.2)	4.0 (36.4)	2.0 (33.3)	3.0 (42.9)	5.0 (27.8)
Number of relatives evaluated	115	65	84	53	44	95
Age-corrected number of relatives at risk for						
– major depression	91.1	51.3	65.3	43.2	32.4	76.1
– mania	95.7	53.9	68.0	45.1	33.4	80.0
– schizophrenia spectrum disorder	105.0	58.8	75.6	49.0	37.8	87.6
– schizophrenia	105.0	58.7	74.9	48.8	37.7	87.3
Number of affected relatives (morbid risk)						
– major depression	18.0 (19.8)	8.0 (15.6)	13.0 (19.9)	4.0 (9.3)	9.0 (27.8)	13.0 (17.1)
– mania	4.0 (4.2)	2.0 (3.7)	2.0 (2.9)	0	1.0 (3.0)	3.0 (3.8)
– schizophrenia spectrum disorder	6.0 (5.7)	2.0 (3.4)	4.0 (5.3)	2.0 (4.1)	1.0 (2.6)	7.0 (8.0)
– schizophrenia[a]	4.0 (3.8)	2.0 (3.4)	0	1.0 (2.0)	0	3.0 (3.4)

[a] <4 μg/dl vs >6 μg/dl, $z = 1.71$, $P < 0.05$ (1-tailed).

contravening effects arising from the admixture of actual schizophrenics among schizoaffective probands, the lower morbid risk for affective disorder among schizophrenic patients (Coryell and Zimmerman 1988), and the greater likelihood of recovery among true affective disorder patients.

We must also question whether the relationship between neuroendocrine test results and outcome necessarily support the heterogeneity hypothesis. The fact that DST nonsuppression similarly predicted recovery among patients with DSM-III major depression with mood-congruent psychotic features (Coryell and Zimmerman 1989) is relevant here. In that comparatively homogeneous group, patients with post-dexamethasone cortisol values greater than 6 were almost three times as likely to recover as those with post-dexamethasone cortisol values less than 4 (11 of 12, or 91.7%, vs 3 of 9, or 33.3%; Fisher's exact test, $P = 0.009$). It appears, then, that the presumed specificity of DST nonsuppression to affective disorder cannot account entirely for a relationship between nonsuppression and recovery seen here. Rather, as suggested earlier (Coryell and Zimmerman 1989), DST nonsuppression may connote a relatively unstable phase of psychotic major depression – one in which chronicity has not become established and recovery is more likely.

DST diagnostic specificity may account in part for these findings, nevertheless. A family history of schizophrenia was seen predominantly among DST suppressors. Moreover, among 18 patients given an RDC diagnosis of schizophrenia at baseline and reevaluated at 1 year, five were given a new diagnosis of schizoaffective disorder (Coryell et al. 1988); four of these five had been nonsuppressors at baseline compared with only one of the remaining 13 diagnostically stable schizophrenic patients ($P = 0.008$, Fisher's exact test).

In summary, neuroendocrine test results and outcome interacted in predicted ways among patients with schizoaffective depression, though these interactions may exist for other than the hypothesized reasons. Family history correlated with these other two factors in only a very limited way.

Targum (1983) found similar relationships between abnormal DST or TRH-ST results and outcome among DSM-III schizophreniform patients, and Langer et al. (1986) found a better response to antipsychotics among patients with schizophrenia or schizoaffective disorder and blunted TRH-ST results. Otherwise, the findings described here have little support in the literature, simply because such comparisons have not been made. Instead, studies of schizoaffective disorder are still largely limited to comparisons with reference groups using one of the three factors discussed here. Such studies are now sufficiently numerous; the results strongly suggest a move to the next phase, an exploration of heterogeneity within schizoaffective disorder.

References

Akiskal HS (1982) Factors associated with incomplete recovery in primary depressive illness. J Clin Psychiatry 43:266–271

Brockington IF, Meltzer HY (1983) The nosology of schizoaffective psychoses. Psychaitr Dev 4:317–338

Coryell W (1988) Nosology: schizoaffective and schizophreniform disorders. In: Tsuang MT,
    Simpson JC (Ed) Nosology, epidemiology and genetics. Elsevier, Amsterdam, pp 27–39
    handbook of schizophrenia, vol 2.
Coryell W, Zimmerman M (1986) Demographic, historical and symptomatic features of the
    nonmanic psychoses. J Nerv Ment Dis 174:585–592
Coryell W, Zimmerman M (1988) The heritability of schizophrenia and schizoaffective dis-
    order: a family study. Arch Gen Psychiatry 45:323–327
Coryell W, Zimmerman M (1989) Hypothalamic-pituitary-adrenal axis hyperactivity and
    recovery from functional psychoses. Am J Psychiatry 146:473–477
Coryell W, Zimmerman M, Winokur G, Cadoret R (1988) Baseline neuroendocrine function
    and diagnostic stability among patients with a nonmanic psychosis. Eur Arch Psychiatry
    Neurol Sci 237:197–199
Endicott J, Spitzer RJ, Fleiss JL, Cohen J (1976) The Global Assessment Scale: a procedure
    for measuring overall severity of psychiatric disturbance. Arch Gen Psychiatry 33:
    766–771
Keller MB, Lavori PW, Friedman B, Neilsen E, Endicott J, McDonald-Scott P, Andreasen
    NC (1987) The Longitudinal Interval Follow-up Evaluation. Arch Gen Psychiatry 44:
    540–548
Langer G, Koinig G, Hatzinger R, Schonbeck G, Resch F, Aschauer H, Keschaven MS,
    Sieghart W (1986) Response of thyrotropin to thyrotropin-releasing hormone as predictor
    of treatment outcome. Arch Gen Psychiatry 43:861–868
Pfohl B, Stangl D, Zimmerman M (1982) The structured interview for personality disorders
    (SIDP). Department of Psychiatry, University of Iowa, Iowa City
Robins LN, Helzer JE, Croughan J, Ratcliff KS (1981) National institute of mental health
    diagnostic interview schedule. Arch Gen Psychiatry 38:381–389
Spitzer RL, Endicott J, Robins E (1978) Research diagnostic criteria, 3rd edn. Biometrics
    Research, New York State Department of Mental Hygiene, New York
Targum SD (1983) Neuroendocrine dysfunction in schizophreniform disorder: correlation with
    six-month clinical outcome. Am J Psychiatry 140:309–313
Winokur G, Black DW, Nasrallah A (1987) DST nonsuppressor status: relationship to specific
    aspects of the depressive syndrome. Biol Psychiatry 22:360–368

Genetic Relationship Between the Psychoses – Implications for Genetic Modeling

P. PROPPING[1]

In contrast to psychiatry, genetics has a powerful theory to offer which can explain various phenomena of the biological basis of many diseases. Genetics uses information from different fields (epidemiology; onto- and phylogeny; formal, biochemical, and molecular genetics; population genetics) and can integrate this information into a general theory of disease etiology and pathogenesis (Vogel 1982). Genetics is becoming the general theory of medicine.

The problem with psychiatry is that we do not know the best parameters to apply to genetic models. Many studies have shown that genetic factors are involved in the development of most psychiatric diseases. It is sometimes forgotten, however, that it is not the psychiatric symptomatology, but the neurophysiological substrate – the brain – the development and differentiation of which is influenced by genetic factors. Psychiatric symptoms and syndromes (sometimes conceptualized to "diagnoses") are certainly only epiphenomena which at best in a very indirect way reflect the structure and function of the neurophysiological substrate. It is therefore of heuristic value to apply the general experiences of medical genetics to psychiatry.

Lessons from Medical Genetics

The great progress that has been made in medical genetics – gene mapping, molecular understanding of gene defects, diagnosis, pathogenesis, and therapy of inherited diseases – refers mainly to monogenic disorders. A simple mode of inheritance points to a specific abnormality at the gene level and thus to a specific biochemical defect. The great majority of monogenic disorders are rare.

In contrast, disorders that are common in the general population usually have a complex etiology, with respect both to genetics and to exogenous influences. Several general rules can be formulated that emerge from the genetic analysis of common disorders such as atherosclerosis, convulsive disorders, and mental retardation (see Propping 1989):

1. The clinical phenotype may be variable; clinical "types" do not correspond to etiological entities.
2. The morbidity risk in relatives cannot be theoretically explained. Empirical risk figures in first-degree relatives are usually on the order of magnitude of 5% – 15%.

---

[1] Institut für Humangenetik, Universität Bonn, Wilhelmstraße 31, D-5300 Bonn 1, FRG

Affective and Schizoaffective Disorders
Edited by A. Marneros and M.T. Tsuang
© Springer-Verlag Berlin Heidelberg 1990

3. Twin concordance rates lie at around 50% in MZ and at around 10% in DZ pairs.
4. The clinical phenotype may be the result of a variety of etiological factors, including genetic and exogenous ones, that lead to a final common pathway.
5. The relationship between genotype and phenotype may be easier to understand when parameters from the final common pathway are used instead of the usual clinical phenotype.

Thus, in psychiatry a clinician's diagnosis cannot be expected to represent a phenotype suitable to be related to a genotype.

Empirical Findings in Schizoaffective Psychoses

Since Kraepelin dichotomized the major psychoses into the two main forms schizophrenia and affective disorder, most studies in psychiatric genetics have been based on this concept. Kraepelin's dichotomy was supported essentially by genetic studies: Among the afflicted relatives of either schizophrenic or affective index patients there is certain tendency for homotypic clinical syndromes.

A certain proportion of familial secondary cases, however, do not present the same symptomatology as the index cases. Instead, some secondary cases appear to show psychoses of the opposite type (Crow 1986). This fact is convincingly demonstrated by a study of Angst and Scharfetter (1985). Having collected schizophrenic, affective, and schizoaffective index cases, the authors determined the morbidity risk for schizophrenia and affective psychoses in the first-degree relatives. Then they calculated the ratio of the morbidity risk for the two types of psychoses in the relatives (Fig. 1). A clear gradient emerged. Thus, there is obviously a genetic relationship between "neighboring" types of psychoses.

Diagnosis in probands	UP	BP	A–SA	S–SA	S
No. of probands	58	31	34	35	105
No. of first-degree relatives	405	219	236	172	574

| Ratio $\dfrac{\text{schizophrenia}}{\text{affective psychoses}}$ in first-degree relatives | 0.30 | 0.47 | 0.92 | 2.99 | 5.05 |

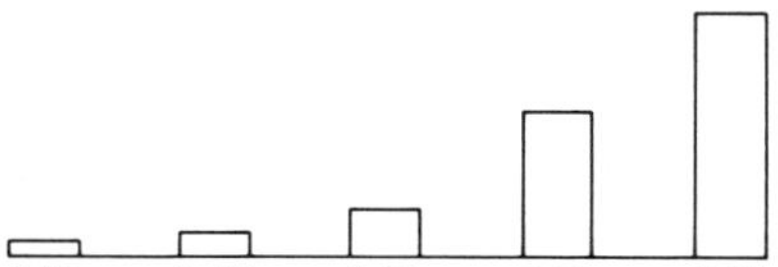

Fig. 1. Ratio of morbidity risk for schizophrenia and affective psychosis in first-degree relatives of index patients with the various types of psychoses. (From data of Angst and Scharfetter 1985)

Table 1. Morbidity risk for the various psychoses among first-degree relatives of index patients with schizoaffective psychoses in different studies

	Diagnostic criteria	Number of probands	Morbidity risk (%) for first-degree relatives			
			Schizo-affective psychoses	Schizo-phrenia	Affective psychoses	
					Unipolar	Bipolar
Tsuang et al. (1977)	DSM-III	53		0.9	11.8	
Angst et al. (1979)	ICD	150	3.0	5.3	5.6	1.1
Scharfetter and Nüsperli (1980)	ICD	40	2.5	13.5	4.4	4.4
Gershon et al. (1982)	RDC	11	6.5	4.8	14.5	16.8
Kendler et al. (1986)	DSM-III	27 mainly bipolar,	9.0	3.8	7.1	3.9
		15 mainly unipolar	3.3	8.1	7.5	3.5

A number of family studies that started from index cases with schizoaffective psychoses pointed in the same direction (Table 1). First-degree relatives of schizoaffective probands show an increase not only of the same disorder but of schizophrenia and affective psychoses as well.

Even more interesting are observations in monozygotic twins. Usually, twin studies are carried out in order to compare concordance rates in monozygotic and dizygotic twins. The variation in monozygotic pairs is also important, however, (Table 2): A bipolar disorder has been observed to develop concordantly to schizophrenia. Monozygotic twins or triplets varied with respect to the type of their psychoses. These observations show that the same genetic basis may lead to different psychopathological syndromes.

Genetic Models

There exists no consistent genetic concept that can explain the empirical findings. All attempts of biometrical genetics aimed at explaining the empirical data have failed so far (McGuffin 1989). It appears at least plausible that schizophrenia is the result of a disturbance in a final common pathway for which there may be various etiologies (Propping 1983). Thus, the majority of cases are thought to be based on a multifactorial system, whereas a certain proportion of cases may be due to monogenic disorders, major gene effects, or clearly exogenous etiologies (Gottesman and Shields, 1982). The empirical findings in the different types of psychoses suggest that there is a certain overlap between genetically controlled predispositions (Fig. 2).

Such an overlap presumably exists in other groups of complex disorders such as allergy as well (Lubs 1972): Atopia may present as asthma, hay fever, or

Table 2. Findings in single twin pairs or triplets that are important for genetic concepts of the psychoses

McGuffin et al. (1982): Varying psychotic symptomatology in male MZ triplets	*Triplet 1:*	Manic and depressive episodes between 14 and 21 years; schizoaffectie episode, manic type, at 26 years
	Triplet 2:	Schizoaffective episodes, both manic and depressive type, between 15 and 20 years; chronic schizophrenia after 20th year
	Triplet 3:	Schizoaffective episodes, both manic and depressive type, between 15 and 17 years; chronic schizophrenia after 17th year
Kendler and Tsuang (1982): Concordant evolvement of schizophrenia after bipolar onset	*Twin 1:*	At age 31 depressive, 10 months later manic; 1 year later hallucinations, change of diagnosis to hebephrenia, afterwards chronic course
	Twin 2:	At age 31 depressive, later agitated depression; at age 37 change of diagnosis to schizophrenia; at age 40 hallucinations and delusions of persecution, afterwards chronic course
Dalby et al. (1986): Male MZ Pair Discordant for Type of psychosis	*Twin 1:*	At age 16, some marihuana abuse; psychotic development at age 20, afterwards typical schizophrenia
	Twin 2:	No drug abuse; during teens changing emotions up to aggressivity; no hallucinations; finally diagnosis of mania

neurodermatitis. First-degree relatives of index patients have an increased risk for atopic diseases. Within families, there is a clear tendency for homotypic symptoms, but the morbidity risk for another form of allergic disease is increased as well. These findings can most easily be explained by overlapping predisposing systems.

The hypothesis of overlapping systems in the different psychoses implies that disturbances in the same neurophysiological systems can be responsible for one or the other form of psychosis. Obviously – as hypothesized above – the psychotic symptoms are epiphenomena that only indirectly reflect dysfunctions of the responsible neurophysiological systems. This consequence is of high importance for research into the etiology of the psychoses, including molecular genetic approaches.

Finally, another argument can be brought forward that also questions the genotype-phenotype relationship in psychiatric disorders. Genetic defects of lysosomal enzymes with onset in adult life frequently present with various neuropsychiatric symptoms. Examples are the adult forms of metachromatic leukodystrophy or of GM 2 gangliosidosis. The latter is due to hexosaminidase-A deficiency. Clinically, it may appear as a muscle disease, but psychiatric symptoms may precede somatic signs. Navon et al. (1986) found hebephrenic schizophrenia in nine of 33 cases of GM 2 gangliosidosis. In about ten case reports a bipolar symptomatology was described (see Propping 1989), and Lichtenberg et al. (1988) observed a case of puerperal psychosis. It is unclear so far which factors are responsible for the varying symptomatology on the basis of

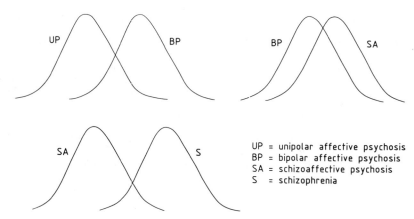

Fig. 2. Hypothesis of overlapping polygenic systems that predispose to the various forms of psychoses. The distributions are not necessarily one-dimensional

the same enzymatic defect. Possible explanations might be the topographical distribution of the central lesions, or the existence of compensating mechanisms.

At present, there is much hope that molecular genetic methods will lead to a better understanding of the psychoses. When applying these techniques, however, one should not forget to take the relationship between the psychoses into account.

References

Angst J, Scharfetter C (1985) Familial aspects of schizoaffective disorder. World Psychiatric Association, Regional Symposium Athens, October 13–17

Angst J, Felder W, Lohmeyer B (1979) Schizoaffective disorders. Results of a genetic investigation, I. J Affective Disord 1:139–153

Crow TJ (1986) The continuum of psychosis and its implication for the structure of the gene. Br J Psychiatry 149:419–429

Dalby JT, Morgan D, Lee ML (1986) Schizophrenia and mania in identical twin brothers. J Nerv Ment Dis 174:304–308

Gershon ES, Hamovit JH, Guroff JJ et al. (1982) A family study of schizoaffective, bipolar I, bipolar II, unipolar, and normal control probands. Arch Gen Psychiatry 39:1157–1167

Gottesmann II, Shields J (1982) Schizophrenia. The epigenetic puzzle. Cambridge University Press, Cambridge

Kendler KS, Tsuang MT (1982) Identical twins concordant for the progression of affective illness to schizophrenia. Br J Psychiatry 141:563–566

Kendler KS, Gruenberg AM, Tsuang MT (1986) A DSM-III family study of the nonschizophrenic psychotic disorders. Am J Psychiatry 143:1098–1105

Lichtenberg P, Navon R, Wertman E, Dasberg H, Lerer B (1988) Post-partum psychosis in adult GM gangliosidosis. Br J Psychiatry 153:387–389

Lubs M-LE (1972) Empiric risks for genetic counseling in families with allergy. J Pediatr 80:26–31

McGuffin P (1989) Models of heritability and genetic transmission. In: Häfner H, Gattaz WF (eds) Search for the causes of schizophrenia. Springer, Heidelberg Berlin New York Tokyo

McGuffin P, Reveley A, Holland A (1982) Identical triplets: non-identical psychosis? Br J Psychiatry 140:1–6

Navon R, Argov Z, Frisch A (1986) Hexosaminidase-A deficiency in adults. Am J Med Genet 24:179–196

Propping P (1983) Genetic disorders presenting as "schizophrenia". Karl Bonhoeffer's early view of the psychoses in the light of medical genetics. Hum Genet 65:1–10

Propping P (1989) Psychiatrische Genetik. Befunde und Konzepte. Springer, Berlin Heidelberg New York Tokyo

Scharfetter C, Nüsperli M (1980) The group of schizophrenias, schizoaffective psychoses, and affective disorders. Schziophr Bull 6:586–591

Tsuang MT, Dempsey GM, Dvoredsky A, Struss A (1977) A family history study of schizoaffective disorder. Biol Psychiatry 12:331–338

Vogel F (1982) Die Bedeutung der Humangenetik für eine Theorie der Krankheit. Verh Dtsch Ges Pathol 66:1–15

Morbid Risks in Relatives of Affective, Schizoaffective, and Schizophrenic Patients – Results of a Family Study

W. Maier, J. Hallmayer, J. Minges, and D. Lichtermann[1]

Introduction

Affective disorders have been the major focus of recent family studies; the results of many family studies agree as regards the increased morbid risks for family members of patients with affective disorders and the distinction between unipolar and bipolar affective disorders. However, in spite of the large number of family studies that have been done there are still some unsettled problems, such as the association of delusional unipolar depression and bipolar depression (Weissman et al. 1986), the relationship of anxiety disorders and depressive disorders in families (Leckman et al. 1983), and the modeling of the association between depression and alcoholism in families (Merikangas et al. 1985; Winokur et al. 1979). Except for these problems, the patterns of affective disorders in families are quite well understood.

In contrast to affective disorders, the situation for schizoaffective disorders and schizophrenia is less clear. Although the enhancement of the morbid risk for affective disorders in relatives of schizoaffective patients is an often replicated finding, there is no general consensus on a significant enhancement of the lifetime risk for schizoaffective and schizophrenic disorders in consecutively recruited families of patients with these disorders (Coryell and Zimmerman 1988; Kendler 1988).

Even more controversial is the problem of overlap of affective and schizophreniform psychopathology in families: some researchers report an increased morbid risk for affective disorders in relatives of schizophrenic patients (Crow 1986; Gershon et al. 1988), whereas others have not been able to replicate these findings; however, only a few family studies have addressed this issue (Gershon et al. 1988).

The classical studies and some recent family studies of schizophrenic and affective disorders are in favor of the Kraepelinean dichotomy between schizophrenic and affective disorders or of a trichotomy between affective, schizoaffective, and schizophrenic disorders (Kendler 1984); another body of data can be interpreted as an argument against the validity of a strict demarcation between different diagnostic classes and point to a unitary or continuum model for the range of affective, schizoaffective, and schizophreniform disorders (Crow

[1] Abteilung für Psychiatrie, Universität Mainz, Untere Zahlbacher Straße 8, 6500 Mainz, FRG

Affective and Schizoaffective Disorders
Edited by A. Marneros and M.T. Tsuang
© Springer-Verlag Berlin Heidelberg 1990

1986; Angst 1984). A more sophisticated model was rcently proposed by Gershon et al. (1988).

Because of the lack of controlled studies examining the families of affective, schizoaffective, and schizophrenic patients these controversial issues can hardly be settled. Therefore, we carried out a family study tapping the broad range of affective and schizophrenic probands in order to obtain more information about these controversional issues.

Methods

A blind family study was carried out involving 300 consecutive inpatients with unipolar or bipolar-II major depression (RDC), bipolar disorder (RDC), or schizoaffective or schizophrenic disorder (RDC). Selection criteria were:

1. Age 20–70
2. No history of primary alcohol or drug dependency (RDC)
3. No history of seizure
4. Consent of the patient to participate in the family study
5. At least one living first-degree relative willing to be interviewed for the family study.

The diagnostic assessments of the patients and all their living and participating first-degree relatives were based on an interview by the Schedule of Affective Disorders and Schizophrenia – life-time version (SADS-LA, 1985); all other available information (from case reports, family history, and telephone interviews with physicians treating the patients or their relatives) were combined with the SADS-LA data by the procedure of Best Estimate Diagnosis (Leckman et al. 1982). The sample of patients and relatives personally interviewed is characterized in Table 1.

Fifty healthy controls were selected by a private company; these probands were matched by age, sex, social status, and level of education to a random subsample of the inpatients included in this family study. An additional criterion of selection was that the proband had never visited a psychiatrist or a physician asking for help with psychiatric or psychological problems. The probands and their first-degree relatives were interviewed with the SADS-LA. If a proband reported a history of any psychiatric disorder according to RDC or DSM-III (including minor disorders such as minor depression or personality disorders), the proband and his or her family were excluded from the control group.

The family-history method was used for the diagnostic assessment of relatives not able or not willing to participate in the study. We are reporting here only data for relatives who were interviewed personally; data collected by the family-history method will be reported else where.

The lifetime morbid risks in the first-degree family members for different diagnostic categories of the probands were calculated by the Weinberg-Strömgren method (modification by Gershon et al. 1982). These coefficients were con-

Table 1. Description of the family study sample

Diagnosis (RDC) of probands	Controls	Unipolar major depression	Bipolar-I disorder, bipolar-II major depression	Schizo-affective disorder	Schizo-prenia
Probands					
Number	50	98	60	75	67
Mean age	41.9	47.8	39.1	46.5	33.2
Sex ratio men:women	21:29	38:60	34:26	41:34	36:31
*First-degree relatives**					
Number	142	265	159	229	185
Mean age	39.9	39.6	35.4	40.4	38.7
Sex ratio men:women	79:63	130:135	79:80	110:119	96:89

*Relatives personally interviewed by SADS-LA/SCID-II.

trolled for age and variation in the age at onset distributions. The age at onset frequency distributions is modeled by a log normal curve.

Results

The morbid risks for the disorders listed in Table 2 in families of normal controls are within the range defined by the most recent epidemiological studies (Gershon et al. 1988). Consequently, the control sample constitutes a valid comparison group.

The lifetime risk for unipolar major depression in male relatives in all groups of probands is nearly 50% lower than that in female relatives; the familial morbid risks for the other disorders listed in Table 2 are very similar for both sexes; these results are in agreement with the majority of family and epidemiological studies.

Table 2 reports that the frequency of secondary cases with unipolar major depression is enhanced for all diagnostic groups of patients (including those with schizophrenia). The frequencies for bipolar disorders are mainly enhanced in families of bipolar disorder patients. Schizoaffective disorders and schizophrenia are most frequent in families of patients with schzioaffective and schizophrenic disorders. All these familial lifetime risks mentioned are significantly different from the lifetime risks in first-degree relatives of the control probands (modified chi-square test with $P \leq 0.05$).

Table 3 reports the impact of the psychotic/nonpsychotic distinction in unipolar depression, and of the bipolar I/bipolar II distinction and the unipolar/

Table 2. Lifetime risks (in percent) in first-degree relatives of psychiatric inpatients according to probands' diagnoses – Strömgren-Weinberg morbid risks

Relative's diagnosis (RDC)	Proband diagnosis (RDC)				
	Controls	Major depression unipolar	Bipolar (I, II) disorder	Schizoaffective disorder	Schizophrenia
Male relatives					
Major depression unipolar	6%	15%	17%	17%	14%
Bipolar (I, II) disorder	1%	2%	7%	4%	1%
Schizoaffective disorder	0%	1%	2%	3%	5%
Schizophrenia	1%	2%	1%	5%	6%
Female relatives					
Major depression unipolar	11%	25%	26%	23%	23%
Bipolar (I, II) disorder	0%	2%	8%	5%	1%
Schizoaffective disorder	1%	0%	3%	5%	6%
Schizophrenia	0%	0%	2%	3%	4%

bipolar distinction on schizoaffective disorders on the familial loading. Psychotic unipolar depression is associated with an enhanced risk of bipolar-I disorders in first-degree relatives; conversely, the frequency of psychotic unipolar depression is enhanced in relatives of bipolar-I, -II, and schizoaffective probands. Psychotic unipolar depression was not breeding true in families.

Bipolar disorders in probands increase the lifetime risk for bipolar affective and bipolar schizoaffective disorders in family members. Bipolar affective disorders are most frequent among relatives of probands with this diagnosis, and bipolar schizoaffective disorders are most frequent in relatives of bipolar schizoaffective probands.

Schizoaffective (unipolar) psychosis is associated with moderately elevated familial risks for schizoaffective disorders, bipolar disorder and psychotic depression. Schizoaffective disorder also more frequent among relatives of schizoaffective unipolar probands. Schizoaffective bipolar psychosis is characterized by the maximal familial risk for schizoaffective (especially bipolar) disorders.

Discussion

A major finding is the nonspecificity of the familial risk for unipolar depression across the different diagnostic categories of the probands. There is one family

Table 3. Lifetime (in Perent) risks for major psychiatric disorders in first-degree relatives of affective/schizoaffective probands

Relatives	Probands					
	Nonpsychotic major depression – unipolar	Psychotic major depression – unipolar	Bipolar-II major depression	Bipolar-I disorder	Schizoaffective disorder – unipolar	Schizoaffective disorder – bipolar
Nonpsychotic major depression – unipolar	19.0	21.1	19.9	23.9	20.2	19.3
Psychotic	0.5	0.7	1.6	1.9	1.6	1.2
Bipolar II	1.3	0.9	3.8	4.8	1.6	3.1
Bipolar I	1.9	4.5	2.8	6.8	2.1	3.6
Schizoaffective disorder – unipolar	0.0	0.5	0.0	0.9	1.8	1.6
Schizoaffective disorder – bipolar	0.0	0.0	2.3	1.3	0.9	4.5

study (Gershon et al. 1988) reporting an enhancement of lifetime risk for unipolar major depression in relatives of schizophrenic probands; all other family studies examining this relationship are at variance with this finding (Gershon et al. 1988; Coryell and Zimmerman 1988). The Kraepelin dichotomy and all kinds of trichotomy of endogenous mental disorders are challenged by this result.

Another peculiar result is the relationship between psychotic unipolar depression and bipolar disorders. A single study in the literature (Weissman et al. 1984) reports an increased risk for bipolar (I) disorders in families of probands with psychotic unipolar depression without examining the reverse direction; the present family study reaffirms this report and simultaneously comes up with an increased risk for psychotic unipolar depression in bipolar depression.

Other findings are supported by a broad range of family studies. Schizophrenia and schizoaffective disorders can hardly be discriminated by family study data on psychotic disorders (Scharfetter and Nüsperli 1980); unipolar and bipolar depression differ as regards the risk in families; the risk for bipolar disorders is especially high in families of probands with the same disorder (Coryell et al. 1982). Psychotic unipolar depression is associated with an enhanced risk for unipolar depression in the family (Weissman et al. 1986). The findings of the present study are in contrast to the Collaborative Study on the psychobiology of Depression (Andreasen et al. 1986) with regard to the risk for schizophrenia in schizoaffective probands: we found a very similar morbid risk for schizophrenia in families of bipolar schizoaffective probands as compared with those of unipolar schizoaffective probands. However, the low absolute number of schizophrenic relatives in both family studies may induce a high degree of variance which may explain this finding.

The similarities between affective and schizoaffective disorders are (a) the risks are nearly equal for unipolar major depression in first-degree family members of patients with all diagnostic categories investigated; and (b) bipolar affective symptomatology is associated with highest risks for bipolar and psychotic disorders. The discrepancies between these two disorders are: (a) bipolar affective disorders carry a higher risk for psychotic unipolar depression than bipolar schizoaffective disorders; (b) families of probands with schizoaffective disorders have a higher risk for schizoaffective/schizophrenic disorders, and families of probands with bipolar affective disorders have a higher risk for bipolar affective disorders; (c) Generally bipolar affective disorders are generally more similar to bipolar schizoaffective disorders than to unipolar affective disorders, and unipolar affective disorders (with the exception of psychotic unipolar depression) are more similar to schizoaffective (unipolar) disorders than to bipolar affective disorders.

The risk for unipolar major depression in families is enhanced in patients samples and does not discriminate between different diagnostic groups of patients; this nonspecific finding clearly supports the continuum model and contradicts any dichotomous or trichotomous model of endogenous psychoses. On the other hand, the familial aggregation of bipolar disorders (affective and schizoaffective) is relatively specific: maximal familial rates for bipolar disorders are found among probands with bipolar disorders; the specificity of this finding is limited by an increased risk for bipolar disorders in families of probands with psychotic unipolar disorder and schizoaffective unipolar disorder. Neither a simple categorical nor a one-dimensional continuum model is able to fit these findings of nonspecificity and relative specificity. A two-dimensional spectrum concept is able to model the risk for bipolar, schizoaffective, and schizophrenic disorders. Both proposed dimensions can be discrimineted by:

Dimension 1: a bipolar spectrum related to the affective symptomatology comprising also unipolar psychotic depression and bipolar schizo-affective disorders.

Dimension 2: the schizoaffective/schizophrenic spectrum related to productive symptomatology comprising psychotic unipolar depression as well.

Unipolar depression is tapped by goth dimensions equally.

References

Andreasen NC, Rice J, Endicott J, Reich T (1987) Familial rates of affective disorders. Arch Gen Psychiatry 44:461–472

Angst J, Felder W, Lohmeyer B (1979a) Schizoaffective disorders: results of a genetic investigation, I. J Affective Disord 1:139–153

Angst J, Felder W, Lohmeyer B (1979b) Are schizoaffective psychoses heterogeneous? Results of a genetic investigation, II. J Affective Disord 1:155–165

Angst J, Scharfetter C, Stassen HH (1983) Classification of schizoaffective patients by multidimensional scaling and cluster analysis. Psychopathology 16:254–264

Baron M, Gruen R, Asnis L, Kane J (1982) Schizoaffective illness, schizophrenia and affective disorders: morbidity risk and genetic transmission. Acta Psychiatr Scand 65:253–262

Coryell W, Endicott J, Andreasen N, Keller M (1985) Bipolar I, bipolar II and nonbipolar major depression among relatives of affectively ill probands. Am J Psychiatry 142: 817–821

Crow TJ (1986) The continuum of psychosis and its implication for the structure of the gene. Br J Psychiatry 149:419–429

Gershon ES, DeLisi LE, Hamovit J, Nurnberger JI Jr, Maxwell ME, Schreiber J, Dauphinais D, Dingman CW, Groff JJ (1988) A controlled family study of chronic psychoses. Arch Gen Psychiatry 45:328–336

Rice J, Reich T, Andreasen NC, Endicott J, Van Eerdewegh M, Fishman R, Hirschfeld RMA, Klerman GL (1987) The familial transmission of bipolar illness. Arch Gen Psychiatry 4:441–447

Scharfetter C, Nüsperli M (1980) The group of schizophrenias, schizoaffective psychoses and affective disorders. Schizophr Bull 6:586–591

Weissman MM, Prusoff BA, Merikangas KR (1984) Is delusional depression related to bipolar disorder? Am J Psychiatry 141:892–893

Weissman MM, Merikangas KR, Wichramaratne P, Kidd KK, Prusoff BA, Leckman JF, Pauls DL (1986) Understanding the clinical heterogeneity of major depression using family data. Arch Gen Psychiatry 43:430–434

Dexamethasone Suppression Test in Schizoaffective Disorders

K.R.R. Krishnan, K. Rayasam, and B.J. Carroll[1]

Introduction

The concept of schizoaffective disorder as a distinctive diagnostic entity is controversial (Maj et al. 1987). At one time, schizoaffective disorder was viewed primarily as a variant of schizophrenia. Wellner et al. (1974, 1977, 1979) reported that patients with schizoaffective disorder have a prognosis similar to that for patients with schizophrenia. They also found no prognostic significance for affective symptoms in patients with marked schizophrenic psychopathology.

However, other studies have suggested that schizoaffective disorder is probably a variant of affective disorder. Sovner and McHugh (1976) thought that, because of the time-honored tradition of giving more weight to schizophrenic symptoms when the clinical picture is ambiguous, many bipolar patients were misdiagnosed as schizophrenic. Follow-up studies by several groups have found no difference in clinical outcome between groups of patients with mania and with schizoaffective disorder, manic type. Patients with schizoaffective mania had a family history of bipolar disorder with a frequency similar to that found in bipolar disorder (Abrams and Taylor 1976). Pope et al. (1980) suggest that all types of schizophrenic symptoms are quite common in affective disorder and that individuals with a mixed presentation of schizophrenic and affective symptoms should be considered to be suffering from an affective disorder.

Recent studies regard schizoaffective disorder as a heterogeneous diagnostic entity. In a number of studies, Tsuang et al. (Tsuang and Dempsey 1979; Tsuang and Simpson 1984) have noted that schizoaffective patients have an earlier age at onset than bipolar patients and a course that is better than that of schizophrenic patients, but worse than that of affective disorder patients. Some authors have reported a greater familial risk for schizoaffective disorder in schizoaffective probands compared with probands with affective disorders (Tsuang and Dempsey 1979; Tsuang and Simpson 1984).

Biological studies related to schizoaffective disorder are relatively rare in the literature. This is partly because patients with schizoaffective disorder are usually seen in clinical settings where research is not conducted, and partly because of the difficulty in standardizing the diagnosis. Recent studies of schizo-

---

[1] Duke University Medical Center, Department of Psychiatry, Box 3215, Durham, NC 27710, USA

Affective and Schizoaffective Disorders
Edited by A. Marneros and M.T. Tsuang
© Springer-Verlag Berlin Heidelberg 1990

affective disorder have utilized the Research Diagnostic Criteria for schizoaffect-ive disorder (Meador-Woodruff et al. 1988). The dexamethasone suppression test, a surrogate test widely used to investigate neuroendocrine abnormalities in affective disorders, has been utilized to study the issue of diagnostic hetero-geneity in schizoaffective disorder. In their initial studies on the DST, Greden et al. (1981) and Schlesser et al. (1981) suggested that the DST might allow for the identification of a homogeneous subtype of schizoaffective disorder probably more related to the affective spectrum. In this chapter we review various studies of the DST in schizoaffective disorder and consider the potential utility of this test in characterizing a homogeneous subgroup of schizoaffective patients.

Dexamethasone Suppression Test

Abnormalities of the hypothalamo-pituitary-adrenal (HPA) axis are frequently seen in patients with depression. Carroll et al. (1981) showed that the DST is a sensitive instrument for measuring the disturbance of the hypothalamo-pitu-itary-adrenal axis function in patients with depression. The standardized DST assesses early escape of cortisol following dexamethasone suppression of the HPA axis. The test is conducted as follows: 1 mg dexamethasone is given orally at 11 pm. Plasma cortisol is measured the following day at 4 pm and 11 pm. Our early studies showed that 50% of endogenous depressed patients failed to show suppression of cortisol below the threshold criterion at either the 4 pm or the 11 pm measurement. In contrast, 95% of healthy controls suppressed cortisol. The DST was also noted to be abnormal in patients with schizoaffective disorder and schizophreniform disorder.

A significant number of patients with bipolar disorder, manic phase, or mixed bipolar disorder were also found to have abnormal DST results. Table 1 summarizes the DST data from studies of schizoaffective disorders. Early studies of schizoaffective disorder patients with the DST focused primarily on the depressed subtype. Carman et al. (1981) reported that 51% of the schizoffective patients in their study were DST nonsuppressors. Aguillar et al. (1984) found that nine of 13 schizoaffective patients were also DST nonsuppressors. Sauer et al. (1984) reported that 89% of a group of schizoaffective patients, depressed subtype, were DST nonsuppressors. Coccaro et al. (1985) studied the DST in a group of patients with coexisting depression and psychosis as well as in patients with nondepressive psychosis. The frequency of dexamethasone nonsuppression among the non-depressed psychotic group was 90% (nine of ten patients), significantly greater than among either the schizoaffective depressed, 22% (two of nine patients) or the nondepressed 17% (two of 12). They suggested that the DST was specific for primary major depressive disorders, especially of the psychotic subtype. The schizoaffective patients studied were primarily of the schizophrenic subtype. Rothschild et al. (1982) found that 25% of schizoaffect-ive patients were DST nonsuppressors. Schlesser et al. (1981) reported abnor-mal dexamethasone suppression primarily in schizoaffective depressives with a family history of affective disorder in contrast to those schizoaffective depres-

Table 1. Results of dexamethasone suppression test in various studies

Reference	Diagnosis	No. of patients	DST Non-suppressors (%)	Remarks
Coccaro et al. (1985)	MDP	10	90	11 pm and 4 pm post-dexamethasone mean plasma cortisol values higher in depressed psychotic group – schizoaffective group mainly schizophrenic
	SAD	9	22	
	ND	12	17	
Meador-Woodruff et al. (1988)	MD	49	40	Moderate correlation between severity of illness and post-dex cortisol levels in all diagnostic groups
	MDP	10	60	
	SAD	25	32	
Greden et al. (1981)	SAD	30	24	
Katona and Roth (1985)	SAD	30	30	Patients not medication free
Carman et al. (1981)	SA	Unknown	51	
Aguilar et al. (1984)	SAD	13	69	
Sauer et al. (1984)	SAD	18	89	
	SAM	12	66.7	
Meltzer et al. (1984)	SAD	14	28.6	Patients primarily affective in both groups. Nonsuppression occurred in schizoaffective patients more than in schizophrenic group, but less than in depression group
	SAM	7	28.6	
Rothschild et al. (1982)	SA	4	25	
Targum (1983)	SA	10	30	
Maj (1986)	SAD	20	25	
Coryell et al. (1985)	SAD	42	40	
Kiriike et al. (1987)	SAM	10	50	
Stokes et al. (1976)	SA	9	33	

MD, Major depression; MDP, major depression with psychotic features; SAD, schizoaffective, depressed type; SAM, schizoaffective, manic type; ND, nondepressed.

sives with a family history of schizophrenia. Meltzer et al. (1984) found that 28.6% of schizoaffective depressed patients were DST nonsuppressors, a rate intermediate between those of major depression and schizophrenia. Katona and Roth (1985) studied 17 patients with schizoaffective disorder. They found six of the 17 depressed subtype patients and one of six schizophrenic patients to be DST nonsuppressors. Their findings were similar to the data reported by Greden et al. (1981). Meador-Woodruff et al. (1988) studied 25 patients with schizoaffective disorder, depressed subtype. They found that 30% of the patients were DST nonsuppressors. The rate of nonsuppression was lower than that reported in patients with psychotic depression and in agreement with the findings of Coccaro et al. (1985). Meador-Woodruff et al. (1988) did not find a relationship between age and weight loss and DST nonsuppression in schizoaffective disorder patients. They showed a positive correlation between severity ratings of psychosis and the DST nonsuppression and no correlation between the DST and severity of depression. Maj (1986) studied 20 schizoaffective depressed patients with the DST. He found that 25% were DST nonsuppressors. There was no significant difference between suppressor and nonsuppressor schizodepressives with respect to demographic, historical, clinical, and family history variables.

Schizoaffective Disorder, Manic Subtype

Considerable attention has been focused on schizoaffective disorder, depressed subtype, but there has been only limited research into the schizoaffective disorder, manic subtype, with regard to the DST. Early studies of bipolar disorder suggested that the DST was normal in patients with bipolar disorder, manic phase. However, recent studies, including those conducted by us, have shown DST nonsuppression in the manic phase as well as in the mixed phase of bipolar disorder. In a group of 26 manics, 85% were DST nonsuppressors (Krishnan et al. 1987). Studies conducted by Winokur et al. (1985) and others have noted few, if any, differences between schizoaffective manic patients and bipolar disorder manic patients with regard to demographic, clinical, historical, prognostic, and family history variables. Meltzer et al. (1984) reported that two of seven schizoaffective manic patients were DST nonsuppressors. Sauer et al. (1984) reported that eight of 12 schizoaffective manic patients were DST nonsuppressors. Kiriike et al. (1987) compared DST results in patients with schizoaffective mania, mania, and schizophrenia. They noted that the frequency of DST nonsuppression was 50%, 22%, and 9% respectively in these groups. DST nonsuppression was significantly higher in schizoaffective mania than in schizophrenic patients.

DST as a State Marker in Schizoaffective Disorder

We have studied the frequency of nonsuppression on the DST in patients with schizoaffective disorder and psychotic major depression in a state hospital

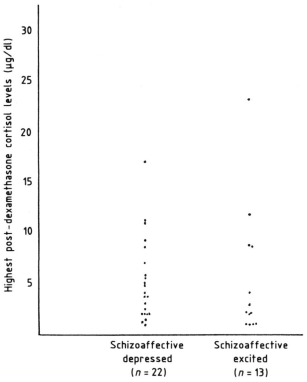

Fig. 1. Highest post-dexamethasone cortisol concentrations in patients with schizoaffective disorder, depressed subtypes, and schizoaffective disorder, excited subtypes

setting. All patients were evaluated by the attending psychiatrist and by one of the study psychiatrists. Detailed psychiatric, family, and social histories were obtained from medical records and by direct interview of patients. The diagnoses were made based on a detailed review of all available information and using RDC criteria. The dexamethasone suppression test was conducted as follows: 1 mg of dexamethasone was given at 11:00 pm and plasma cortisol was measured at 4:00 pm and 11:00 pm the following day by a radioimmunoassay method (Krishnan et al. 1983). The threshold criterion was 5 µg/dl. The exclusion criteria listed by Carroll et al. (1981) were applied in all cases. In a subgroup of patients the DST was repeated at the end of the treatment period. Results are presented in Fig. 1.

Thirteen patients with schizoaffective mania and 22 patients with schizoaffective depression as defined by RDC were studied. The mean age of the schizoaffective manic patients was 37.5 ± 10.9 years. The mean post dexamethasone cortisol concentration was 4.56 ± 3.95 µg/dl. There was no significant relationship between age and the highest post-dexamethasone cortisol concentration. Five of the 13 patients with schizoaffective mania (38%) were nonsuppressors on the DST. Nine of 22 schizoaffective depressed patients (41%) were nonsuppressors on the DST. The mean age of the schizoaffective depressed patient population was 32.86 ± 11.2 years. The highest post-dexamethasone cortisol concentration was 5.23 ± 4.08 µg/dl. There was no significant relationship between age and highest post-dexamethasone cortisol concentration. The percentage of nonsuppressors in the schizophrenic population was 13%. The percentage of nonsuppressors in the psychotic depressive population was 56% (Krishnan et al. 1987). The percentage of DST nonsuppression in patients with schizoaffective disorder was higher than in patients with schizophrenia, but lower than in patients with psychotic depression.

Pretreatment and post-treatment DSTs were conducted in four schizoaffective depressed patients. The severity of depression was assessed using the Montgomery Asberg Depression Rating Scale (MADRS) in both phases (Table 2). The initial MADRS score was 33. Post-treatment scores were 19.5. The mean post-dexamethasone cortisol concentration declined from 7.6 to 3.5 µg/dl (Table 2). Three of the four depressed patients improved after treatment (Table 1). Seven of the schizoaffective manic patients were studied before and after treatment. The severity of the mania was assessed by the Bech Rafaelsen Scale. The initial pretreatment mean score was 12.67. It declined to 7.6 after treatment, and the post-dexamethasone cortisol concentration changed from 2.92 to 1.33 µg/dl (Table 2). The change in post-dexamethasone cortisol concentration pre- and post-treatment in the schizoaffective patient population is illustrated in Fig. 2. This study shows that the change in cortisol is similar to that in the depressed patient population. There is a decline in the highest post-dexamethasone cortisol concentrations following treatment, suggesting that the DST abnormality is a state marker in this population as well.

Diagnostic Stability and the DST

The wide range in the frequency of nonsuppression seen in patients with schizoaffective disorder, depressed subtype, suggests that the entity is heterogeneous. Early open studies by Evans and Nemeroff (1987) have noted that when patients who present with an abnormal DST and nonaffective diagnosis are followed up over time, the diagnosis changes to one of affective disorder in significant numbers. The separation of psychotic depression from and schizoaffective dis-

Table 2. Results of DST in schizoaffective depressed patients

Initial depression score (MADRS)	33	± 10.25
Final depression score (MADRS)	19.5	± 12.68
Mean post-dex cortisol concentration (initial)	7.6	± 3.9
Mean post-dex cortisol concentration (final)	3.5	± 3.3
Initial schizoaffective manic (Beck Rafaelsen scale)	12.67	± 2.76
Final schizoaffective manic	6.5	± 3.09
Mean post-dex cortisol concentration (initial)	2.92	± 2.70
Mean post-dex cortisol concentration (final)	1.33	± 0.65

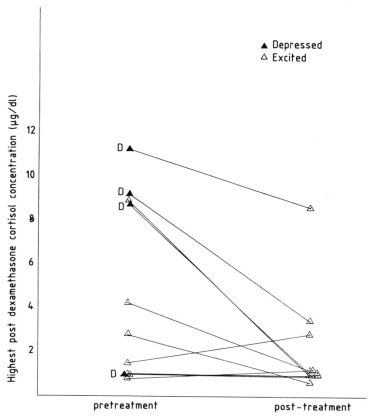

Fig. 2. Highest post-dexamethasone cortisol concentration in pre- and post-treatment patients with schizoaffective disorders

order and schizophrenia is often difficult, and diagnostic certainty increases when patients are followed up over time. Coryell et al. (1988) studied the DST blind to diagnostic stability in a group of patients. Ninety-seven patients who met the criteria for depression, schizoaffective disorder, depressed type, or schizophrenia were entered into a longitudinal follow-up study. The DST was performed in a standard fashion. The authors reinterviewed all patients at 6 month and 1-year intervals to review diagnostic stability. Initially, six (33%) of 18 patients with schizophrenia were nonsuppressors on the DST. In five of these patients the diagnosis was changed to schizoaffective disorder on follow-up. Four of these five patients were DST nonsuppressors on the DST initially. Twenty-six patients met the criteria for major depression, psychotic subtype, initially. In seven of these patients the diagnosis changed to schizoaffective depression over time. Of these seven, only two patients were DST nonsuppressors initially. The specificity of the DST increased from 66% to 84.6% when initial DST results were correlated with the longitudinal follow-up diagnosis. Based on this, only 15.4% of patients with schizophrenia were DST nonsuppressors whereas 63% of the patients with psychotic depression and 42% of the schizoaffective depressed were nonsuppressors on the DST. The study clearly suggests that nonsuppression at baseline was associated with diagnostic instability in schizophrenic patients, and appeared to indicate a change toward schizoaffective diagnosis over time. When patients present with a mixture of affective symptoms as well as psychosis, DST nonsuppression in indicates the possibility of an affective disorder.

TRH Stimulation Test

Another neuroendocrine marker, the thyrotropin-releasing hormone stimulation test, has been studied in a very small number of patients with schizoaffective disorder. Loosen and Prange (1980) studied five schizoaffective patients, primarily of the schizophrenic subtype. All these patients had normal TSH responses. Gold et al. (1981) studied five schizoaffective depressed patients and none had abnormal TRH Stimulation Test results. Meltzer et al. (1984) found blunted TSH responses to TRH in five of 13 schizoaffective depressed patients. Targum (1983) reported that five of ten schizoaffective patients had a blunted TSH response. Wolkin et al. (1984) demonstrated blunted TSH response in one of four schizoaffective patients. Sauer et al. (1984) reported that schizoaffective depressed patients had a lower mean delta max TSH, and that there was an increased rate of blunted TSH responses in schizoaffective depressed patients compared with schizophrenic patients.

The TRH Stimulation Test has not been well studied in schizoaffective manic patients. Gold et al. (1981) reported that three of ten schizoaffective manic patients had blunted TSH responses to TRH; Kiriike et al. (1987) obtained the same results. All studies have used the standard 500-µg dose of TRH administered in the morning. The only study which used a different dose was that of Sauer et al. (1984), who used a 200-µg dose.

Sleep EEG

A number of abnormalities in sleep EEG have been reported in patients with endogenous depression. These include shortened REM latency, low overall sleep efficiency, and an increased REM activity. Kupfer et al. (1979) studied schizoaffective depressed patients and reported that there was shortening of the REM latency and alternations in REM density, with an increase during the earlier part of the night. They also had sleep discontinuity and a reduction of delta sleep similar to that seen in patients with psychotic depression.

In summary, neuroendocrine markers may be a helpful tool in identifying a homogeneous subgroup of patients who carry a diagnosis of schizoaffective disorder, especially the depressed subtype. However, more studies of larger numbers of patients are needed with not only the DST, but also other measures such as platelet imipramine binding, sleep EEG, and the TRH stimulation test.

These studies need to be carried out in relation to follow-up diagnosis, prognosis, family history, and treatment response. Such studies coupled with statistical techniques such as Grade of Membership analysis may provide insights into the biology of schizoaffective disorder.

References

Abrams R, Taylor MA (1976) Manic and schizoaffective disorder manic type: a comparison. Am J Psychiatry 133:1445–1447

Aguilar MT, Lemaire M, Castro P, Libohee M, Reynder SJ, Herchnelz (1984) A study of diagnostic value of dexamethasone suppression test in endogenous depression. J Affective Disord 6:33

Carman J, Wyatt E, Crewe E, Hall K, Sealise BBG, Walt D, Hoppers L (1981) Dexamethasone suppression test – predictor of thymoleptic response in catatonic paranoid, hebephrenic and schizoaffective patients. In: Perris C, Struwe G, Jansson B (eds) Biological psychiatry: developments in psychiatry, vol 5. Elsevier, North Holland

Carroll BJ, Feinberg M, Greden JF, Tarika J, Albala AA, Haskett RF, James NM, Kronfol Z, Lohr W, Steiner M, deVigne JP, Young E (1981) A specific laboratory test for diagnosis of melancholia: standardization, validation and clinical utility. Arch Gen psychiatry 38:15–22

Coccaro EF, Prudic J, Rothpearl A, Nurnberg HG (1985) The dexamethasone suppression test in depressive, non-depressive and schizoaffective psychosis. J Affective Disord 9:107–113

Coryell W, Zimmerman M, Winokur G, Cadoret R (1988) Baseline neuroendocrine function and diagnostic stability among patients with a non-manic psychosis. Eur Arch Psychiatry Neurol Sci 237:197–199

Evans DL, Nemeroff B (1987) The clinical use of dexamethasone suppression test in DSM-III affective disorders; correlations with the severe depressive subtype of melancholia and psychosis. J Psychiatr Res 21:185–194

Gold MS, Pottash ALC, Extein I, Martin DM, Howard E, Mueller, Sweeney DR (1981) The TRH test in diagnosis of major and minor depression. Psychoneuroendocrinology 6:159–169

Greden J, Kronfol Z, Gardner R, Feinberg M, Carroll BJ (1981) Neuroendocrine evaluation of schizoaffectives with dexamethasone suppression test. In: Perris C, Struwe G, Jansson B (eds) Biological psychiatry: developments in psychiatry, vol 5. Elsevier, North Holland

Katona CLE, Roth M (1985) The dexamethasone suppression test in schizo-affective depression. J Affective Disord 8:107–112

Kiriike N, Izumiya Y, Nishiwaki S, Maeda Y, Nagata T, Kawakita Y (1987) TRH test and DST in schizoaffective mania, mania and schizophrenia. Biol Psychiatry 24:415–422

Krishnan KRR, Davidson JRT, Rayasam K, Tanas KS, Shope GS, Pelton S (1987) Diagnostic utility of dexamethasone suppression test. Biol Psychiatry 22:618–628

Krishnan RR, Maltbie AA, Davidson JRT (1983) Abnormal cortisol suppression in bipolar patients with simultaneous manic and depressive symptoms. Am J Psychiatry 140:2:203–205.

Kupfer DJ, Broudy D, Spiker DG, Neil JF, Coble PA (1979) EEG sleep and affective psychoses I. Schizoaffective disorders. Psychiatry Res 1:173–178

Loosen PT, Prange AJ (1980) Thyrotropin-releasing hormone (TRH). A useful tool for psychoneuroendocrine investigation. Psychoneuroendocrinology 5:63–80

Maj M (1986) Response to the dexamethasone suppression test in schizoaffective disorder, depressed type. J Affective Disord 11:63–67

Maj M, Starace F, Kemali D (1987) Prediction of outcome by historical, clinical and biological variables in schizoaffective disorder, depressed type. J Psychiatr Res 21:289–295

Meador-Woodruff JH, Greden JF, Grunhaus L, Haskett RP (1988) Plasma post dexamethasone cortisol levels in schizoaffective disorders. Psychiatry Res 26:35–42

Meltzer HY, Arora RC, Metz J (1984) Biological studies of schizoaffective disorders.

Schizophr Bull 10:49–70

Pope HG Jr, Lipinski JF, Cohen BM, Axelrod DT (1980) "Schizoaffective disorder": an invalid diagnosis? A comparison of schizoaffective disorder, schizophrenia, and affective disorder. Am J Psychiatry 1980:921–927

Rothchild AJ, Saltzberg AF, Rosenbaum AH, Stahl JB, Cole JO (1982) The dexamethasone suppression test as a discriminator among subtypes of psychotic patients. Br J Psychiatry 141:471

Sauer H, Koehler KG, Sass H, Hornstein C, Minne HW (1984) The dexamethasone suppression test and thyroid-stimulating hormone response to TRH in RDC schizoaffective patients. Eur Arch Psychiatry Neurol Sci 234:264–267

Schlesser MA, Winokur G, Sherman BM (1980) Hypothalamic pituitary adrenal axis in depressive illness. Arch Gen Psychiatry 37:737

Schlesser MA, Winokur G, Rush AJ (1981) Dexamethasone suppression test. In: Schizoaffective psychosis, abstracts of the 3rd World Congress of Biological Psychiatry, Stockholm

Sovner RD, McHugh PR (1976) Bipolar course in schizoaffective illness. Biol Psychiatry 195:205

Stokes PE, Stoll PM, Mattson MR, Sollod RN (1976) Diagnosis and psychopathology in psychiatric patients resistant to dexamethasone. In: Sachar EJ (ed) Hormones, behavior and psychopathology. Raven, New York, pp 225–229

Targum SD (1983) Neuroendocrine dysfunction in schizophreniform disorders: correlation with six-month clinical outcome. Am J Psychiatry 140:309–313

Tsuang MT (1979) Schizoaffective disorder: dead or alive? Arch Gen Psychiatry 36:633–634

Tsuang MT, Dempsey GM (1979) Long-term outcome of major psychoses. II. Schizoaffective disorder compared with schizophrenia, affective disorders, and a surgical control group. Arch Gen Psychiatry 36:1302–1304

Tsuang MT, Simpson JC (1984) Schizoaffective disorder: concept and reality. Schizophr Bull 10:14–25

Wellner A, Croughan JL, Robins E (1974) The group of schizoaffective and related psychoses – critique, record, follow-up and family studies. I. A persistent enigma. Arch Gen Psychiatry 31:628–631 (Review)

Wellner A, Croughan J, Fishman R, Robins E (1977) The group of schizoaffective and related psychoses: a follow-up study. Compr Psychiatry 18:413–422

Wellner A, Welner Z, Fishman R (1979) The group of schizoaffective and related psychoses. IV. A family study. Compr Psychiatry 20:21–26

Winokur G, Scharfetter C, Angst J (1985) A family study of psychotic symptomatology in schizophrenia, schizoaffective disorder, unipolar depression, and bipolar disorder. Eur Arch Psychiatry Neurol Sci 234:295–298

Wolkin A, Peselow ED, Smith M, Lantin A, Kahn IY, Rotrosen J (1984) TRH test abnormalities in psychiatric disorders. J Affective Disord 6:273–281

Neuroleptic-Induced and Postremissive Depression in Schizophrenics

K. Heinrich and J. Tegeler[1]

Introduction

States of depressive disorder occur frequently in the course of schizophrenic diseases and are very complex syndromes as regards their etiology, phenomenology, and clinical prognosis. There is some controversy about to what extent an increase of depressive disorder can be established following the introduction of neuroleptics and whether they are of any significance for the various pathogenetic factors. Individual authors proceed from different theoretical concepts and emphasize difficulties of diagnostic differentiation from anxiety syndromes, dysphoria, sedation, chronic residual schizophrenic states, and akinesia.

Depressions as a prodromal syndrome and in the course of schizophrenia were described by E. Bleuler (1911), Kraepelin (1913), and Gruhle (1922) long before the introduction of neuroleptics. According to Conrad (1958), an "initial depression" precedes a developing schizophrenia; Mayer-Gross (1920) described the "post-psychotic depression," and Meyer (1950) emphasized that the further development of schizophrenia may also involve "cyclothymic waves."

Prevalence of Depressive Syndromes in Schizophrenia

In the Bonn Study of Schizophrenia (Huber et al. 1979), Gross and Huber (1980) noted depressive premonitory symptoms in 8% of 502 mainly untreated patients and prodromes of endomorph-depressive appearance in 8.2% of the patients. Adding the depressive-asthenic-cenesthesic syndromes, the rate increased to 22.3%. Johnson (1981) found depressive prodromes in 29% of patients prior to the first schizophrenic illness and without neuroleptic medication. Within the scope of neuroleptic interval therapy, Donlon and Blacker (1973), Docherty et al. (1978), Herz and Melville (1980), and Heinrichs and Carpenter (1985) emphasized the particular significance of apparently depressive prodromes for a psychotic relapse. Heinrich (1967, 1969) described a "postremissive exhaustion syndrome" in schizophrenics after remission of the florid symptoms, which was characterized by lack of drive, depressive mood, anxiety, restlessness, tiredness, loss of contacts, loss of self-confidence, dysphoria, and the feeling of impaired functioning. There is a connection between "reduction of

---

[1] Psychiatrische Klinik der Universität, Bergische Landstraße 2, 4000 Düsseldorf 12, FRG

Affective and Schizoaffective Disorders
Edited by A. Marneros and M.T. Tsuang
© Springer-Verlag Berlin Heidelberg 1990

the energetic potential" (Conrad 1958), "dynamic voiding" (Janzarik 1959), "exhaustion syndrome" (Weitbrecht 1959) and "exhaustive depression" (Kielholz 1960). Heinrich (1967) discussed as causal factors the neuroleptics, the reaction of the vital personality to the psychotic breakdown, and the primarily chronic schizophrenic hypoergasia. The etiological unspecifity and principal reversibility of this syndrome in particular should be noted. In the context of recent survey results, the multiconditional concept of this syndrome, as stipulated by Heinrich, deserves special consideration; it entails the suggestion of a multidimensional therapeutic concept. Helmchen and Hippius (1967, 1969) assumed a relation of the neuroleptic medication in patients to initial depression, since these patients were pretreated more frequently and complained about inner restlessness, sleep disturbances, and akathisia. For a second group a peak of depressive symptoms was found in the 4th–7th and the 20th week of treatment. The early manifestation was mainly brought into causal connection with psychoreactive factors, whereas for later manifestations pharmacogenic as well as pathogenic factors were assumed to be causal. Gross and Huber (1980) reported endogenous depressive syndromes in 18.7% of 502 mainly untreated patients. In 25% of the patients this syndrome appeared during the first year of illness, whereas it was distributed equally at a rate of 14%–17% for medium- and long-term courses of illness. In the International Pilot Study of Schizophrenia (IPSS), 15% of the patients showed depressive paranoid signs at admission, 39% showed special features of depression, 78% other symptoms of depression, and 81% the characteristics of a simple depression (WHO 1973).

McGlashan and Carpenter (1976a) also emphasized in their concept of "postpsychotic depression" the multiconditionality of the etiology. The insight into the psychotic breakdown and its negative social consequences and the withdrawal of the defense mechanism after remission of the florid symptoms are supposed to influence to some extent the pathogenesis of this syndrome, whereas the pharmacogenesis is apt to be of minor importance. The authors base their findings on studies of Steinberg et al. (1967), Roth (1970), Stern et al. (1972), and McKinnon (1977).

McGlashan and Carpenter (1976b) carried out a 1-year follow-up of 30 acute schizophrenics who had not been treated with neuroleptics but had undergone intensive socio- and psychotherapy. At the time of discharge a postpsychotic depression was recorded in 50% of the patients, many of these patients having shown depressive symptoms at the beginning of the treatment. Möller and von Zerssen (1981a) investigated 81 acute schizophrenics at the time of admission and at discharge by means by various rating scales. Combining the three IMPS syndromes, i.e., depressive syndrome, apathy, and impaired functioning, in an overall score, 31% of the patients showed significant to severe depressive symptoms on admission but this applied to only 23% at the time of discharge. Patients who showed severe depression at the time of discharge already had these symptoms in most cases on admission. An increase or a recurrence of these symptoms in the course of the inpatient treatment was observed in only 5%–10% of the patients, however. In a second study, 280 acute schizophrenics were investigated (Möller and von Zerssen 1981b). Whereas at the time of admission

48% of the patients showed severe signs of the depressive-apathic syndrome, this was noted for only 17% at the time of discharge. An impairment was recorded in only 3% at the time of discharge, a recurrence of depressive symptoms in only 14%. The authors note that the majority of the patients were not being treated with neuroleptics at the time of admission, and that only 10% of the patients suffered from distinct negative symptoms. The authors concluded that the depressive symptoms initially went unnoticed in favor of the more dominant acute psychotic symptoms, and became particularly obvious only after remission of these positive schizophrenic symptoms. Knights and Hirsch (1981) recorded depressive symptoms in 65% of 27 newly admitted schizophrenics by means of the present state examination (PSE) at the time of admission. While the acute psychotic symptoms remitted after 3 months under neuroleptic drugs, depressive and neurotic symptoms persisted. According to the authors' point of view, the initially existing depressive symptoms were revealed after reduction of the positive schizophrenic symptoms ("revealed depression"). The control group of depressive and neurotic patients offered an almost congruent profile of symptoms. In a second group of patients, who were treated with fluphenazine-decanoate or flupenthixol-decanoate, the frequency and severity of depression were measured before discharge and after 6 months on maintenance therapy. Within this period depressive symptoms did not increase and were significantly less severe than in the acute schizophrenics on admission to hospital. The authors took their findings as a proof that neuroleptics do not produce depression, but that these symptoms are an integral part of the schizophrenic syndrome. Shanfield et al. (1970), Siris et al. (1981), and Lerner and Moscovich (1985) also found that depressive symptoms were more prevalent at the time of admission than after remission of the acute schizophrenic symptoms on neuroleptic treatment.

Johnson (1981, 1985) investigated patients with a first episode of schizophrenia without medication, as well as chronic patients on maintenance therapy with fluphenazine decanoate or flupenthixol decanoate. Twenty percent of the first-admission patients without medication and 30% each of the long-term patients who experienced an acute relapse either under continuous therapy or after discontinuation of the neuroleptics showed depressive symptoms. The lowest rate of depression (10%) was noted for patients in stable remission under maintenance treatment with depot neuroleptics. To be able to judge the consequences of a depressive syndrome, Johnson (1981) conducted a 2-year follow-up of chronic schizophrenics who had relapsed on long-term therapy with depot neuroleptics. In 70% of these patients a depressive syndrome was observed, and in 60% the corresponding symptoms were prevalent at times of readmission to the hospital. The depression lasted twice as long as the schizophrenic symptoms. On the other hand, schizophrenic symptoms had significantly more negative consequences for the patients and their families (loss of employment, compulsory hospital admissions, arguments with relatives/family).

In a later, 3-year follow-up study, Johnson (1988) found early postpsychotic depression in 30% of 80 patients within 1 year after the last remission, in 40% a late depression during the 2nd or 3rd year. Of the patients who had a psychotic relapse on long-term neuroleptic treatment, 96% developed a depression during the 3-year period; these were mainly late depressions. For the patients with a late depression the risk of an acute relapse within the 3 years was significantly higher than for the patients with an early depression (72% versus 29%). Johnson (1988) suggested that the two types of depression have different etiologies; the late form may represent underlying schizophrenia prior to an early relapse.

Phenomenology and Problems of Differential Diagnosis

It can be difficult to separate this depressive syndrome from apathy, negative features of schizophrenia, and parkinsonism. Describing the postremissive exhausation syndrome, Heinrich (1967) stressed the dim sadness of the depressive state and the impaired functioning. Helmchen and Hippius (1967) observed transitions of a dim sadness up to a severe depression with vital symptoms, marked daily fluctuations, and depressive delusions. According to McGlashan and Carpenter (1976a) and to Müller (1981), agitation occurs rather seldom, affective lability more frequently, whereas Heinrich (1969) was of the opinion that an emotional incontinence with increased irritability and vivid affective expression is missing in almost all cases. According to Gross and Huber (1980), depressive syndromes in pure and mixed defect states are often perceivable and accompanied by an impairment of conductivity of the thought process, increased exhaustion, and disturbance of general feeling, along with performance deficiency and a loss of energy and perseverance. Whereas the majority of authors assume that a depressive syndrome is reversible, negative symptoms are rather related to a chronic course. There are special differential diagnostic difficulties between a depression in schizophrenia and a schizoaffective psychosis (Wellner et al. 1974; Tsuang et al. 1979; Vogl and Zaudig 1983, Berner and Lenz 1986, Marneros and Tsuang 1986).

According to Goplerud and Depue (1978) the diagnosis of schizophrenia is made too frequently; often it is a case of mania, and a postpsychotic depression is often the depressive phase of a bipolar psychosis.

Depressive Syndromes Induced by Neuroleptics

It is commonly supposed that neuroleptics can cause depression. This assumption is based mainly upon considerations of a possible "pharmacogenetic shift of symptoms" and on anecdotal experiences, but less on results of controlled studies. Neuroleptics are supposed to produce depression either directly ("pharmacogenetic depression") or via the akinesia of parkinsonism ("akinetic depression").

Huber (1964, 1966, and 1967) Glatzel (1967), Schmitt (1967), and Battegay and Gehring (1968) compared the symptoms of schizophrenics before and after the introduction of neuroleptics. Huber (1966, 1967) and Glatzel (1967) suggested that there was, a reduced frequency of first-rank symptoms in patients with neuroleptics and a "depressive shifting" of psychosis in the direction of a residual state. The question is whether this change is an improvement in the prognosis of schizophrenia with current therapeutic approaches, or a real increase of depression after the use of neuroleptics. Angst and Dinkelkamp (1974), Ananth and Chadirian (1980), Müller (1981), Hirsch and Knights (1982), Hirsch (1982), and Johnson (1985) disconfirmed the hypothesis of pharmacogenetic depression. They raised methodological objections against anecdotal experiences and uncontrolled studies with no distinction between acute or long-term medication, no standardized evaluation of symptoms, no specification of medication, and no placebo control group.

Many uncontrolled studies have been published supporting the argument that depot neuroleptics carry a higher risk of producing depression (Alarcon and Carney 1969; Keskiner 1973). In our hospital Floru et al. (1975) found that 16% of 161 schizophrenics who had been treated with fluspirilene for 1 year developed a depressive syndrome. Nineteen percent of these were readmitted; for the remaining patients a reduction of the neuroleptics or prescription of antidepressants led to an improvement of depression. Forty-seven percent of these syndromes occurred within 4–19 weeks, 53% within 20–52 weeks. During a 1-year treatment with penfluridol 25% of the patients experienced a depression, 24% in 4–19 weeks and 76% in 20–52 weeks. The 20% prevalence of postpsychotic depression in patients on long-term therapy with depot neuroleptics was not higher than that in patients on the oral form of the drug. Results of placebo-controlled studies support this evidence. Hirsch et al. (1973) found that two of 12 patients who did not suffer any relapse under placebo in 9 months needed an antidepressant, whereas to only one of the 33 patients treated with fluphenazine decanoate had an antidepressant been prescribed. One can object critically that there was a lack of data about the criteria for prescribing antidepressants. Mueller et al. (1978), Hartmann et al. (1979), and Mueller (1981) noted that 19 of 25 patients treated with fluphenazine decanoate had a depression, but only three of 25 patients on placebo showed similar symptoms. Sixteen of 20 patients with extrapyramidal side effects also showed depressive syndromes. The authors interpreted these syndromes as pharmacogenetic depression. In the study of Rifkin et al. (1977), eight of 23 patients (35%) treated with fluphenazine decanoate were withdrawn from the study at an early stage due to akinetic depression, as opposed to only two of 26 patients who received fluphenazine dihydrochloride. The fluphenazine decanoate dosage was considerably higher than that of fluphenazine dihydrochloride. Falloon et al. (1978) reported that a depressive syndrome was the main factor for readmission to hospital (four of 20 patients receiving fluphenazine decanoate and three of 24 receiving pimozide). During therapy with fluphenazine decanoate, 11 of 20 patients (55%) had depressive symptoms after 1 month of treatment and 14 of 20 patients (70%) after 1 year. In only eight of 24 patients (33%) treated with pimozide did depression occur after 1 month, and in eight of 24 patients (33%) after 1 year ($P<0.059$). The validity of these findings is diminished by the small number of patients and the variable and nonequivalent dosages. Hogarty et al. (1979) reported a higher incidence of affective symptoms in patients relapsing under fluphenazine decanoate, whereas in those patients who relapsed under fluphenazine dihydrochloride, acute psychotic symptoms were recorded more often, a factor which was associated with the early discontinuation of oral medication. Depressive dysphoric symptoms of neurotic appearance along with apathy, akinesia, and akathisia were identified as the most important predictors of a relapse. One could object to this study as well by pointing out that the fluphenazine decanoate dosage exceeded the fluphenazine dihydrochloride dosage. Mandel et al. (1982) published results of a study by Schooler et al. (1980). In 25% of the patients on fluphenazine dihydrochloride and in 22% of those on fluphenazine decanoate, depressive symptoms were noted; these occurred mainly during the 6th month after discharge. Patients with depression, compared with patients without, experienced a psychotic relapse more frequently and had to be readmitted more often (64% versus 19%).

Concerning an association with the neuroleptic dose, only a few studies exist. Johnson (1981) found a positive relation between the dosage of fluphenazine decanoate and fluphenthixol decanoate and the incidence of depressive syndromes. On the other hand, Siris et al. (1981) and Roy (1984) established no such association. Kane et al. (1983) found that the scores of the BPRS items "emotional withdrawal," "affective blunting," "tension," and "motor retardation" were significantly lower for the low-dose group of patients than for those receiving a standard dosage of fluphenazine decanoate at the end of 1 year. Marder et al. (1984, 1987) established a close relation between motor retardation and akathisia on the one side and depression and anxiety on the other side with standard dosages. Goldstein et al. (1978) reported that schizophrenics with a good premorbid personality who were treated with 25 mg fluphenazine decanoate for 6 weeks seemed to be more anxious and depressive, compared with those who received 6.25 mg fluphenazine decanoate. For patients with a poor premorbid personality this correlation was the reverse. In their preliminary reports, Carpenter and Heinrichs (1983) and Pietzcker et al. (1986) did not find any essential difference in the frequency of depressive syndromes with long-term and interval therapy. According to Hirsch et al. (1986), patients of the early intervention group estimated themselves more favorably on the SCL-90 and showed a lower score on the affective-balance scale as regards a better sense of well-being.

Only a few trials with high doses have studied the occurrence of depressive syndromes. Steiner (1984) recorded a postremissive exhaustion syndrome in 50% of the 206 patients during a period of 3.5 years and a prevalence rate of 7% at a fixed day evaluation. Four percent of 54 patients showed significant depressive syndromes while under fluphenazine decanoate and 9% of 152 patients after discontinuation of the medication. van Putten and May (1978) analyzed the results of double-blind studies. In 12 studies with mainly chronic schizophrenics depressive syndromes were no more frequent with high doses than with standard dosage. In contrast to this, in three studies of acute schizophrenics a depressive syndrome was recorded more often with high doses. In the double-blind studies with depot neuroleptics of McClelland et al. (1976), McCreadie et al. (1979), Platz and Hinterhuber (1981), and Langner and Stoessl (1984), the frequency of depressive syndromes was no higher with a high dose than with a standard dose. We found in a controlled study that after reduction of the high dosage, patients with an initially lower score for the catatonic and the hostility syndromes showed (in comparison with patients with higher scores in these syndromes) an improvement of the hallucinatory-disintegrative syndrome, apathy, and the neurological syndrome of the AMP, as well as an increased subjective anxiousness and depression on the EWL-K scale (Lehmann et al. 1980). The depression that occurred after florid psychotic symptoms had decreased may be interpreted as a revealed depression (Knights and Hirsch 1981; Hirsch 1982).

Rifkin et al. (1975, 1977), Rifkin (1981), Rifkin and Siris (1986), and van Putten and May (1978) emphasized the close relation between parkinsonism, e.g., akinesia, and a depressive syndrome. Many patients did not complain about a depressive mood, but rather about apathy, and were socially withdrawn and silent. Galdi et al. (1981) and Galdi (1983) used the term "pharmacogenetic depression" after they had observed that depression and parkinsonism occurred more often in those schizophrenics who had depressed relatives, irrespective of the neuroleptic used. Galdi (1983) discussed an interaction between neuroleptics and a genetic deficiency, which is supposed to lead to a disturbance in the nigrostriatal dopaminergic system. The validity of these genetic factors cannot be judged yet, due to the low number of cases studied.

The complexity of problems of depressive syndromes in schizophrenic illness is also a result of the antidepressive efficacy of some neuroleptics. Extensive experience has been gained, especially with flupenthixol vs. placebo and amitriptyline (Young et al. 1976) or nortriptyline (Johnson 1981) and vs. tetracyclic antidepressants, in patients with neurotic or moderate endogenous depressions. Positive results have been reported for administration of thioridazine in chronic schizophrenics with depressive symptoms and in neurotic depressive patients. Also, sulpiride in a low dose proved to be effective in depressive patients (Niskanen et al. 1975; Benkert and Holsboer 1984).

In the double-blind studies of Johnson and Malik (1975), Hamilton et al. (1979), and Pinto et al. (1979) with flupenthixol decanoate and fluphenazine decanoate, an antidepressive impact and an anxiolytic effect were only noted with flupenthixol decanoate, but Floru et al. (1975), Kelly et al. (1977), and Knights et al. (1979) did not find any significant difference between these depot neuroleptics. Kielholz et al. (1979), Ahlfors et al. (1981), and Esparon et al. (1986) used flupenthixol decanoate in the prophylactic treatment of affective psychoses. Ahlfors et al. (1981) saw a positive prophylactic effect for manias, but not for depressions, while Esparon et al. (1986) did not find any prophylactic effect with flupenthixol decanoate.

Treatment of Depressive Syndromes

With regard to the treatment of depressive syndromes in schizophrenic psychoses there is more consensus. Hartmann et al. (1979), Mueller (1981) and Hartmann (1987), as well as Rifkin et al. (1977), Rifkin and Siris (1986), and van Putten and May (1978) recommended first reducing the neuroleptics, second administering anticholinergic drugs, and only as a third step, prescribing antidepressants. In practice, neuroleptics and antidepressants are very often administered in combination for such depressive states. It is surprising that there are a great number of positive clinical reports but only a few placebo-controlled studies and double-blind investigations concerning this therapy. According to a survey of the literature by Siris et al. (1978), there are 14 trials were schizophrenics were treated either with only one antidepressant or with a MAO inhibitor. In the majority of studies no difference of efficacy was established between antidepressants and placebo. Also, the majority of the 16 controlled studies did not result in a definite superiority of the combination of a neuroleptic with an antidepressant as opposed to monotherapy. Most of the studies, however, do not concern schizophrenics with depressive syndromes, but rather chronic schizophrenics with residual conditions. Prusoff et al. (1979) treated 35 ambulatory chronic schizophrenics with depressive symptoms with either perphenazine or a combination of this neuroleptic drug and amitriptyline. Only after 4 months was a significant superiority of the combination with regard to an improvement of the depressive symptoms established, but an increase of schizophrenic thought disorders and agitation was also noted. Johnson (1981) treated 50 remitted schizophrenics with acute depressive states with either 150 mg nortriptyline per day or placebo. After 5 weeks no relevant difference was found between the two groups as far as depressive symptoms were concerned. Johnson (1981, 1985) concluded that the combination of a neuroleptic and an antidepressant has only a minor therapeutic effect. In a retrospective study, Siris et al. (1982) noted a remission in 48% of schizophrenics with depressive symptoms, and in 32% a distinct improvement of depression with antidepressants. Rifkin and Siris (1986) first administered benztropine to schizophrenics with depressive symptoms, in order to compensate for akinesia and then, under double-blind conditions, imipramine up to 200 mg daily or placebo. After 6 weeks a significant improvement of depressive symptoms was found with imipramine as opposed to placebo. In a double-blind study of 50 schizophrenic patients with depressive syndromes we noted a significant improvement of these symptoms according to the Hamilton depression scale and the AMP system with administration of maprotiline and imipramine (75–150 mg daily). For the somatic-depressive syndrome there was a significant difference in favor of maprotiline, and for apathy and hypochondriasis a difference in favor of clomipramine was established. Thus, maprotiline seems to have a sedative effect, whereas for clomipramine an activating effect was seen. Tolerability was good in both groups.

Heinrich (1960) was the first to describe the thymoleptic symptom provocation. Under conditions of anergic schizophrenic psychosis with a depressive syndrome, paranoid-hallucinatory phenomena could be provoked with activating antidepressants or monoamine oxydase inhibitors. Bucci and Saunders (1961), Klein and Fink (1962), and Pollack et al. (1965) came to similar conclusions.

The prognostic implications of depressive syndromes are judged differently. Whereas Bleuler (1972), Ciompi and Mueller (1976), Huber et al. (1979), and Vaillant (1962) came to the conclusion that initial depressive syndromes are a good prognostic predictor, other authors, mainly because of the increased suicide risk, the worse social integration, the increased danger of relapse, and long-term hospitalization, are of the opinion that the manifestation of depressive syndromes is associated rather with an unfavorable prognosis (McGlashan and Carpenter 1976a; Glazer et al. 1981; Mandel et al. 1982; Roy et al. 1983).

Conclusion

The differences in opinion and also in the results of controlled studies make it difficult to come to definite conclusions about the true prevalence of depression and its causal factors. Neuroleptic drugs may be a factor producing depression, but they are not the only cause. The risk for depot neuroleptics is not higher than that for short-acting neuroleptics. The results of treatment of depression in schizophrenia are good, but because of the suicide risk and a higher relapse rate, the prognosis can be less favorable.

References

Ahlfors UG, Baastrup PC, Dencker SJ, Elgen K, Linjiaerde O, Pedersen V, Schou M, Aaskoven O (1981) Flupenthixol decanoate in recurrent manic-depressive illness. Acta Psychiatr Scand 64:226–237

Anath J, Chadirian AM (1980) Drug-induced mood disorders. Int Pharmacopsychiatry 15:59–73

Angst J, Dinkelkamp T (1974) Die somatische Therapie der Schizophrenie. Literatur der Jahre 1966–1972. Thieme, Stuttgart

Battegay R, Gehring A (1968) Vergleichende Untersuchungen an Schizophrenen der prä-neuroleptischen und der postneuroleptischen Ära. Pharmacopsychiatry 1:107–119

Becker RE, Colliver JA, Verhulst SJ (1985) Diagnosis of secondary depression in schizophrenia. J Clin Psychiatry 46:48

Benkert O, Holsboer F (1984) Effect of sulpiride in endogenous depression. Acta Psychiatr Scand [Suppl] 311:43–48

Berner P, Lenz G (1986) Definitions of schizoaffective psychosis: mutual concordance and relationship to schizophrenia and affective disorder. In: Marneros A, Tsuang MT (eds) Schizoaffective psychoses. Springer, Berlin Heidelberg New York Tokyo, pp 31–49

Bleuler E (1911) Dementia praecox oder Gruppe der Schizophrenien. In: Aschaffenburg B (ed) Handbuch der Psychiatrie. Deuticke, Leipzig

Bleuler M (1972) Die schizophrenen Geistesstörungen im Lichte langjähriger Kranken- und Familiengeschichten. Thieme, Stuttgart

Bucci L, Saunders JC (1961) A unique monoamine oxidase inhibitor for depression. Am J Psychiatry 118:255–256

Carpenter WT, Heinrichs DW (1983) Early intervention, time-limited, targeted pharmacotherapy of schizophrenia. Schizophr Bull 9:533–542

Ciompi L, Müller C (1976) Lebensweg und Alter der Schizophrenen. Eine katamnestische Langzeitstudie bis ins Senium. Springer, Berlin Heidelberg New York

Conrad K (1958) Die beginnende Schizophrenie. Thieme, Stuttgart

de Alarcon R, Carney MWP (1969) Severe depressive mood changes following slow-release intramuscular fluphenazine injection. Br Med J 111:564–567

Docherty JP, Kammen DP van, Siris SG, Marder SR (1978) Stages of onset of schizophrenic psychosis. Am J Psychiatry 135:420–423

Donlon PT, Blacker KG (1973) Stages of schizophrenic decompensation and reintegration. J Nerv Ment Dis 157:200–209

Esparon J, Kolloori J, Naylor GJ, McHarg AM, Smith AHW, Hopwood SE (1986) Comparison of the prophylactic action of flupenthixol with placebo in lithium-treated manic-depressive patients. Br J Psychiatry 148:723–725

Falloon I, Watt DC, Shepherd M (1978) A comparative controlled trial of pimozide and fluphenazine decanoate in the continuation therapy of schizophrenia. Psychol Med 8: 59–70

Floru L, Heinrich K, Wittek F (1975) The problem of postpsychotic schizophrenic depressions and their pharmacological induction. Int Pharmacopsychiatry 10:230–240

Galdi J (1983) The causality of depression in schizophrenia. Br J Psychiatry 142:621–625

Galdi J, Reider RO, Silber D, Bonato RR (1981) Genetic factors in the response to neuroleptics in schizophrenia: a psychopharmacogenetic study. Psychol Med 11:713–728

Glatzel J (1967) Zur Frage der schizophrenen Verläufe unter der Pharmakotherapie. Arch Psychiatr Nervenkr 209:87–100

Glazer W, Prusoff B, John J, Williams D (1981) Depression and social adjustment among chronic schizophrenic outpatients. J Nerv Ment Dis 169:712–717

Goldstein MJ, Rodnick EH, Evans JR, May PRA, Steinberg MR (1978) Drug and family therapy in the after-care treatment of acute schizophrenics. Arch Gen Psychiatry 35: 1169–1177

Goplerud E, Depue RA (1978) The diagnostic ambiguity of postpsychotic depression. Schizophr Bull 4:477–479

Gross G, Huber G (1980) Depressive Syndrome im Verlauf von Schizophrenien. Fortschr Neurol Psychiatr 48:438–446

Gruhle HW (1922) Die Psychologie der Dementia praecox. Z Neur 78:454

Hamilton M, Card IR, Wallis GG, Mahmoud MR (1979) A comparative trial of the decanoates of flupenthixol and fluphenazine. Psychopharmacology 64:225–229

Hartmann W (1987) Neuroleptikabedingte pharmakogene Depressionen. In: Pichot P, Möller HJ (eds) Neuroleptika. Rückschau 1952–1986. Künftige Entwicklungen. Springer, Berlin Heidelberg New York Tokyo, pp 131–138

Hartmann W, Kind J, Meyer JE, Müller P, Steuber H (1979) Die Neuroleptika in der Rückfallverhütung bei schizophrenen Psychosen. Nervenarzt 50:734–737

Heinrich K (1960) Die gezielte Symptomprovokation mit monoaminoxidasehemmenden Substanzen in Diagnostik und Therapie schizophrener Psychosen. Nervenarzt 31:507–512

Heinrich K (1967) Zur Bedeutung des postremissiven Erschöpfungssyndroms für die Rehabilitation Schizophrener. Nervenarzt 38:487–491

Heinrich K (1969) Das postremissive Erschöpfungssyndrom als multikonditionale depressive Reaktionsform Schizophrener. In: Hippius H, Selbach H (eds) Das depressive Syndrom. Urban and Schwarzenberg, Munich, pp 453–456

Heinrichs DW, Carpenter WT Jr (1985) Prospective study of prodromal symptoms in schizophrenic relapse. Am J Psychiatry 142:371–373

Helmchen H, Hippius H (1967) Depressive Syndrome im Verlauf neuroleptischer Therapie. Nervenarzt 38:455–458

Helmchen H, Hippius H (1969) Pharmakogene Depressionen. In: Hippius H, Selbach H (eds) Das depressive Syndrom. Urban and Schwarzenberg, Munich, pp 443–448

Herz M, Melville C (1980) Relapse in schizophrenia. Am J Psychiatry 137:801–805

Hirsch SR (1982) Depression "revealed" in schizophrenia. Br J Psychiatry 140:421–424

Hirsch SR, Knights A (1982) Gibt es die pharmakogene Depression wirklich? Beweismaterial aus zwei prospektiven Studien. In: Kryspin-Exner K, Hinterhuber H, Schubert H (eds) Ergebnisse der psychiatrischen Therapieforschung. Schattauer, Stuttgart, pp 249–260

Hirsch SR, Gaind R, Rohde PD, Stevens BC, Wing JK (1973) Outpatient maintenance of chronic schizophrenic patients with long-acting fluphenazine. Br Med J 1:715–716

Hirsch SR, Jolley AG, Manchanda R, McRink A (1986) Frühzeitige medikamentose Intervention als Alternative zur Depot-Dauermedikation in der Schizophreniebehandlung: ein vorläufiger Bericht. In: Böker W, Brenner HD (eds) Bewältigung der Schizophrenie. Huber, Bern, pp 62–71

Hogarty GE, Schooler NR, Ulrich R, Mussare F, Ferro P, Herron E (1979) Fluphenazine and social therapy in the aftercare of schizophrenic patients. Relapse analyses of a two-year controlled study of fluphenazine decanoate and fluphenazine hydrochloride. Arch Gen Psychiatry 36:1283–1294

Huber G (1964) Grenzen der psychiatrischen Pharmakotherapie bei der Behandlung chronisch Schizophrener. In: Kranz H, Heinrich K (eds) Begleitwirkungen und Mißerfolge der psychiatrischen Pharmakotherapie. Thieme, Stuttgart, pp 167–170

Huber G (1966) Reine Defektsyndrome und Basisstadien endogener Psychosen. Fortschr Neurol Psychiatr 34:409

Huber G (1967) Symptomwandel der Psychosen und Pharmakopsychiatrie. In: Kranz H, Heinrich K (eds) Pharmakopsychiatrie und Psychopathologie. Thieme, Stuttgart

Huber G, Gross G, Schüttler R (1979) Schizophrenie. Eine verlaufs- und sozialpsychiatrische Langzeitstudie. Springer, Berlin Heidelberg New York

Janzarik W (1959) Dynamische Grundkonstellationen in endogenen Psychosen. Ein Beitrag zur Differentialtypologie der Wahnphänomene. Springer, Berlin Göttingen Heidelberg

Johnson DAW (1979) A double-blind comparison of flupenthixol nortriptyline and diazepam in neurotic depression. Acta Psychiatr Scand 59:1–8

Johnson DAW (1981) Studies of depressive symptoms in schizophrenia. Br J Psychiatry 139:89–101

Johnson DAW (1985) Depression in schizophrenia. In: Schiff AA, Roth M, Freeman HL (eds) New pharmacological and clinical developments. Royal Society of Medicine Services, London, pp 15–25

Johnson DAW (1988) The significance of depression in the prediction of relapse in chronic schizophrenia. Br J Psychiatry 152:320–323

Johnson DAW, Malik NA (1975) A double-blind comparison of fluphenazine decanoate and flupenthixol decanoate in the treatment of acute schizophrenia. Acta Psychiatr Scand 51:257–267

Kane JM, Rifkin A, Woerner M, Reardon G, Sarantakos S, Schiebel D, Ramos-Lorenzi J (1983) Low-dose neuroleptics in the treatment of outpatient schizophrenics. I. Relapse rates, preliminary results. Arch Gen Psychiatry 40:893–896

Kelly HB, Freeman HL, Banning B, Schiff AA (1977) Clinical and social comparison of fluphenazine decanoate and flupenthixol decanoate in the community maintenance therapy of schizophrenia. Int Pharmacopsychiatry 12:54–64

Keskiner A (1973) A long-term follow-up fluphenazine enanthate treatment. Curr Ther Res 15:305–313

Kielholz P (1960) Diagnostik und Therapie der erschöpfungsdepressiven Zustandsbilder. Wien Med Wochenschr 1960:714

Kielholz P, Terzani S, Pöldinger W (1979) The long-term treatment of periodical and cyclic depressions with flupenthixol decanoate. Int Pharmacopsychiatry 14:305–309

Klein DF, Fink M (1962) Psychiatric reaction patterns to imipramine. Am J Psychiatry 119:432–438

Knights A, Hirsch SR (1981) Revealed depression and drug treatment for schizophrenia. Arch Gen Psychiatry 38:806–811

Knights A, Okash MS, Salih MA, Hirsch SR (1979) Depressive and extrapyramidal symptoms and clinical effects: a trial of fluphenazine versus flupenthixol in maintenance of schizophrenic outpatients. Br J Psychiatry 135:515–523

Kraepelin E (1913) Psychiatrie, 8th edn. Johann Ambrosius Barth, Leipzig

Langner E, Stössl J (1984) Analyse der Wirkungsmodalitäten einer Standard- und Hochdosierung von Fluphenazin-Decanoat aufgrund einer Doppelblindstudie. In: Kryspin-Exner K, Hinterhuber H, Schubert H (eds) Langzeittherapie psychiatrischer Erkrankungen. Schattauer, Stuttgart

Lehmann E, Quadbeck H, Tegeler J, Fararuni M, Heinrich K (1980) Wirkungsdifferenzen bei Hoch- und Standarddosierung von Fluphenazin-Decanoat in Abhängigkeit von Patienten-Merkmalen. Pharmacopsychiatry 13:117–120

Lerner Y, Moscovich D (1983) Depressive symptoms in acute schizophrenic hospitalized patients. J Clin Psychiatry 46:483–484

Mandel MR, Severe JB, Schooler NR, Gelenberg AJ, Mieske M (1982) Development and prediction of postpsychotic depression in neuroleptic-treated schizophrenics. Arch Gen Psychiatry 39:197–203

Marder SR, van Putten T, Mith J, McKenzie J, Lebell H, Faltico G, May PRA (1984) Costs and benefits of two doses of fluphenazine. Arch Gen Psychiatry 41:1025–1029

Marder SR, van Putten T, Mintz J, Lebell M, McKenzie J, May PRA (1987) Low- and conventional-dose maintenance therapy with fluphenazine decanoate. Two-year outcome. Arch Gen Psychiatry 44:518–521

Marneros A, Tsuang MT (eds) (1986) Schizoaffective psychoses. Springer, Berlin Heidelberg New York Tokyo

Mayer-Gross W (1920) Über die Stellungnahme zur abgelaufenen akuten Psychose. Z Neurol Psychiatr 60:160–212

McClelland HA, Farquharson RG, Leyburn P, Furness JA, Schiff AA (1976) Very high dose fluphenazine decanoate. Arch Gen Psychsatry 33:1435–1439

McCreadie RG, Flanagan WL, McKnight J, Jorgensen A (1979) High-dose flupenthixol decanoate in chronic schizophrenia. Br J Psychiatry 135:175–179

McGlashan TH, Carpenter WT (1976a) An investigation of the postpsychotic depressive syndrome. Am J Psychiatry 133:14–19

McGlashan TH, Carpenter WT (1976b) Postpsychotic depression in schizophrenia. Arch Gen Psychiatry 33:231–239

McKinnon BL (1977) Postpsychotic depression and the need for personal significance. Am J Psychiatry 134:427–429

Meyer HH (1950) Zyklothyme Wellen in schizophrenen Psychosen. Zbl Neurol Psychiatr 108:314

Möller HJ, von Zerssen D (1981a) Depressive Symptomatik bei Aufnahme und Entlassung stationär behandelter schizophrener Patienten. Nervenarzt 52:525–530

Möller HJ, von Zerssen D (1981b) Depressive Symptomatik im stationären Behandlungsverlauf von 280 schizophrenen Patienten. Pharmacopsychiatry 14:172–179

Müller P (1981) Depressive Syndrome im Verlauf schizophrener Psychosen. Enke, Stuttgart

Müller P, Kind J, Steuber H (1978) Pharmakogene depressive Syndrome im Verlauf schizophrener Psychosen. Arzneimittelforschung 28:1501–1502

Niskanen P, Tamminen T, Viukari M (1975) Sulpiride vs amitriptyline in the treatment of depression. Curr Ther Res 17:281–286

Pietzcker A, Gaebel W, Köpcke W, Linden M, Müller P, Müller-Spahn F, Schüssler G, Tegeler J (1986) A German multicenter study on the neuroleptic long-term therapy of schizophrenic patients. Preliminary report. Pharmacopsychiatry 19:161–166

Pinto A, Bannerjee A, Gosh N (1979) A double-blind comparison of flupenthixol decanoate and fluphenazine decanoate in the treatment of chronic schizophrenia. Acta psychiatr Scand 60:313–322

Platz T, Hinterhuber H (1981) Die hochdosierte Neuroleptikatherapie. Pharmacopsychiatry 14:141–147

Pollack M, Klein DF, Willner A (1965) Imipramine-induced behavioral disorganization in schizophrenic patients: physiological and psychological correlates. Rec Adv Biol Psychiatry 7:53–61

Prusoff BA, Williams DH, Weissman MM, Astrachan BA (1979) Treatment of secondary depression in schizophrenia. Arch Gen Psychiatry 36:569–575

Rifkin A (1981) The risks of long-term neuroleptic treatment of schizophrenia: especially depression and akinesia. Acta Psychiatr Scand [Suppl] 291:63–75

Rifkin A, Siris SG (1986) Zum heutigen Erkenntnisstand der Problematik: Depression bei der Schizophrenie. In: Hinterhuber H, Schubert H, Kulhanek F (eds) Seiteneffekte und Störwirkungen der Psychopharmaka. Schattauer, Stuttgart, pp 67–78

Rifkin A, Quitkin F, Klein DF (1975) Akinesia: a poorly recognized drug-induced extrapyramidal disorder. Arch Gen Psychiatry 32:672–674

Rifkin A, Quitkin F, Rabiner CJ, Klein DF (1977) Fluphenazine decanoate, fluphenazine hydrochloride given orally and placebo in remitted schizophrenics. Arch Gen Psychiatry 34:43–47

Roth S (1970) The seemingly ubiquitous depression following acute schizophrenic episodes: a neglected area of clinical discussion. Am J Psychiatry 127:51–58

Roy A (1984) Do neuroleptics cause depression? Biol Psychiatry 19:777–781

Roy A, Thompson R, Kennedy S (1983) Depression in chronic schizophrenia. Br J Psychiatry 142:465–470

Schmitt W (1967) Zur Frage des psychopathologischen Strukturwandels pharmakotherapierter endogener Psychosen. In: Kranz H, Heinrich K (eds) Pharmakopsychiatrie und Psychopathologie. Thieme, Stuttgart

Schooler NR, Levine J, Severe JB (1980) Prevention of relapse in schizophrenia: an evaluation of fluphenazine decanoate. Arch Gen Psychiatry 37:19–24

Shanfield S, Tucker GJ, Harrow M, Detre T (1970) The schizophrenic patient and depressive symptomatology. J Nerv Ment Dis 151:203–210

Siris SG, Kammen DP van, Docherty JP (1978) Use of antidepressant drugs in schizophrenia. Arch Gen Psychiatry 35:1368–1377

Siris SG, Harmon GK, Endicott J (1981) Postpsychotic depressive symptoms in hospitalized schizophrenic patients. Arch Gen Psychiatry 38:1212–1223

Steinberg HR, Green R, Durell J (1967) Depression occurring during the course of recovery from schizophrenic symptoms. Am J Psychiatry 124:699–702

Steiner S (1984) MODELL VIII – Konzept und Verwirklichung einer neuroleptischen Intensivbehandlung bei schizophrenen Patienten. Facultas, Vienna

Stern MJ, Pillsbury JA, Sonnenberg SM (1972) Post-psychotic depression in schizophrenics. Compr Psychiatry 13:591–598

Tsuang MT, Woolson RF, Fleming JA (1979) Long-term outcome of major psychoses. I. Schizophrenia and affective disorders compared with psychiatrically symptom-free surgical conditions. Arch Gen Psychiatry 36:1295–1301

Vaillant G (1962) The prediction of recovery in schizophrenia. J Nerv Ment Dis 135:534–543

van Putten T, May PRA (1978) Akinetic depression in schizophrenia. Arch Gen Psychiatry 35:1101–1107

Vogl G, Zaudig M (1983) Zur Frage der operationalisierten Diagnostik schizoaffektiver und zykloider Psychosen. Arch Psychiatr Nervenkr 233:385–396

Weitbrecht HJ (1959) Zur Psychopathologie der sogenannten Erschöpfung. Med Klin 26: 1136–1144

Welner A, Croughan L, Robins E (1974) The group of schizoaffective and related psychoses – critique, record, follow-up and family studies. I. A persistent enigma. Arch Gen Psychiatry 31:628–631

World Health Organization (1973) The international pilot study of schizophrenia. WHO, Geneva

Young JPR, Hughes WC, Lader MH (1976) A controlled comparison of flupenthixol and amitriptyline in depressed outpatients. Br Med J 1:1116–1118

Antidepressants and Neuroleptics in Treatment and Prophylaxis of Schizoaffective Psychoses

H.-J. Möller[1]

Introduction

Over the past 20 years, the schizoaffective psychoses have become an extremely interesting and intensively researched area (Marneros and Tsuang 1986). Despite variations in the definition of this diagnostic group, attempts have been made to investigate genealogical, genetic, biological, and case-specific aspects of schizoaffective psychoses and to classify them by placing them either among the schizophrenic psychoses (Detre and Jarecki 1971), among the affective psychoses (Pope and Lipinski 1978), or in a separate diagnostic category between these two broad areas of endogenous psychoses (Klein et al. 1981).

Despite this interest, the pharmacologic treatment of this group of endogenous psychoses, which are characterized by a mixture of affective and schizophrenic symptoms, has until now received little attention in carefully designed studies. It seems that the transfer of empirically determined treatment approaches from the areas of affective psychoses and the schizophrenias appeared theoretically sensible and was not regarded as requiring complicated empirical justification. Investigations dealing specifically with the treatment of schizoaffective disorders have been carried out only in more recent years. It is possible that the establishment of more specific diagnostic concepts, e.g., the Research Diagnostic Criteria (RDC), has created necessary diagnostic tools which were previously lacking.

Of course, in the forefront of the efforts to determine which pharmacologic treatment strategy has the best therapeutic effect is the issue of immediate therapeutic relevance. In addition, it has been postulated by several authors that the response to specific medications may enable nosologically relevant conclusions to be drawn: for example, a positive response of a schizodepressive disorder to antidepressants or lithium would indicate that this disorder belongs among the affective psychoses (Forssman and Walinder 1970; Sicignano and Lichtenstein 1978). This position has been rejected by other authors (Shopsin et al. 1970; Dunner and Fieve 1978; Braden et al. 1982).

---

[1] Psychiatrische Klinik und Poliklinik der Universität, Sigmund-Freud-Straße 25, 5300 Bonn 1, FRG

Affective and Schizoaffective Disorders
Edited by A. Marneros and M.T. Tsuang
© Springer-Verlag Berlin Heidelberg 1990

Nosologic and Syndromic Approaches in Psychopharmacology

In order to elucidate the theoretical background of the different approaches in psychopharmacology and the consequences for therapy arising from them, I will now give a very general description of the nosologic and syndromic approaches in current clinical pharmacology and of the corresponding positions held regarding some disorders relevant for our discussion: depressive illness, delusional depression, depressive disorders in the context of schizophrenic illnesses, and schizo-depressive syndromes in the context of schizoaffective psychoses. Only when these basic theoretical positions and the practical approaches to the various types of disorder derived from these positions have been examined and understood can the relevant facts be analyzed sensibly.

Two basic positions can be discerned in current clinical psychopharmacology (Möller 1987a). The symptomatic/syndromic approach (Freyhan 1957; Van Praag 1978) considers particular symptoms or groups of symptoms to be the targets of psychopharmacologic interventions; expressed in the simplest terms, this approach involves the administration of "sedating" psychoactive agents to agitated/hyperactive patients and of "stimulating" agents to apathetic/anergic patients. This means that, for example, relatively sedating neuroleptics would be recommended for treating not only agitated schizophrenics but also agitated depressives, in the latter either in combination with sedating antidepressants or as a monotherapy. Similarly, stimulating antidepressants would be indicated for anhedonic depressives and schizophrenics. By contrast, the nosologic approach views the diagnosis as being the decisive criterion for determining which medication should be used (Simpson and Watts 1965; Klein 1968), so neuroleptics would be indicated to treat the various schizophrenic disorders and antidepressants to treat the various syndromes associated with (endogenous) depression.

These different clinical-psychopharmacologic positions are by no means insignificant in their effects on practical clinical strategies, for they contribute to the formation of basic theoretical attitudes and associated stereotypic patterns in prescribing medication. The syndrome-oriented psychiatrist will in general be prepared to employ a single psychoactive agent in treating a specific target symptom or syndrome even the patients involved may come from different diagnostic groups, while the nosologically oriented psychiatrist would assume a more "purist" position, according to which neuroleptics would be administered essentially only to schizophrenics, and antidepressants only to (endogenous) depressives. At a more sophisticated level, it is obvious that when the nosologic approach is being used a syndromic perspective, which provides to a certain extent a secondary decision-making criterion, can also be employed.

The difference between the two positions is most clearly seen in a comparison of their views on the significance of neuroleptics in the treatment of depressive disorders. On the basis of experiences indicating that the syndromic spectrum of effects of some neuroleptics include antidepressant effects, several authors working during the early phase of psychopharmacology reported that certain neuroleptics were as effective as antidepressants in the treatment of depression (Overall et al. 1964, 1966). Other researchers have criticized these findings, pointing out that the term "depression" was not defined uniformly and that this was the source of the unexpected results (Raskin et al. 1970; McConaghy 1970). If treatment is addressing the symptom "depressivity," which can occur in any diagnostic group, then it may be that neuroleptics are just as effective as antidepressants. In this regard one must bear in mind that these depressive states may often be characteristic of illnesses for which neuroleptics are usually indicated. If, however, endogenous depression is considered, i.e., the illness which from a nosologic point of view represents the main indication for antidepressants, then more distinct differences in efficacy in favor of the antidepressants can be expected (Simpson et al. 1972).

This controversy, which first arose shortly after the discovery of antipsychotic agents, has to this day not been settled by verifiable conclusions drawn from empirical data. That these agents were named "neuroleptic" or "antidepressant" reflects their classification according to primary indication, a classification to which agreement – especially during the early phase of psychopharmacology – was slow in coming (Arnold et al. 1970; Bobon 1973). It was particularly unclear whether the "antianxiety" effect of the neuroleptics was being confused with an "antidepressive" effect in a more strict sense (Robertson and Trimble 1982). Later empirical findings supplied arguments and counterarguments regarding the use of neuroleptics in the treatment of depressive illnesses (Simpson et al. 1972; Raskin et al. 1970; Paykel 1977; Pöldinger and Sieberns 1983; Overall et al. 1969; Menter and Mandel 1979). However, it gradually became clear that circumstances were more complex than was originally assumed: both pharmacologically and clinically, it appeared that the effect of the neuroleptics changed as a function of dosage, i.e., at the usual clinical dosages antipsychotic tranquilization took place, while at substantially lower dosages antidepressive stimulation occurred (Simpson 1969). More recently, this difference has been explained by postulating different points of attack at the dopaminergic receptors in the CNS: a postsynaptic attack for tranquilization, a presynaptic one for stimulation (Puech et al. 1984).

The differences between the nosologic and syndromic approaches to establishing medication indications also become evident when it comes to deciding whether a neuroleptic is indicated in addition to an antidepressant in delusional depression in order to resolve ego-syntonic delusional symptoms. From the nosologic position, which takes the ego-syntonic delusion to be a result of the depressed state, the use of a neuroleptic here would not necessarily make sense, while from the syndromic position, which views neuroleptics as a means to combat delusions, such use makes complete sense. These clinical considerations, however, are independent from the still open question of the extent to which ego-syntonic delusions and schizophrenic symptoms may be related to functional disturbances of central dopaminergic synapses or explained by the types of malfunctions in the noradrenergic and serotonergic systems which serve as the bases for biological models of depression. There are some empirical findings from clinical studies which appear to confirm that neuroleptics can be sensibly employed alone or in combination with antidepressants in the treatment of delusional depression: as regards global therapeutic effect, this treatment mode is superior to monotherapy using antidepressants (Spiker et al. 1982, 1985; Nelson and Bowers 1978). Nevertheless, it is not completely clear whether such positive findings are indeed always related to mood discordant delusions or even whether mood discrepant delusions are predominantly implicated. Inclusion of the latter would then from the point of view of traditional psychiatry in the German-speaking countries speak more for a diagnosis of schizoaffective psychosis, thus possibly implying the implementation of treatment with neuroleptics (see below).

The reverse problem is presented by the existence of depressed or apathetic states in the context of schizophrenic illness (Prusoff et al. 1979; Siris 1978). The more nosologically inclined clinician would, at least initially, regard the use of neuroleptics as being indicated in such cases, since he views symptoms of depression as a component of an underlying disorder which should be treated with neuroleptics (Hirsch 1983; Möller and von Zerssen 1986). The more syndrome-oriented clinician, on the other hand, would in such cases tend more towards the use of antidepressants, although he might be concerned about the – probably overestimated (Prusoff et al. 1979) – risk of provoking schizophrenic symptoms with this kind of stimulation. Neither approach appears to be especially successful, at least not when residual symptoms rather than actual depressed states are concerned (Klein and Rüther 1983). In acute depressed and/or apathetic states within the context of schizophrenic psychoses, one must differentiate between etiologically different but clinically hardly distinguishable forms (Möller and von Zerssen 1986). Depression accompanying an acute schizophrenic illness for the most part resolves, albeit with a certain time lag, as the neuroleptic treatment reduces the schizophrenic symptoms and thus, in contrast to endogenous depression, does not require the use of antidepressants. Precisely this fact represents an important argument against the "target syndrome" approach, since although schizophrenics are just as "depressed" as endogenous depressives, the treatment of schizophrenic symptoms with a neuroleptic suffices. One can discern here a psychopharmacologic variation of Jaspers' "*Schichtenregel*": the treatment of the deepest layer of disturbance suffices, as all of the more superficial layers will then normalize automatically. The (pharmacologically triggered?) depressions observed particularly in long-term treatment with neuroleptics are often viewed as "akinesia" or "akinetic depression" in the sense of a Parkinson-like syndrome (Rifkin et al. 1975) and as such should respond well to anticholinergic agents or dose reduction; alternatively, they may be interpreted as specific neuroleptic-induced depressions, analogous to reserpine depression, and in this case would require treatment with antidepressants. On the whole, however, the success of antidepressant therapy of depressed states in the context of schizophrenic illness is not comparable to the significant effects shown for endogenous depression (Klein and Rüther 1983).

How problematic the issues under discussion here are becomes more evident when one considers schizodepressive states. If one views these conditions (from an extreme nosologic viewpoint, then, depending on the diagnostic category a particular case is assigned to, a schizodepressive state might have to be treated with neuroleptics, with antidepressants, or with a combination of both, in the first case the state being ascribed to a schizophrenic disorder, in the second to an affective psychosis, and in the third to a mixture somewhere between schizophrenia and affective psychosis. To the syndrome-oriented clinician it will at least initially be apparent that he must prescribe neuroleptics to treat the schizophrenic syndrome and antidepressants to treat the depressive syndrome, possibly needing to adjust the dosages according to which range of symptoms is predominant. However, if one compares the empirical profile of patients with schizophrenia and schizoaffective psychosis, the similarity can be seen and one questions the validity of the latter approach: both are characterized by depressive and schizophrenic symptoms. There is no conclusive empirical evidence showing that one of these approaches is superior to the other, but if one for the moment uncritically accepts the position presented by Nedopil and Rüther (1983), then this would seem to indicate that neuroleptics are more effective and more often prescribed as monotherapies than antidepressants. It also appears that many clinicans' decisions to add an antidepressant are influenced not so much by the depressive symptoms presented but rather seem to follow another rationale. It is possible that anamnestic data (e.g., history of manic or depressive episodes) or other factors play a greater role in this decision-making process.

Diagnosis in Schizoaffective Illness and Clinical Psychopharmacology

The results of research on treatment of schizodepressive illness are strongly dependent on the diagnostic concepts employed. For this reason the results of older studies of pharmacologic therapy of this disorder are difficult to interpret, since the studies distinguish, if anything, only between mood-congruent and mood-incongruent delusions in the context of psychotic depression. The introduction of ICD-8 and ICD-9 and particularly of operationalized diagnostic systems has only partially relieved this situation. Although various operationalized diagnostic systems have been used to establish relatively unambiguous definitions of some illnesses, it must be pointed out that the various definitions of a particular illness may be based on different theoretical ideas about the illness. It is not possible to provide an outline of current pharmacologic treatment of schizoaffective syndromes without giving sufficient attention to the problem of diagnosis.

The differences between the various diagnostic concepts for schizoaffective psychoses are a result of different viewpoints regarding the following:

1. *The definitions of schizophrenic and affective symptomatologies.* The question of affective symptomatology in schizoaffective illness is especially relevant: Are all the clinical symptoms of an endogenous depression required, or do symptoms of major depression suffice?
2. *The temporal relationship of depressive and schizophrenic symptoms.* Must both be present simultaneously or does the (separate) occurrence of affective and schizophrenic symptoms in different phases throughout the course of the

illness suffice? In the case of mixed symptoms which symptoms, arise first, and which dominate over time and in relative intensity?

3. *Drawing the line between affective and schizophrenic psychoses.* For example, does Jaspers' *Schichtenregel* apply, i.e., does the presence of schizophrenic symptoms always indicate schizophrenic illness even if affective symptoms are also present, or is the inverse position (as formulated in DSM-III) where affective symptoms support the diagnosis of an affective psychosis despite the presence of schizophrenic symptoms true?

Diagnostic systems which follow the *Schichtenregel* (as is the case in the classical psychiatry of the German-speaking countries) or DSM-III basically do not allow for the existence of schizoaffective psychosis as a nosologically distinct entity, since these systems prefer to classify a particular case in one of the two categories according to their respective algorithms. Because of this, the concept of schizoaffective psychosis was introduced relatively late into classical German psychiatry and in DSM-III was defined only as a residual group, a position which was altered in DSM-III-R. That schizoaffective psychosis is not a subgroup of the schizophrenic or affective disorders, but most probably represents an independent diagnostic group, is a position that is becoming more firmly established and one which will be reflected in ICD-10.

If one employs a polydiagnostic instrument, as was done in Berner's study (1987), it can be seen that, in keeping with the different diagnostic concepts presented above, patients presenting with functional psychoses will, according to the respective diagnostic system, be classified as belonging in the group of schizoaffective psychoses or another diagnostic group. The same diagnosis can be reached for different reasons. In Berner's study, of 200 patients who were admitted for the first time with a functional psychosis, 37 were classified as "schizoaffective" by RDC, 33 by ICD-9, 6 by DSM-III, and 4 by Vienna Research Criteria (VRC). The agreement between the two broader (RDC and ICD-9) and the two narrower (DSM-III and VRC) definitions was relatively good ($\kappa = 0.69$ and 0.59, respectively). Nevertheless, it is notable that nearly one-third of the RDC schizoaffectives were not assigned to this category under ICD criteria and that half of the DSM schizoaffectives were not diagnosed as such using the VRC. Although most of the cases diagnosed under the narrower definitions were also diagnosed using the broader criteria, they only comprise a small proportion of the latter. When schizomanic and schizodepressive cases are differentiated, classification of the depressive cases appears to be much more problematic. Of the 16 patients diagnosed by RDC to be schizodepressive, nearly one-third were designated by DSM-III as pure schizophrenics and one was diagnosed as having a paranoid disorder; the VRC left the diagnosis open in more than one-third of these cases, and two others were viewed as schizophrenia.

Our experiences in the context of a large follow-up project carried out in the Max Planck Psychiatric Institute have been similar (Möller et al. 1989). Data from this study make it clear that the concepts of schizoaffective illness which provide the basis of the various diagnostic systems are very different from each other, and that only the broader definitions are acceptable for therapy studies since the narrow ones allow very few patients with functional psychoses to be diagnosed as schizoaffective.

Empirical Studies on Treatment and Prophylaxis of Schizoaffective Disorders

As mentioned above, several problems complicate interpretations of psychopharmacological studies in this field. In early psychopharmacological studies the subcategory schizoaffective psychoses was not in general used, and when it has been used in more recent studies, the definitions have differed (ICD, RDC, DSM-III, etc.; Möller and Morin, 1989). Other methodological pitfalls concern differences in design, ex post subgrouping, small numbers of patients, discrepancies in treatment procedures, lack of differentiation between the relative strengths of schizophrenic and depressive symptoms in each case, etc. Prospective controlled double-blind studies focusing only on treatment of schizoaffective disorders are quite seldom.

In spite of these methodological problems some general conclusions can be drawn based on the empirical evidence communicated in the literature.

Acute Treatment of Schizodepressive Patients

In discussing therapy of delusional depressions Kantor and Glassman (1977) came to the conclusion that delusional depressives are much less responsive to antidepressants than nondelusional depressives. This overall conclusion seemed true to the authors independent of whether the delusions were mood-congruent or mood-incongruent. An important point was that a high percentage of patients with delusional depressions who did not respond to antidepressants improved significantly with electroconvulsive therapy (ECT).

Further important steps in this field were the publications of Spiker (1981), Spiker et al. (1982, 1985), and Nelson and Bowers (1978). They concluded that in delusional depressions better results are achieved by combining antidepressants with neuroleptics.

A recent review on the pharmacological treatment of schizoaffective patients was published by Goodnick and Meltzer (1984). The authors described 12 studies on schizodepressive patients, although only six of them were double-blind (see Table 1). Most patients were treated with tricyclic antidepressants and only in a few studies with neuroleptics.

Four of these studies investigated the response rate of depressives and schizodepressives undergoing treatment with antidepressants (Angst 1961; Greenblatt et al. 1962; Hordern et al. 1963; Avery and Winokur 1977). On average, the response rate of the schizodepressives was lower (41%) than that of the depressives (48%). If we exclude two studies reporting on fewer than 10 cases of schizoaffective psychoses, this becomes much more evident: the response rate for the schizodepressives amounts only to about 28%, in comparison to 45% in the depressives. Three studies using the RDC for diagnosing schizodepressive psychoses (Avery and Winokur 1977; Brockington et al. 1978, 1980) reported a response rate of 37%. These response rates are all quite low in comparison to the response rates of depressions generally found in the many psychopharmacological studies done in this diagnostic group.

Table 1. Acute treatment of schizoaffective depression and major depression (from Goodnick and Meltzer 1984)

Study	Subjects	Diagnostic criteria	Response measures	Medication	Duration	Condition	Results
Angst (1961)	41 MD 17 RD 7 SA	Author's	Author's	Imipramine 200 mg	2 weeks	Open	% Improved MD 63.4 RD 58.8 SAD 57.1
Greenblatt et al. (1962)	25 MD 24 "Psycho-neurotic" 10 Psychotic 31 SA	Authors'	Global (authors') Mental status score Depression rating	ECT (≥9 treatments) Isocarboxazid 40–50 mg Phenelzine 60–75 mg Imipramine 150–187 mg	8 weeks	DB	% Marked improvement AD ECT Total MD 40.0 80.0 48.0 Psycho- neurotic 87.0 71.0 84.0 Psychotic 30.0 50.0 33.0 SAD 23.0 60.0 29.0
Hordern et al. (1963)	110 N-DD 23 DD 4 "S" D	Authors'	HAMD	Amitriptyline 200 mg Imipramine 200 mg Nonresponders receive ECT (all SA on amitriptyline)	4–6 weeks	DB	% Improvement to amitriptyline Nondelusional 88.0 Delusional 67.0 SAD 50.0
Small et al. (1975)	14 S 4 SAD	Feighner & authors'	BPRS GGI NOSIE	Continued neuroleptic Lithium 0.6–1.0 mEq/l Placebo	4 weeks	DB	% Positive response S 43.0 SAD 25.0

		Feighner diagnosis RDC (SA)	Clinical global (MD notes)			Retrospective	% Improved after treatment
Avery and Winokur (1977)	444 UP 47 BP 54 SA	RDC (SA)	(MD notes)	Amitriptyline 150 mg Imipramine 150 mg Desipramine 150 mg Nortriptyline 150 mg Protriptyline 45 mg Phenelzine 45 mg Tranylcypramine 30 mg Isocarboxazid 30 mg ECT 5 treatments	4 weeks (minimum 2 weeks at indicated drug dose)	UP BP SAD	ECT AD 52 26 43 33 41 33
Brockington et al. (1978)	41 SA (36 studied)	PSE + authors'	BPRS PSE	Amitriptyline 150–250 mg (13) CPZ 450–750 mg (11) Combined (12)	1 month	DB	(all SAD) Amitriptyline 45 CPZ 54 Amitriptyline + CPZ 75
Alexander et al. (1979)	5 S 5 SAD	RDC DSM-II	Bunney-Hamburg	Lithium mean 1600 mg 0.7–1.2 mEq/l plasma Placebo	3 weeks	DB	Improved: S 40% SA 40%
Van Kammen, et al. (1980)	1 S 10 SAD	RDC	Bunney-Hamburg	Lithium 900–2100 mg 0.7–1.3 mEq/l plasma	3 weeks	DB	Improvement in depression rating (more than 1.5) 60% of SAD

Table 1. (continued)

Study	Subjects	Diagnostic criteria	Response measures	Medication	Duration	Condition	Results
Prusoff et al. (1979)	40 Dep S	DSM-II NHSI + authors'	NHSI BPRS HAM depression Raskin SCL-90 SAS II	Continued perphenazine Amitriptyline 100–200 mg Placebo	1–6 months	DB	Symptom improvement of 0.05 significance BPRS thought disorder (6 months) HAMD somatization (2 months) HAMD anxiety-depression (4 months) Raskin depression (4 months)
Hirschkowitz et al. (1980)	20 S 9 SAD 2 SAM	RDC	NHSI ADRS	Lithium 1.1–1.4 mEq/l	2 weeks	Open	% Improved: S 25.0 SA 36.0
Brockington et al. (1980)	4 S 8 MD 60 SAD 4 Other	RDC	Authors'	Tricyclic anti-depressants, various neuroleptics ECT	Variable	Open	% Improved of SAD Tricyclic 33 Neuroleptic 55 ECT 62
Carman et al. (1981)	11 S 2 SAD	RDC	IBRS	Continued neuroleptic Lithium 0.75–1.3 mEq/l Placebo	4 weeks	DB	% improved Psychosis Depression S 18 36 SAD 0 50

MD, manic-depressive; SA, schizoaffective; S, schizophrenic; SAM, schizoaffective manic (used when schizoaffective depressed also present); SAD, schizoaffective depressed; RD, recurrent depressive; N-DD, nondelusional depression; DD, delusional depression; UP, unipolar; BP, bipolar; BPRS, Brief Psychiatric Rating Scale; IMPS; Inpatient Multidimensional Psychiatric Scale; CGI, Clinical Global Impression; HAM, Hamilton; PIP, Psychotic Inpatient Profile; NOSIE, Nurses Observation Scale for Inpatient Evaluation; RDC, Research Diagnostic Criteria; WHO, World Health Organization; DSM, Diagnostic and Statistical Manual; PSE, Present State Examination; SCL-90, Symptom Checklist-90; NHSI, New Haven Schizophrenia Index; IBRS, Inpatient Behavioral Rating Scale; SADS, Schedule for Affective Disorders and Schizophrenia; CPZ, chlorpromazine; ECT, electro-convulsive therapy; "S"D, "Schizophrenic mixture" depression; SAS II, Social Adjustment Scale; ADRS, Affective Disorder Rating Scale.

The review by Goodnick and Meltzer (1984) points out that neuroleptics have been investigated very seldom in schizodepressive episodes. One of the more informative investigations is the double-blind study by Brockington et al. (1978) comparing chlorpromazine, amitriptyline, and the combination of these two. The worst result (46%) was obtained by amitriptyline alone, whilst 54% responded to chlorpromazine treatment. The best result was obtained by the combination therapy (75% responders). Because of the small sample size, these results must be considered with caution but it should be mentioned that in a non randomized open study on a large sample (Brockington et al. 1980) the results were in favor to neuroleptics: 55% response rate with neuroleptics, 33% with antidepressants. This tendency was also confirmed in an open study by Good-nick and Meltzer (1984) who investigated 99 schizodepressives.

Four studies came to the conclusion that ECT is more effective in schizode-pressive patients than psychopharmacotherapy (Greenblatt et al. 1962; Hordern et al. 1963; Avery and Winokur 1977; Brockington et al. 1980). On average the response rate was 55% with ECT and only about 30% with antidepressants.

To summarize:
1. Antidepressants seem in general not effective enough for treatment of schizodepressive patients.
2. Especially in patients who do not respond to antidepressants, neuroleptics or, perhaps better, the combination of antidepressants and neuroleptics seem to be indicated.

These are, however, only hypotheses which need to be tested in randomized, controlled studies. Such new studies should focus among other things on the prognostic implications of the ratio between schizophrenic and depressive symptoms.

Acute Treatment of Schizomanic Patients

Psychopharmacotherapy for acute schizomanic patients is less controversial. Neuroleptics are known from classical studies on treatment of schizophrenics (including schizoaffectives) to be effective and have long been indicated for these patients. Research has concentrated more on the questions of whether neuroleptics are as potent as lithium and whether the combination of lithium and neuroleptics would be superior.

Five double-blind controlled studies have compared the therapeutic effi-cacies of neuroleptics and lithium in schizomanic patients (see the review by Bandelow and Rüther, 1989). Overall, it seems from these studies that neuro-leptics are as effective as or more effective than lithium (Braden et al. 1982; Brockington et al. 1978; Johnson et al. 1968, 1971; Prien et al. 1972a). Especially in agitated cases, neuroleptics seem to be superior.

Three double-blind controlled studies compared monotherapy with neuro-leptics with combined neuroleptics and lithium in schizomanic patients (Bieder-man et al. 1979; Carman et al. 1981; Small et al. 1975). The results of these

Table 2. Acute treatment of schizoaffective mania and mania (from Goodnick and Meltzer 1984)

Study	Subjects	Diagnostic criteria	Response measures	Medication	Dose	Duration	Condition	Results
Rice (1956)	37 MD 9 SA 12 S	Author's	Author's	Lithium	0.4–2.4	1 month	Open	% Improved + recovered MD 92 SA 78 S 25
Gottfries (1968)	32 MD 19 SA 10 S	Unstated	Unstated	Lithium Placebo	Blood level 1.0 mEq/l	6 weeks	Open	% Improved MD 94 SA 84 S 0
Zall et al. (1968)	33 MD 10 SA	Authors'	Authors'	Lithium Placebo	Maximum blood level 1.5 mEq/l	2 weeks	Open	% Improved MD 79 SA 90 (little effect on S type symptoms)
Aronoff and Epstein (1970)	12 MD 6 SA	Authors'	Authors'	Lithium	Minimum blood level 0.9 mEq/l	10–14 days	Various	% Improved MD 100 SA 67
Johnson (1970)	19 MD 11 SA	Author's	BPRS CGI	Lithium Placebo	Blood level 1.0–2.5 mEq/l	21 days	Double blind	% Improved MD 95 SA 45
Prien et al. (1972a, 1972b)	255 MD 83 SA	DSM-II Mayer-Gross	BPRS IMPS PIP	Lithium CPZ	Blood level 0.6–2.0 mEq/l 1000 mg	3 weeks	Double-blind	Improvement averaged over entire group Lithium = CPZ "Highly active," CPZ better
Small et al. (1975)	4 SAM 4 SAD 14 S	Feighner Authors'	BPRS CGI NOSIE	Continued neuroleptic Lithium Placebo	Blood level 0.6–1.0 mEq/l	4 weeks	Double-blind	% Improved SAM 100 SAD 25 S 43

Study				Drugs	Therapeutic blood levels / dose	Duration	Design	Results
Brockington et al. (1978)	19 SAM	PSE Authors'	BPRS	Lithium / CPZ	Therapeutic blood levels Minimum 400 mg	1 month	Double-blind	% Improved Lithium 83 CPZ 80
Megrabyan et al. (1979)	23 SA	Authors'	Authors'	Lithium / Placebo	Blood levels 1.5–2.0 mEq/l	Unknown	Unknown	% Improved Lithium 83
Alexander et al. (1979)	3 SAM 5 SAD 5 S	RDC DSM-II	Bunney-Hamburg	Lithium / Placebo	Blood levels 0.7–1.2 mEq/l	3 weeks	Double-blind	% Improved SAM 100 SAD 40 S 40
Biederman et al. (1979)	36 SA	RDC	BPRS CGI Beigel-Murphy	Continued neuroleptic Lithium Placebo	Minimum 1200 mg	4 weeks	Double-blind	Lithium better than placebo in 5 subscales of BPRS
Pope et al. (1980)	34 MD 52 SA 41 S	RDC	Physician notes	Lithium Neuroleptics	Unknown	Variable	Open	% Moderately improved Mania: Lithium 100 ($n = 13$) Lithium + neuroleptic 100 ($n = 17$) Neuroleptic 67 ($n = 3$) Schizomanic: Lithium 95 ($n = 20$) Lithium + neuroleptic 86 ($n = 14$) Neuroleptic 83 ($n = 12$) Schizophrenia: Neuroleptic 55 ($n = 40$)

Table 2. (continued)

Study	Subjects	Diagnostic criteria	Response measures	Medication	Dose	Duration	Condition	Results
Carman et al. (1981)	11 S 5 SAM 2 SAD	RDC	IBRS	Continued neuroleptic Lithium Placebo	Blood level 0.75–1.3 mEq/l	4 weeks	Double-blind	% Improved Psychosis: SAM 60 S 18 Arousal: SAM 80 S 36
Hirschkowitz et al. (1980)	20 S 11 SA	RDC	NHSI ADRS	Lithium	Blood level 1.1–1.4 mEq/l	2 weeks	Open	% Improved S 25.0 SA 36.0
Goodnick and Meltzer (1983)	41 MD 30 SA	RDC	SADS-C BPRS	Lithium Neuroleptic	Blood Levels 0.8–1.5 mEq/l Equivalent CPZ 800 mg	Variable	Open	% Improved MD 100 SA 100 Differences only in degree and rate of response

MD, manic-depressive; SA, schizoaffective; S, schizophrenic; SAM, schizoaffective manic (used when schizoaffective depressed also present); SAD, schizoaffective depressed; RD, recurrent depressive; N-DD, nondelusional depression; DD, delusional depression; UP, unipolar; BP, bipolar; BPRS, Brief Psychiatric Rating Scale; IMPS; Inpatient Multidimensional Psychiatric Scale; CGI, Clinical Global Impression; HAM, Hamilton; PIP, Psychotic Inpatient Profile; NOSIE, Nurses Obsevation Scale for Inpatient Evaluation; RDC, Research Diagnostic Criteria; WHO, World Health Organization; DSM, Diagnostic and Statistical Manual; PSE, Present State Examination; SCL-90, Symptom Checklist-90; NHSI, New Haven Schizophrenia Index; IBRS, Inpatient Behavioral Rating Scale; SADS, Schedule for Affective Disorders and Schizophrenia; CPZ, chlorpromazine; ECT, electroconvulsive therapy; "S"D, "Schizophrenic mixture" depression; SAS II, Social Adjustment Scale; ADRS, Affective Disorder Rating Scale.

Table 3. Prophylactic treatment of schizoaffective disorders (from Goodnick and Meltzer 1984)

Study	Subjects	Diagnostic criteria	Response measures	Medication	Dose	Duration	Condition	Results
Hofmann et al. (1970)	46 MD 54 RD 19 SA	DSM-II Authors'	Authors'	Lithium	Unknown	Unknown	Open	% At least moderate prevention MD 72 SA 53
Aronoff and Epstein (1970)	12 MD 6 SA	Authors'	Authors'	Lithium	Minimum blood level 0.6 mEq/l	3 years	Open	% Moderate prevention MD 58 SA 83
Angst et al. (1970)	114 MD 58 RD 72 SA	WHO Authors'	Hospital admission Change in treatment	Lithium	0.8–1.2 mEq/l blood level	1–4 years	Open	% With decreased frequency of episodes MD 67 RD 57 SA 49
Prien et al. (1973, 1974)	192 MD 6 SA	DSM-II Mayer-Gross	IMPS Global affective KAS	Lithium Placebo	0.5–1.4 mEq/l blood level	2 years	Double-blind	% Severe relapse after discontinuing lithium MD 31 SA 60
Smulevitch et al. (1974)	50 MD 49 SA	WHO DSM-II	Authors'	Lithium Placebo	0.6–0.8 mEq/l blood level	1–3 years	Open	Effective % MD 88 SA 83

Table 3. (continued)

Study	Subjects	Diagnostic criteria	Response measures	Medication	Dose	Duration	Condition	Results
Hullin et al. (1975)	9 M, 47 MD, 36 RD, 3 SA	Authors'	Hospital admissions, Time in hospital	Lithium Placebo	0.6–1.4 mEq/l blood level	18–75 months	Open	% Readmission during treatment M 0, MD 45, RD 19, SA 33
Perris (1978)	18 "Cycloid psychosis"	Author's (similar to DSM-II "schizo-affective")	Episodes, Months of hospitalization	Lithium Placebo	0.6–0.8 mEq/l blood level	1–8.5 years	Open	% Reduction after treatment Episodes 76, Months hospitalization 90
Tress and Haag (1979)	21 MD, 22 SA	Leonhard Authors'	Episodes	Lithium	Unknown	MD: 2.8 ± 1.8 years, SA: 2.4 ± 1.4 years	Open	% Reduction in relapse/patient/year MD 51, SA 69
Rosenthal et al. (1980)	46 MD, 25 SA	RDC	Mood scale, Treatment change	Lithium	Therapeutic blood levels	4 weeks	Combined Open + double-blind	% Likelihood of staying well at 1 year MD 55, SA 68
Sarantidis and Waters (1981)	37 MD, 9 SA	RDC	Days hospitalized, Authors'	Lithium	0.7 mEq/l mean blood level	2 years-51 months (mean)	Open	% Positive response MD 78, SA 89

MD, manic-depressive; RD, recurrent depressive; SA, schizoaffective; M, manic only; DSM, Diagnostic and Statistical Manual; WHO, World Health Organization; RDC, Research Diagnostic Criteria; KAS, Katz Adjustment Scale.

studies showed that combination therapy seems to give better results than neuroleptic monotherapy in agitated cases (Table 2).

Prophylactic Treatment of Schizoaffective Psychoses

An important point is whether neuroleptics or lithium should be used for the prophylactic treatment of schizoaffective psychoses. Some empirical data derived from prospective controlled studies (Table 3) have shown lithium to be efficacious (Goodnick and Meltzer 1984), but perhaps not as effective as in pure affective psychoses (Nedopil and Rüther 1983).

Neuroleptics are also efficacious in treating schizoaffective psychoses, as is well known from classical investigations on long-term treatment of schizophrenics, including schizoaffectives (Möller 1987b). Unfortunately, there is a lack of investigations comparing lithium and neuroleptics directly as regards their efficacy in preventing relapse. One controlled study has demonstrated that in patients with a predominantly schizophrenic schizoaffective psychosis, neuroleptics are more effective (Mattes and Nayak 1984). For these patients neuroleptics seem to be indicated as prophylactic treatment of first choice.

One problem of long-term treatment with neuroleptics, especially for schizoaffective psychoses, is the risk of neuroleptic-induced depressions. Another problem of therapy tolerability is the well-known risk of tardive dyskinesia. Taking these two problems into account, prophylactic treatment with lithium seems to be in general preferable, even though it might not be as effective. If this drug proves not to be efficacious in a particular case, neuroleptics or a combination of lithium and neuroleptics are indicated. Schizoaffective psychoses with predominantly schizophrenic symptoms (perhaps misdiagnosed schizophrenias?) should be treated with neuroleptics as the drug of first choice. All these suggestions, however, need empirical confirmation.

References

Alexander PE, van Kammen DP, Bunney WR (1979) Antipsychotic effects of lithium in schizophrenia. Am J Psychiatry 136:283–287

Angst J (1961) A clinical analysis of the effects of tofranil in depression. Psychopharmacologia 2:381–407

Angst J, Weis P, Grof P, Baastrup PC, Schou M (1970) Lithium prophylaxis in recurrent affective disorders. Br J Psychiatry 116:604–613

Arnold OH, Collard J, Deniker P, Ginestet D, Hippius H, Itil TM, Labhardt F, Leeds AA, Montanini R, Morozov G, Simon P, Villeneuve A (1970) Definition and classification of neuroleptics. Mod Probl Pharmacopsychiatry 5:141–147

Aronoff MS, Epstein RS (1970) Factors associated with poor response to lithium carbonate: a clinical study. Am J Psychiatry 127:472–480

Avery D, Winokur G (1977) The efficacy of electroconvulsive therapy and antidepressants in depression. Biol Psychiatry 12:507–523

Bandelow B, Rüther E (1989) Neuroleptika in der Behandlung schizoaffektiver Psychosen. In: Marneros A (ed) Schizoaffektive Psychosen. Diagnostik, Therapie und Prophylaxe. Springer, Berlin Heidelberg New York pp 149–158

Berner P (1987) Neuroleptika zur Behandlung schizoaffektiver Psychosen. In: Pichot P, Möller HJ (eds) Neuroleptika, Rückschau 1952–1986 – Künftige Entwicklungen. Springer, Berlin Heidelberg New York, pp 103–110

Biederman J, Lerner Y, Belmaker RH (1979) Combination of lithium carbonate and haloperidol in schizoaffective disorder. Arch Gen Psychiatry 36:327–333

Bobon DP (1973) Classification and terminology of psychotropic drugs. Pharmacopsychiatry 6:1–12

Braden W, Fink EB, Qualls CB, Ho CK, Samuels WO (1982) Lithium and chlorpromazine in psychotic patients. Psychiatry Res 7:69–81

Brockington IF, Kendell RE, Kellett JM, Curry SH, Wainwright S (1978) Trials of lithium, chlorpromazine and amitriptyline in schizoaffective patients. Br J Psychiatry 133:162–168

Brockington IF, Kendell RE, Wainwright S (1980) Depressed patients with schizophrenic or paranoid symptoms. Psychol Med 10:665–675

Carman JS, Bigelow LB, Wyatt RJ (1981) Lithium combined with neuroleptics in chronic schizophrenic and schizoaffective patients. J Clin Psychiatry 42:124–128

Detre TP, Jarecki HP (1971) Modern psychiatric treatment. Lippincott, Philadelphia

Dunner DL, Fieve RR (1978) The lithium ion: its impact on diagnostic practice. In: Akiskal HS, Wells WL (eds) Psychiatric diagnosis: exploration of biological predictors. SP Medical and Scientific Books, New York, pp 233–246

Forssman H, Walinder J (1970) Lithium as an aid in psychiatric diagnostics. Acta Psychiatr Scand (Suppl) 219:59–66

Freyhan FA (1957) Psychomotilität, extrapyramidale Syndrome und Wirkungsweisen neuroleptischer Therapie (Chlorpromazin, Reserpin, Prochlorperazin). Nervenarzt 28:504–509

Goodnick PJ, Meltzer HY (1983) Lithium treatment of schizomania and mania. Presented at the Annual Meeting of the American Psychiatric Association, May 1–6, 1983

Goodnick, PJ, Meltzer HY (1984) Treatment of schizoaffective disorders. Schizophr Bull 10:30–48

Gottfries CS (1968) Effect of lithium salts on various kinds of psychiatric disorders. Acta Psychiatr Scand (Suppl) 203:157–167

Greenblatt M, Grosser GH, Wechsler H (1962) A comparative study of selected antidepressant medications and ECT. Am J Psychiatry 119:144–153

Hirsch SR (1983) The causality of depression in schizophrenia. Br J Psychiatry 142:624–625

Hirschkowitz J, Casper R, Garver DL, Chang S (1980) Lithium response in good prognosis schizophrenia. Am J Psychiatry 137:916–920

Hofmann G, Kremser M, Katschnig H, Scheiber V (1970) Prophylaktische Lithiumtherapie bei manisch-depressivem Krankheitsgeschehen und bei Legierungspsychosen. Int Pharmacopsychiatry 4:187–193

Hordern A. Holt NF, Burt CG, Gordon WF (1963) Amitriptyline in depressive states. Br J Psychiatry 109:815–825

Hullin RP, McDonald R, Allsopp MNE (1975) Further report on prophylactic lithium in recurrent affective disorders. Br J Psychiatry 126:281–284

Johnson G (1970) Differential response to lithium carbonate in manic depressive and schizoaffective disorders. Dis Nerv Syst 31:613–615

Johnson G, Gershon S, Hekimian LJ (1968) Controlled evaluation of lithium and chlorpromazine in the treatment of manic states: an interim report. Compr Psychiatry 9:563–573

Johnson G, Gershon S, Burdock EI, Floyd A, Hekimian LJ (1971) Comparative effects of lithium and chlorpromazine in the treatment of acute manic states. Br J Psychiatry 119:267–276

Kantor SJ, Glassman AH (1977) Delusional depressions: natural history and response to treatment. Br J Psychiatry 131:351–360

Klein DF (1968) Importance of psychiatric diagnosis in prediction of clinical drug effect. Psychopharmacology 13:359–368

Klein DF, Rüther E (1983) Klinisch bedeutsame Wechselwirkungen der Psychopharmaka. In: Langer G, Heimann H (eds) Psychopharmaka. Grundlagen und Therapie. Springer, Vienna New York, pp 617–635

Klein DF, Gittelman R, Quitkin F, Rifkin A (1981) Diagnosis and drug treatment of psychiatric disorders. Williams and Wilkins, Baltimore

Marneros A, Tsuang MT (eds) (1986) Schizoaffective psychoses. Springer, Berlin Heidelberg New York

Mattes JA, Nayak D (1984) Lithium vs fluphenazine for prophylaxis in mainly schizophrenic schizoaffectives. Biol Psychiatry 19:445–449

McConaghy N (1970) Actuarial v. clinical prediction. Br J Psychiatry 117:122

Megrabyan, AA, Khachaturyan AM, Amadyan MG, Burnazyan GA (1979) The treatment of schizoaffective psychoses with lithium carbonate. Zh Eksp Klin Med 19 (4):54–58

Menter RE, Mandel MR (1979) The treatment of psychotic major disorder with drugs and electroconvulsive therapy. J Nerv Ment Dis 12:726–733

Möller HJ (1987a) Konsequenzen aus der klinischen Psychopharmakologie für die nosologische und syndromatologische Klassifikation funktioneller psychischer Störungen. In: Simhandl C, Berner P, Luccioni H, Alf C (eds) Klassifikationsprobleme in der Psychiatrie. Medizinisch-pharmazeutische Verlagsgesellschaft, Purkersdorf, pp 163–188

Möller HJ (1987b) Indikation und Differentialindikation der neuroleptischen Langzeitmedikation. In: Pichot P, Möller HJ (eds) Neuroleptika, Rückschau 1952–1986 – Künftige Entwicklungen. Springer, Berlin Heidelberg New York, pp 63–79

Möller HJ, Morin C (1989) Behandlung schizodepressiver Syndrome mit Antidepressiva. In: Marneros A (ed) Schizoaffektive Psychosen. Diagnose, Therapie und Prophylaxe. Springer, Berlin Heidelberg New York, pp 159–178

Möller HJ, von Zerssen D (1986) Depression in schizophrenia. In: Burrows GD, Norman TR, Rubinstein G (eds) Handbook of studies in schizophrenia. Part I. Elsevier, Amsterdam, pp 183–191

Möller HJ, Schmid-Bode W, Cording-Tömmel C, Wittchen HU, Zaudig M, von Zerssen D (1988) Psychopathological and social outcome in schizophrenia vs affective/schizoaffective psychoses and prediction of poor outcome in schizophrenia: Results from a 5–8 years follow-up. Acta Psychiatr Scand 77:379–389

Möller HJ, Hohe-Schramm M, Cording-Tömmel C, Schmidt-Bode W, Wittchen HU, Zaudig M, von Zerssen D (1989) The classification of functional psychoses and its implications for prognosis. Br J Psychiatry 154:467–472

Nedopil N, Rüther E (1983) Psychopharmakotherapie bei schizoaffektiven Psychosen. In: Langer G, Heimann H (eds) Psychopharmaka. Grundlagen und Therapie. Springer, Vienna New York, pp 467–476

Nelson IC, Bowers MB (1978) Delusional unipolar depression. Description and drug response. Arch Gen Psychiatry 35:1321–1328

Overall JE, Hollister LE, Meyer F (1964) Imipramine and thioridazine in depressed and schizophrenic patients: Are there specific antidepressant drugs? JAMA 189:605–608

Overall JE, Hollister LE, Johnson M (1966) Nosology of depression and differential response to drugs. JAMA 195:946–948

Overall JE, Hollister LE, Shelton J (1969) Broad-spectrum screening of psychotherapeutic drugs: thiothixene as an antipsychotic and antidepressant. Clin Pharmacol Ther 10:36–43

Paykel ES (1977) Response to treatment and depressive classification. In: Burrows GD (ed) Handbook of studies on depression. Excerpta Medica, Amsterdam, pp 21–47

Perris C (1978) Morbidity suppressive effect of lithium carbonate in cycloid psychosis. Arch Gen Psychiatry 35:328–331

Pöldinger W, Sieberns S (1983) Depression-inducing and antidepressive effects of neuroleptics. Experiences with flupenthixol and flupenthixol decanoate. Neuropsychobiology 10:131–136

Pope HG, Lipinski JF (1978) Diagnosis in schizophrenia and manic-depressive illness. Arch Gen Psychiatry 35:811–828

Pope HG, Lipinski JF, Cohen BM, Axelrod DT (1980) "Schizoaffective disorder": an invalid diagnosis? A comparison of schizoaffective disorder, schizophrenia, and affective disorder. Am J Psychiatry 137:921–927

Prien RF, Caffey EM, Klett CJ (1972a) A comparison of lithium carbonate and chlorpromazine in the treatment of excited schizoaffectives. Arch Gen Psychiatry 27:182–189

Prien RF, Caffey EM, Klett CJ (1972b) Comparison of lithium carbonate and chlorpromazine in the treatment of mania. Arch Gen Psychiatry 26:146–153

Prien RF, Caffey EM, Klett CJ (1973) Prophylactic efficacy of lithium carbonate in manic-depressive illness. Arch Gen Psychiatry 28:337–341

Prien RF, Caffey EM, Klett CJ (1974) Factors associated with treatment success in lithium carbonate prophylaxis. Arch Gen Psychiatry 31:189–192

Prusoff BA, Williams DH, Wiesman MM, Astrachan BA (1979) Treatment of secondary depression in schizophrenia. Arch Gen Psychiatry 36:569–575

Puech AJ, Lecrubier Y, Simon P (1984) Pharmacological classification of benzamides. Acta Psychiatr Scand (Suppl) 311:139–145

Raskin A, Schulterbrandt JG, Reating N, Chase C, McKeon JJ (1970) Differential response to chlorpromazine, imipramine, and placebo. A study of subgroups of hospitalized depressed patients. Arch Gen Psychiatry 23:164–173

Rice D (1956) The use of lithium salts in the treatment of manic states. J Ment Sci 102:604–611

Rifkin A, Quitkin F, Klein DF (1975) Akinesia, a poorly recognized drug induced extrapyramidal disorder. Arch Gen Psychiatry 32:672–674

Robertson MM, Trimble MR (1982) Major tranquilizers used as antidepressants. A review. J Affective Disord 4:173–193

Rosenthal NE, Rosenthal LN, Stallone F, Dunner DL, Fieve RR (1980) Toward the validation of RDC schizoaffective disorder. Arch Gen Psychiatry 37:804–810

Sarantidis D, Waters B (1981) Predictors of lithium prophylaxis effectiveness. Prog Neuropsychopharmacol 5:507–510

Shopsin B, Johnson G, Gershon S (1970) Neurotoxicity with lithium: Differential drug responsiveness. Int Pharmacopsychiatry 5:170–182

Sicignano JR, Lichtenstein J (1978) Rediagnosis of schizophrenia as bipolar affective illness. Hosp Commun Psychiatry 29:112–114

Simpson GM (1969) Experiences with thioxanthenes. Mod Probl Pharmacopsychiatry 2:76–79

Simpson GM, Watts TPS (1965) Antidepressant drugs. Am J Psychiatry 121:1028–1029

Simpson GM, Amin M, Angus JWS, Edwards JG, Hing Go S, Lee JH (1972) Role of antidepressants and neuroleptics in the treatment of depression. Arch Gen Psychiatry 27:337–345

Siris SG, van Kammen DP, Docherty JP (1978) Use of antidepressant drugs in schizophrenia. Arch Gen Psychiatry 35:1368–1377

Small JG, Kellams JJ, Milstein V, Moore J (1975) A placebo-controlled study of lithium combined with neuroleptics in chronic schizophrenic patients. Am J Psychiatry 132:1315–1317

Smulevitch AB, Zavidovskaya GI, Igonin AL, Mikhailova NM (1974) The effectiveness of lithium in affective and schizoaffective psychoses. Br J Psychiatry 125:65–72

Spiker DG (1981) Schizoaffective disease and atypical psychosis. Psychopharmacol Bull 17:75–78

Spiker DG, Hanin I, Perel JM, Cofsky AJ, Rossi AJ, Sorisio D (1982) Pharmacological treatment of delusional depressives. Psychopharmacol Bull 18:184–186

Spiker DG, Weiss JC, Dealy RS, Griffin SJ, Hanin I, Neil JF, Perel JM, Rossi AJ, Soloff PH (1985) The pharmacological treatment of delusional depression. Am J Psychiatry 142:430–436

Tress W, Haag H (1979) Vergleichende Erfahrungen mit der rezidivprophylaktischen Lithium-Langzeitmedikation bei schizoaffektiven Psychosen. Nervenarzt 50:524–526

Van Kammen DP, Alexander PE, Bunney WE (1980) Lithium treatment in post-psychotic depression. Br J Psychiatry 136:479–485

Van Praag HM (1978) Psychotropic drugs. A guide for the practitioner. Van Gorum, Amsterdam

Zall H, Therman PG, Myers JM (1968) Lithium carbonate. A clinical study. Am J Psychiatry 125:549–555

Lithium in Treatment and Prophylaxis of Affective and Schizoaffective Disorders

B. MÜLLER-OERLINGHAUSEN, K. THIES, and J. VOLK[1]

Introduction

Interest in the treatment and prophylaxis of schizoaffective patients with lithium salts seems to be related to two different aspects: First, there is an ongoing search for optimized therapeutic strategies, which always implies the question: Is it possible to replace neuroleptics, or to reduce their dosage in such patients in order to attenuate the risk of extrapyramidal motoric side effects (EPMS)? This is an important issue, since some authors have recently suggested that the risk of neuroleptic-induced EPMS may be particularly high in patients with affective psychosis (Kane 1988, Nasrallah et al. 1988, Waddington and Joussef 1988). Second, it is hoped or presumed that the response or nonresponse to lithium salts would provide a decisive a argument in favor of or against the classification of schizoaffective psychoses among the group of affective disorders (Goodnick and Meltzer 1984, Taylor 1986).

Regarding the latter aspect, however, we feel that some of the straight-forward reasoning in various papers appears to be premature, if not naive, in view of the fact that the mode of action and the specificity of lithium in various indications has remained a matter of controversy and still must be examined in more detail on various descriptive levels and by different approaches e.g., biological and psychological (Müller-Oerlinghausen 1988). It should also be mentioned that at least some evidence exists for a – not too well defined – antipsychotic activity of lithium salts. Delva and Letemendia (1982) reviewed the corresponding literature up to 1980. They reported on two controlled and a dozen uncontrolled studies of schizophrenic patients and came to the conclusion that lithium may be effective in about 30%–50% of schizophrenics. In one controlled study, however, lithium or placebo was added to an ongoing neuro-leptic treatment, and lithium was found to be significantly more effective (Small et al. 1975). In the study by Alexander et al. (1979), from the NIMH group, lithium alone was compared with placebo in a small group of patients; some antipsychotic activity was demonstrated within 7 days in about half of the sample, though full remission of symptoms was not obtained. Zemlan et al. (1984a) confirmed that core symptoms of schizophrenia (hallucinations, delu-sions, and formal thought disorders) showed the greatest change in the first 7

---

[1] Freie Universität Berlin, Psychiatrische Klinik, Klinische Psychopharmakologie, Eschenallee 3, 1000 Berlin 19, FRG

Affective and Schizoaffective Disorders
Edited by A. Marneros and M.T. Tsuang
© Springer-Verlag Berlin Heidelberg 1990

days; this fast reduction of symptoms in some patients could be used for an early prediction of lithium response with sensitivity and specificity of about 90%. Lithium has also been used successfully in the treatment of periodically occurring catatonic arousal states in schizophrenic patients (Weizsäcker et al. 1984). Shalev et al. (1987) reported a clear response to lithium by three schizophrenic patients, for whom neuroleptics had to be withdrawn due to severe akathasia. Prakash (1985) describes two cases of schizophrenic patients effectively treated with lithium where its withdrawal resulted in psychotic relapses.

From some publications, one gets the impression that, in contrast to common belief, the existence of affective symptoms might not be conditional for a positive response to lithium treatment in schizophrenics. Donaldson et al. (1983), who reviewed the more recent literature on this issue, also hold this point of view, which, however, has been contradicted by others (for review, see Taylor 1986). It is mostly argued in this respect that despite the use of modern diagnostic criteria, such as DSM-III, some studies may suffer from severely biased diagnoses and thus include patients with affective disorders.

In our opinion, there is no way out of this rather obscure area at present other than, on the one hand, to do sufficiently large well-controlled comparative studies on various psychotropic agents using polydiagnostic instruments and a clear separation of affective and psychotic features. On the other hand, the action and the specificity of the mental effects of lithium must be further elucidated, such as effects on mood, aggression, cognition, and perception. Lithium responders and nonresponders among various psychiatric diagnoses must be exactly described concerning psychological, physiological, and biological (including genetic) variables.

In this paper we first discuss the available evidence for acute therapeutic effects of lithium in schizoaffective psychoses, based mainly on more recent studies and reviews, and then summarize in more detail the relevant studies on lithium prophylaxis. We will add some results of ongoing retrospective evaluations at the Lithium Clinic of West Berlin.

Acute Treatment

Even when lithium was first used in psychiatry, it was observed by several investigators that lithium was also effective in more or less "atypical" cases of affective disorders, and that lithium acted on both affective and schizophrenic symptoms (Taylor 1986). The open and controlled clinical studies published up to 1984 have been extensively reviewed by Goodnick and Meltzer (1984), Taylor (1986), and Lenz and Wolf (1986).

Studies in this field can be grouped according to various criteria:

1. Diagnostic criteria (authors, DSM-III, RDC)
2. Study design (open/blind; study drugs administered alone or added to ongoing neuroleptic treatment)
3. Control medication (neuroleptics, placebo)
4. Number of cases ($n > 10$?)

Some studies have included only a very small number of schizoaffective patients; thus, their conclusions can be seen only in the context of other findings.

From the present point of view, it appears most essential that the results obtained in schizoaffective-manic patients can be discriminated from those in schizoaffective-depressive patients.

A comparison of the average rate of acute response to lithium in schizo-affective-manic patients with that in pure manic patients (manic-depressive disorder) shows that the efficacy is nearly equal, i.e., about 80% or 90%, respectively. Various studies also indicate that the efficacy of lithium was greater in schizomanic than in schizophrenic patients. However, the number of schizo-manic patients studied using RDC criteria and comparing lithium with neuro-leptics or placebo in double-blind designs is very small (e.g., Alexander et al. 1979, $n = 3$; Carmen et al. 1981, $n = 5$; Braden et al. 1982, $n = 5$; Garver et al. 1984, $n = 1$). It is suggested from those studies using RDC criteria that overall improvement with lithium is not inferior to that obtained with neuroleptics. It is still difficult to say to what extent psychotic symptoms such as thought dis-orders, hallucinations, or delusions respond to lithium. Its seems that here as well those studies including RDC diagnostics found at least some evidence for antipsychotic effects of lithium. Garver et al. (1984) demonstrated a marked reduction of the Serial New Haven Schizophrenia Index scores in four of 15 patients with schizoaffective mania, schizophreniform disorder, or schizophrenia, who had not shown a corresponding response to placebo. In a more recent in-vestigation on the psychiatric life histories of first-degree family members of lithium-responsive and -nonresponsive psychotic patients the same group of authors found some evidence that familial and genetic factors may be involved in lithium responsiveness, since no case of schizophrenic spectrum diseases was found among the relatives of lithium-responsive patients (Sautter and Garver 1985). Also, the results of the open study by Goodnick and Meltzer (1984) in-dicate effects of lithium on more than just affective symptoms. Interpretation of this study, however, suffers from the fact that only one third of the patients were treated with lithium alone, others with neuroleptics or both drugs combined. The authors declare that "no differences among treatment categories were found for thought disorders, hallucinations, or delusions."

An interesting observation was made by Zemlan et al. (1984b): They dem-onstrated a fast and marked antipsychotic effect in eight of 24 inpatients with "mood-incongruent psychosis" (RDC schizophrenic symptoms) resulting in a 50% improvement within 1 week of lithium treatment, whereas reduction of manic symptoms was less marked and slower in patients with mood-incongruent and mood-congruent (mania) disorders as well.

Recently, favorable effects of lithium were also reported in a group of ten children (6–12 years old) who had a DSM-III diagnosis of manic episodes with psychotic features. Reduction of both manic and psychotic symptoms was observed in all children (Varanka et al. 1988).

Concerning possible acute effects of lithium on patients with schizoaffective-depressive disorder, the data base is even less satisfactory than in the case of schizoaffective-manic disorders. Very few controlled studies exist where the action of lithium on schizoaffective-depressed patients was examined. One can agree with the opinion expressed by Goodnick and Meltzer (1984) and Taylor (1986) that only about one third of these patients appear to benefit from lithium treatment, and that this response rate is about equal to that observed in reliably diagnosed schizophrenic patients.

Lithium Prophylaxis

Although the prophylactic efficacy of lithium in the treatment of schizoaffective disorders has been investigated in a relatively large number of studies, the literature is far from being conclusive. Whereas some authors report an equivalent efficacy of lithium in preventing relapses of schizoaffective disorders, as in classical bipolar disorder, other authors found lithium less effective or scarcely useful. These conflicting results reflect at least partly the discrepancy among the diagnostic criteria used for the selection of schizoaffective patients. Thus, some studies included patients with more prominent schizophrenic features (especially chronic thought disorder and deterioration), whereas other studies involved patients whose symptomatology (mood-incongruent delusions or hallucinations together with a full manic or depressive syndrome and full recovery between the episodes) was closer to the spectrum of affective illness. In view of this heterogeneity of the schizoaffective research population, the incongruent results are not surprising.

Especially in the earlier studies up to 1979, the authors usually used their own clinical experience or only very broadly defined diagnostic criteria. From a clinical-pharmacological point of view, the development of the Research Diagnostic Criteria (Spitzer et al. 1975), which included specific criteria for schizoaffective disorder, represented great progress. Through the use of operational criteria, it has become much easier to compare the results of treatment studies and to single out which groups of patients benefit from lithium treatment. Here we briefly review studies including a sufficiently large number of patients, which compare the prophylactic efficacy of lithium in schizoaffective and pure affective disorders (Table 1).

Angst et al. (1970) reported a significant decrease in the frequency of episodes and in the number of hospital admissions of schizoaffective patients during long-term lithium treatment. Nevertheless, the reduction of relapses was less marked than in pure affective disorder. In a study involving patients with chronic thought disorder and deterioration, Hofmann et al. (1970) found lithium prophylaxis better in bipolar than in schizoaffective disorder. In contrast to these results, Smulevitch et al. (1974) – in a comparative study of schizoaffective and affective disorder – found lithium equally effective in both diagnostic groups.

Perris (1978) found lithium to reduce the morbidity of patients with cycloid psychosis. In 1983, Perris and Smigan were able to reproduce this result for cycloid psychosis, but they found lithium scarcely useful for a group of schizoaffective patients who never recovered from their first episode.

Tress and Haag (1979) report a similar reduction in the frequency of relapses for both diagnostic groups.

Table 1. Studies without operational diagnostic criteria

Author	No. of patients	Diagnostic criteria	Response criteria	Study design	Duration	Outcome
Hofmann et al. (1970)	19 SA 46 Bi 54 D	Authors'	Authors'	Open	Mean 19.6 months	At least moderate prevention: Bi 72% SA 53% D 80%
Angst et al. (1970)	72 SA 114 Bi 58 D	Authors' WHO	Hospital admissions, frequency of episodes	Open	1–4 years	Decrease in frequency of episodes: Bi 67% SA 49% D 57%
Smulevitch et al. (1974)	50 Bi 49 SA	WHO DSM-II	Authors'	Open	1–3 years	Effective: Bi 88% SA 83%
Perris (1978)	18 Cy	Authors' (cycloid psychosis)	Number of episodes, total morbidity, time in hospital	Open	1–8.5 years	Significant reduction of episodes, total morbidity, and time in hospital
Tress and Haag (1979)	22 SA 21 Bi	Authors' (Kurt Schneider)	Hospital admissions	Open	2–3 years	Reduction in hospital admissions: Bi 59% SA 73%
Perris and Smigan (1983)	41 Cy 15 SA	Authors' (cycloid psychosis)	Number of episodes, total morbidity, time in hospital	Open	1–16 years	Significant effect in cycloid but not in schizoaffective patients

SA, schizoaffective patients; Bi, bipolar patients; D, monopolar depressive patients; Cy, cycloid patients; n.s., not significant.

Taking all early studies together, they indicate that schizoaffective patients generally benefit from long-term lithium treatment, but in comparison with typical affective patients, lithium prophylaxis appeared to be less effective.

In the past decade, research in this area has focused on the use of clearly defined operational diagnostic criteria in order to make outcome results more comparable, and to single out subgroups of schizoaffective patients who are good lithium responders. In the DSM-III manual, schizoaffective disorder is treated as a residual group, and no operational criteria are given for it. In contrast to DSM-III, the RDC include specific criteria for schizoaffective disorder and for subtyping into "schizomanic" or "schizodepressive," and into "mainly affective" or "mainly schizophrenic." The use of operational diagnostic criteria allows one to separate lithium-responsive and lithium-nonresponsive schizoaffective patients (Table 2).

Rosenthal et al. (1980) compared the probability of nonrelapse in bipolar and schizoaffective patients who fulfilled the RDC. The schizoaffective patients showed psychotic symptoms during manic or depressive episodes and full recovery between the episodes. After 2 years of lithium prophylaxis, there was no significant differences between the two groups concerning drug response.

In a study of the mirror type, Küfferle and Lenz (1983) used a polydiagnostic approach to describe a schizoaffective research population. They found that a group of patients with schizophrenic axial symptoms, such as specific thought disorder, failed to respond, whereas patients without these features showed a significant reduction in episodes of illness and in hospital admissions during lithium treatment.

Similarly, Maj (1984) applied different diagnostic criteria to the same group of patients fulfilling the broad ICD-9 definition of schizophrenic psychosis, schizoaffective type. In the whole group of patients, a significant reduction in the number of episodes and the total morbidity was found. Especially in patients with psychotic symptoms together with a "full" affective syndrome or with previous manic or schizomanic episodes (according to the RDC) and in cycloid psychoses, lithium was highly effective, whereas schizoaffectives with prominent schizophrenic symptoms did not respond satisfactorily.

In a prospective study, Maj (1988) recently confirmed these findings. In this open study, a previous bipolar course was the only successful predictor of a positive lithium response, whereas patients with a prominent schizophrenic-like component or unipolar schizodepressive patients did not benefit from lithium treatment.

In a double-blind, random-assignment study, Mattes and Nayak (1984) found fluphenazine significantly more effective than lithium in preventing relapses of schizoaffective disorder. But their patients were chronically ill and fulfilled the RDC criteria for the subtype "mainly schizophrenic" of schizoaffective disorder, which includes core schizophrenic symptoms in the absence of affective features. It might be due to this fact that six of the seven patients in the lithium group suffered relapses during the first year after the start of prophylaxis.

Table 2. Studies using operational diagnostic criteria

Author	No. of patients	Diagnostic criteria	Response criteria	Study design	Duration	Outcome
Rosenthal et al. (1980)	15 SA 27 Bi	RDC	Change in medication	Open	2 years	No relapse in 2 years: SA 49% Bi 55%
Maj (1984)	38 SA	RDC, ICD-9 Kendell's, Welner's Perris'	Number of episodes, total morbidity	Open	2 years	Significant reduction of episodes and significant decrease in total morbidity
Küfferle and Lenz (1983)	68 SA	RDC, ICD-9 DSM-III, authors'	Number of episodes, hospital admissions	Open	Mean 5.1 years	Significant decrease in number of episodes and hospital admissions
Mattes and Nayak (1984)	14 SA	RDC	Number of relapsed patients	Double-blind, controlled Li/Flu	1 year	Patients who relapsed during treatment with Li: 86%, with Flu: 14%
Maj (1988)	62 SA	RDC, ICD-9 Kendell's, Welner's Perris'	Number of episodes, total morbidity	Open, prospective	2 years	Significant reduction of episodes and significant decrease in total morbidity

SA, schizoaffective patients; Bi, bipolar patients; Li, lithium, Flu, fluphenazine.

Based on these, and the earlier studies, the following major conclusions regarding the efficacy of lithium prophylaxis in schizoaffective disorders can be drawn:

In broadly defined schizoaffective disorders lithium is effective, but relatively less effective than in pure affective disorders. The majority of schizoaffectives with previous manic episodes will respond well to lithium prophylaxis, whereas only some schizodepressives will benefit.

Schizoaffective patients with psychotic symptoms occurring only during a full manic or depressive syndrome and full recovery between the episodes respond equally as well to lithium as bipolar affective patients. Schizoaffectives with interepisodic schizophrenic features like deterioration and specific thought disorders are poor lithium responders.

Results of Lithium Prophylaxis in Schizoaffective Patients of the Berlin Lithium Clinic

To illustrate this mini review of the literature, our findings in 15 schizoaffective patients (ICD-9) receiving long-term lithium prophylaxis will be described briefly. The lithium clinic of Berlin has existed for more than 20 years, and all evaluations were done of patients treated with lithium for at least 3 years. Fourteen of the 15 schizoaffective patients are schizoaffective-manic, i.e., at least one of their preceding episodes fulfilled the corresponding RDC, and 13 had a bipolar course of their illness. In eight patients, the longitudinal pattern of recurrence was clearly polymorphic. All patients were regularly rated by means of the AMP/AMDP system (Arbeitsgemeinschaft für Methodik und Dokumentation in der Psychiatrie 1971; Bobon et al. 1983); thus, 351 AMP documentations were available for them after their initial 3 years of lithium treatment.

Compared with patients with pure affective disorders, they were younger at the onset of lithium treatment and showed a somewhat lower female-to-male ratio (Table 3). The differences are not significant in a one-way factorial analysis. The percentage of total treatment time during which the patients were found to be without even moderate relapses was over 90% in all diagnostic groups (Table 4). The quality of the interepisodic intervals was also comparable, as can be seen from the mean number of AMP symptoms documented during free intervals.

We were particularly interested in seeing whether and to what extent these patients showed typical schizophrenic symptoms under lithium prophylaxis. The "schizophrenic syndrome," according to Woggon and Dittrich (1979), contains 29 items of the AMP system. It turned out that in 82% of the 351 AMP documentations none, and in another 13% just one of these items could be found. Two or more symptoms of the schizophrenic syndrome were found in only 5% of the total sample of AMP documentations.

Even if one considers only those forms which were assessed during a relapse, schizophrenic symptoms are still missing completely in 60% of the corresponding documentations. The most frequent symptoms occurring during interepiso-

Table 3. Age and sex distribution in 15 schizoaffective patients as compared with patients with other diagnoses at the Lithium Clinic, Berlin

	n	Percent female	Age at onset of prophylaxis
Unipolar	17	70.6	47.4 ($\pm$10.1)
Bipolar	59	62.7	42.9 ($\pm$12.7)
Schizoaffective	15	47.1	37.3 ($\pm$11.0)
Total	91	61.5	42.8 ($\pm$12.2)

Table 4. Percentage of cumulated interepisodic intervals related to total treatment time and average frequency of documented AMP symptoms per routine visit in 15 schizoaffective patients as compared with patients with other diagnoses at the Lithium Clinic, Berlin

	Percentage of interepisodic intervals per treatment time	Average frequency of AMP symptoms per checkup
Unipolar	91.3 ($\pm$12.5)	5.55
Bipolar	93.0 ($\pm$9.2)	4.83
Schizoaffective	93.3 ($\pm$6.1)	3.77

dic intervals in these patients were affective rigidity, parathymia, and tension. The amount of additional psychotropic medication administered did not differ in bipolar and schizoaffective patients.

In schizoaffective and bipolar patients, as compared with unipolar patients, the severity of relapses was greater, whereas the number of relapses did not differ among the diagnostic groups.

In summary, the response of these 15 schizoaffective patients to lithium prophylaxis was obviously favorable and did not differ from that of patients with pure bipolar affective disorders. This positive outcome was probably due to an appropriate preselection of the study population.

Conclusions

To conclude from these preliminary findings, we fully agree with the demand for further research as formulated by Goodnick and Meltzer in 1984: "...there is still considerable need for further studies, which include a large series of subjects diagnosed by RDC or other criteria, which provide for the differentiation of different subtypes of schizoaffective disorder. . . . Carbamazepine or L-trypto-phan, with or without lithium, . . . could be useful agents to include in some such studies. Prophylactic studies with lithium, carbamazepine, etc. with a large cohort of schizoaffective depressed and manic patients, studied over a longer period of time and compared with pure bipolar patients, should identify patients who are nonresponders."

It seems fortunate that at present, a large prospective collaborative study (MAP[2]) covering individual observational periods of at least 3 years and including about 350 patients is under way in the Federal Republic of Germany, a study which has been designed exactly according to these criteria. The prophylactic efficacy of lithium and carbamazepine will be compared in schizoaffective and bipolar patients. Preliminary findings can be expected in 1991/1992.

References

Alexander PE, van Kammen DP, Bunney WE (1979) Antipsychotic effects of lithium in schizophrenia. Am J Psychiatry 136:283–287

AMP (Arbeitsgemeinschaft für Methodik und Dokumentation in der Psychiatrie) (1971) Das AMP-System. Manual zur Dokumentation psychiatrischer Befunde. Springer, Berlin Heidelberg New York

Angst J, Weis P, Grof P, Baastrup PC, Schou M (1970) Lithium prophylaxis in recurrent affective disorders. Br J Psychiatry 116:604–614

Bobon D (1983) Foreign adaptations of the AMDP-system. Mod Probl Pharmacopsychiatry 20:19–34

Braden W, Fink EB, Qualls CB, Ho CK, Samuels WO (1982) Lithium and chlorpromazine in psychotic inpatients. Psychiatry Res 7:69–81

Carmen JS, Bigelow LB, Wyatt RJ (1981) Lithium combined with neuroleptics in chronic schizophrenia and schizo-affective patients. J Clin Psychiatry 42:124–128

Delva NJ, Letemendia FJJ (1982) Lithium treatment in schizophrenia and schizo-affective disorders. Br J Psychiatry 141:387–400

Donaldson SR, Gelenberg AJ, Baldessarini RJ (1983) The pharmacologic treatment of schizophrenia: a progress report. Schizophr Bull 9:504–524

Garver DL, Hirschowitz J, Fleishmann R, Djuric PE (1984) Lithium response and psychoses: a double-blind, placebo-controlled study. Psychiatry Res 12:57–68

Goodnick PJ, Meltzer HY (1984) Treatment of schizoaffective disorders. Schizophr Bull 10 (1):30–48

Hofmann G, Kremser M, Katschnig H, Scheiber V (1970) Prophylaktische Lithiumtherapie bei manisch-depressivem Krankheitsgeschehen und bei Legierungspsychosen. Int Pharmacopsychiatry 4:187–193

Kane JM (1988) The role of neuroleptics in manic-depressive illness. J Clin Psychiatry 49 [Suppl]:12–14

Küfferle B, Lenz G (1983) Classification and course of schizo-affective psychoses. Follow-up of patients treated with lithium. Psychiatria Clin 16:169–177

Lenz G, Wolf R (1986) Prophylaxe der schizoaffektiven Psychosen. In: Müller-Oerlinghausen B, Greil W (eds) Die Lithiumtherapie – Nutzen, Risiken, Alternativen. Springer, Berlin Heidelberg New York Tokyo, pp 164–172

Maj M (1984) Effectiveness of lithium prophylaxis is schizoaffective psychoses: application of a polydiagnostic approach. Acta Psychiatr Scand 70:228–234

Maj M (1988) Lithium prophylaxis of schizoaffective disorders: a prospective study. J Affective Disord 14:129–135

Mattes JA, Nayak D (1984) Lithium vs. fluphenazine for prophylaxis in mainly schizophrenic schizo-affectives. Biol Psychiatry 19 (3):445–449

Müller-Oerlinghausen B (1988) Mental functioning. In: Johnson FN (ed) Depression and mania – modern lithium therapy. IRL Press. Oxford, pp 246–252

Nasrallah HA, Churchill CM, Hamdan-Allan GA (1988) Higher frequency of neuroleptic-induced dystonia in mania than in schizophrenia. Am J Psychiatry 145:1455–56

[2] Multicenter Study on Affective Psychoses (study director: Dr. Greil, Munich. Financial support by the Federal Health Ministry for Research and Technology, Bonn).

Perris C (1978) Morbidity – suppressive effect of lithium carbonate in cycloid psychosis. Arch Gen Psychiatry 35:328–331

Perris C, Smigan L (1983) The use of lithium in the long-term morbidity-suppressive treatment of cycloid and schizoaffective psychoses. 7th World Congress of Psychiatry. Pharmaco-psychiatry 3:375–380

Prakash R (1985) Lithium-responsive schizophrenia: case reports. J Clin Psychiatry 46: 141–142

Rosenthal NE, Rosenthal LN, Stallone F, Dunner DL, Fieve RR (1980) Toward the validation of RDC schizoaffective disorder. Arch Gen Psychiatry 37:804–810

Sautter F, Garver D (1985) Familial differences in lithium-responsive vs. lithium nonrespon-sive psychoses. J Psychiatr Res 19:1–8

Shalev A, Hermesh H, Munitz H (1987) Severe akathisia causing neuroleptic failure: an indication for lithium therapy in schizophrenia? Acta Psychiatr Scand 76:715–718

Small JG, Kellams JJ, Milstein V, Moore J (1975) A placebo-controlled study of lithium combined with neuroleptics in chronic schizophrenic patients. Am J Psychiatry 132: 1315–1317

Smulevitch AB, Zavidovskaya GI, Igonin AL, Mikhailova NM (1974) The effectiveness of lithium in affective and schizoaffective psychoses. Br J Psychiatry 125:65–72

Spitzer RL, Endicott J, Robins E (1975) Research diagnostic criteria (RDC) for a selected group of functional disorders, 2nd edn Biometrics Research, New York State Psychiatric Institute, New York

Taylor MA (1986) The validity of schizoaffective disorders: treatment and prevention studies. In: Marneros A, Tsuang MT (eds) Schizoaffective psychoses. Springer, Berlin Heidelberg New York Tokyo, pp 94–114

Tress W, Haag H (1979) Vergleichende Erfahrungen mit der rezidivprophylaktischen Lithium-Langzeitmedikation bei schizoaffektiven Psychosen. Nervenarzt 50:524–526

Varanka TM, Weller RA, Weller EB, Fristad MA (1988) Lithium treatment of manic episodes with psychotic features in prepubertal children. Am J Psychiatry 145:1557–1559

Waddington JL, Youssef HA (1988) Tardive dyskinesia in bipolar affective disorder: aging, cognitive dysfunction, course of illness, and exposure to neuroleptics and lithium. Am J Psychiatry 145:613–616

Weizsäcker M, Wöller W, Tegeler J (1984) Lithium in der Behandlung periodisch auftretender katatoner Erregungszustände bei Schizophrenen. Nervenarzt 55:382–384

Woggon B, Dittrich A (1979) Konstruktion übergeordneter AMP-Skalen: "manisch-depres-sives" und "schizophrenes Syndrom". Int Pharmacopsychiatry 14:325–337

Zemlan FP, Hirschowitz J, Sautter FJ, Garver DL (1984a) Impact of lithium therapy on core psychotic symptoms of schizophrenia. Br J Psychiatry 144:64–69

Zemlan FP, Hirschowitz J, Garver DL (1984b) Mood-incongruent vs. mood-congruent psychosis: differential antipsychotic response to lithium therapy. Psychiatry Res 11: 317–328

Alternatives to Lithium Prophylaxis for Affective and Schizoaffective Disorders

H.M. Emrich[1]

Introduction

Therapeutically, one of the most fruitful discoveries in pharmacopsychiatry was of the prophylactic effect of chronic lithium administration in patients with affective and schizoaffective disorders. Although this therapy represents an important step, several problems remain as yet unresolved: One is the partial or non-response of about 30% of patients with affective psychoses and of about 50% of patients with schizoaffective psychoses; another is the problem of side effects and, resulting from this, noncompliance. For this reason the introduction of the anticonvulsants valproate and carbamazepine for pharmacological treatment of affective disorders was important since these compounds apparently have a lithium-like clinical profile of action. An especially challenging question regarding alternatives to lithium prophylaxis arises because of the relatively low therapeutic efficacy of lithium in schizoaffective psychoses: from a differential-therapeutic perspective, the question of which alternative to lithium may be regarded as a promising candidate in treatment of lithium-resistant schizoaffective psychoses.

Valproate Prophylaxis

Historically, valproate and carbamazepine were developed as mood stabilizers completely independently of each other. The history of valproate as a therapeutic agent in affective disorders goes back to Lambert et al., who, in 1966, described a mood-stabilizing effect of the amidation product of valproate, namely depamide (dipropylacetamide). After the establishment of the γ-amino-butyric acid (GABA) hypothesis of affective disorders, Emrich et al. (1980) characterized valproate firstly as an antimanic compound and, later, as an agent effective prophylactically in manic depression. Long-term prophylactic treatment with valproate (in one case with dipropylacetamide) was given in 12 patients who had not responded appropriately to lithium. Six of them were patients with pure affective psychoses and six suffered from a schizoaffective disorder (for details see Emrich et al. 1985). The clinical course of the patients receiving long-term valproate therapy (mostly in combination with low lithium

---

[1] Max-Planck-Institut für Psychiatrie, Kraepelinstraße 10, 8000 München 40, FRG

Affective and Schizoaffective Disorders
Edited by A. Marneros and M.T. Tsuang
© Springer-Verlag Berlin Heidelberg 1990

dosages) is shown in Table 1, which gives clinical data and the number of relapse of the affective disorder during therapy. The improvement ratio (r) shown in the table is defined as

$$r = \frac{\text{average phase interval (months) after treatment}}{\text{average phase interval (months) before treatment}}$$

$r = 1$ means no effect; $r < 1$ implies deterioration and $r > 1$ implies improvement by a factor of r. Figure 1 shows the phase chart of a patient with an affective psychosis and Fig. 2 the phase chart of a patient with a schizoaffective psychosis.

Table 2 shows the phase intervals prior to treatment with valproate and the relapse-free time during treatment. The difference is highly significant at the 0.5% level. Table 3 compares the results in the six cases with schizoaffective psychoses with those in the six patients with pure affective disorders. As can be seen, the results are better in patients suffering from affective disorders than in those with schizoaffective disorders.

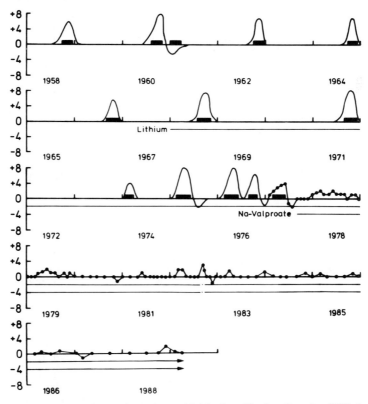

Fig. 1. Time course of the psychopathology of a patient with bipolar affective disorder (ICD-9 296.3) receiving prophylactic long-term medication with valproate combined with low doses of lithium as indicated by the VBS (*Verlaufs-Beurteilungs-Skala*, i.e., "course-assessment scale"; see Emrich et al. 1977). *Symbols:* ■, hospitalization; +8, maximal mania; −8, maximal depression

Table 1. Clinical course of patients receiving long-term valproate/dipropylacetamide therapy

Case	Age (years)	Sex	Diagnosis (ICD-9)	Average interval between phases during the last 5 years before treatment (months)	Duration of therapy (years)	Number of relapses of the affective disorder during therapy	Improvement ratio, r
Valproate (+ low-dosage lithium)							
1	51	m	296.3	9	6.5	0	8.7
2	37	m	295.7	10	6	3[a]	2.4
3	42	m	295.7	5	5.5	0	13.2
4	59	m	296.3	10	4.5	0	5.4
5	36	f	295.7	19	4	2	1.3
6	27	f	295.7	12	4	0	4.0
7	63	f	296.1	7	3.5	0	6.0
8	36	f	296.3	11	1.5[b]	0	1.6
9	28	m	295.7	12	2.5	0	2.5
10	28	m	295.7	15	1.5	0	1.2
11	29	m	296.3	3	2.5	0	10.0
Dipropylacetamide (+ low-dosage lithium)							
12	59	m	296.2	7	4	0	
						$\bar{x}$	6.9 / 5.3
						SD	3.9

[a] Relapses only of schizophrenic symptoms.

[b] Discontinuation of therapy after 1.5 years due to noncompliance.

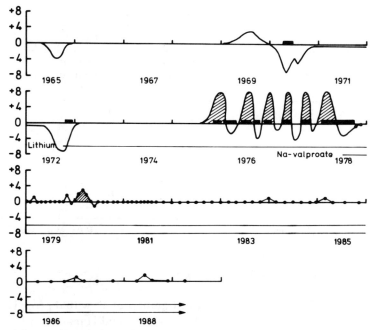

Fig. 2. Time course of the psychopathology of a patient with schizoaffective psychosis (ICD-9 295.7) receiving long-term medication with valproate combined with low doses of lithium. *Symbols* as in Fig. 1. *Hatched areas* represent episodes with admixture of schizophrenic symptoms

Table 2. Statistics (Valproate/dipropylacetamide prophylaxis)

Phase interval prior to treatment (months)	Relapse-free time during treatment (months)
9	78
10	32
5	66
10	54
19	30
12	48
7	42
11	18
12	30
15	18
3	30
7	48
$\bar{x}$ 10.0	41.2
SD 4.3	18.5

$p < 0.005$ (Wilcoxon, 2-tailed).

Table 3. Valproate/dipropylacetamide prophylaxis

ICD 296.1, 296.2, 296.3		ICD 295.7	
Phase interval before treatment (months)	Relapse-free time during treatment (months)	Phase interval before treatment (months)	Relapse-free time during treatment (months)
9	78	10	32
10	54	5	66
7	42	19	30
11	18	12	48
3	30	12	30
7	48	15	18
$\bar{x}$ 7.8	45.0	12.2	37.3
SD 2.9	20.7	4.7	17.0

$p < 0.025$ (Wilcoxon, 2-tailed). $p < 0.03$ (Wilcoxon, 2-tailed).

Carbamazepine Prophylaxis

Independently from the work of Lambert et al. with dipropylacetamide, Okuma et al. (1973), based on work by Takezaki and Hanaoka (1971), investigated the possible prophylactic and acute antimanic effects of carbamazepine in recurrent manic depression. This work has been replicated under double-blind conditions by Post's group at the NIMH (Ballenger and Post 1980) and a great number of studies have in the meantime demonstrated the therapeutic potency of carbamazepine in affective and schizoaffective disorders (for review see Post et al. 1984). A similar study to the above-mentioned study of valproate prophylaxis in problem patients who did not respond sufficiently to lithium has been performed with carbamazepine (Figs. 3, 4). The clinical course of patients receiving long-term carbamazepine prophylaxis (in six patients in combination with low lithium dosages) is shown in Table 4. In this study, which has now lasted 6.5 years, the average improvement ratio reached 4.5. Statistics concerning the phase intervals prior to treatment in comparison to the relapse-free time during treatment are shown in Table 5. A statistically highly significant difference is reached at the 0.5% level.

A comparison between the therapeutic effects of carbamazepine prophylaxis in pure affective disorders and in schizoaffective psychoses is shown in Table 6. In contrast to the findings with valproate, carbamazepine prophylaxis is better in patients with schizoaffective psychoses than in patients suffering from pure affective disorders.

This finding, bearing in mind the study by Dose et al. (1987) which showed that carbamazepine is an effective adjuvant to neuroleptic therapy of schizophrenic psychoses, may indicate that carbamazepine has a slight intrinsic antipsychotic activity.

The present findings are based on a relatively small amount of data. Therefore, no definitive conclusions can be drawn as regards differential therapy. On

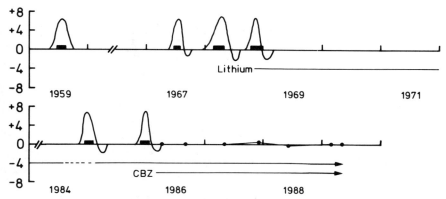

Fig. 3. Time course of the psychopathology of a patient with bipolar affective disorder (ICD-9 296.3) receiving prophylactic long-term medication with carbamazepine (*CBZ*) combined with low doses of lithium. *Symbols* as in Fig. 1.

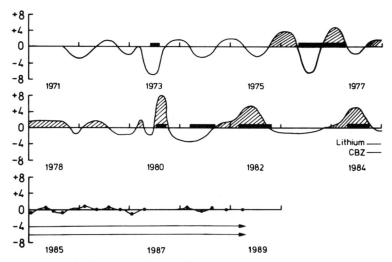

Fig. 4. Time course of the psychopathology of a patient with schizoaffective psychosis (ICD-9 295.7) receiving prophylactic long-term medication with carbamazepine (*CBZ*) combined with low doses of lithium. *Symbols* as in Figs. 1, 2

the other hand, the present findings may be interpreted as a hint indicating that carbamazepine in combination with lithium may be of advantage in the treatment of lithium-resistant cases of schizoaffective psychosis.

Psychopharmacology of Rapid Cycling

Rapid cycling is a rather rare course in patients with bipolar affective disorders. By definition they have four or more affective phases per year. Dunner and

Table 4. Clinical course of patients receiving long-term carbamazepine therapy

Case	Age (years)	Sex	Diagnosis (ICD-9)	Average interval between phases during the last 5 years before treatment (months)	Duration of therapy (years)	Number of relapses of the affective disorder during therapy	Improvement ratio, r
1	38	f	296.2	11	6.5	0[a]	7.1
2	40	f	295.7	17	6	1[a]	1.9
3	49	m	295.7	13	6	0	5.5
4	46	f	295.7	4	5.5	0[a]	16.5
5	47	f	295.7	10	5.5	1	3.3
6	38	f	295.7	16	4.5	0	3.4
7	53	f	296.6	11	4.5	1	3.0
8	40	f	296.3	6	4	8	1.0
9	46	m	296.3	10	5	0	6.0
10	67	f	296.3	6	3	1	3.0
11	62	m	296.3	30	3.5	0	1.4
12	61	f	295.7	27	3.5	0	1.6
							$\bar{x}$ 4.5
							SD 4.2
Rapid cyclers							
1	48	f	296.2	1	5.5	0	66.0
2	23	m	296.3	1	4.5	0	54.0

[a] Withdrawal induced manic phases.

Table 5. Statistics (carbamazepine prophylaxis)

Phase interval prior to treatment (months)	Relapse-free time during treatment (months)
11	78
17	32
13	72
4	66
10	33
16	54
11	33
6	6
10	60
6	18
30	42
27	43
$\bar{x}$ 13.4	44.8
SD 8.1	21.9

$p < 0.005$ (Wilcoxon, 2-tailed).

Table 6. Carbamazepine prophylaxis

ICD 296.2, 296.3, 296.6		ICD 295.7	
Phase interval before treatment (months)	Relapse-free time during treatment (months)	Phase interval before treatment (months)	Relapse-free time during treatment (months)
11	78	17	32
11	33	13	72
6	6	4	66
10	60	10	33
6	18	16	54
30	42	27	43
$\bar{x}$ 12.3	39.5	14.5	50.0
SD 9.0	26.6	7.7	16.8

$p < 0.05$ (Wilcoxon, 2-tailed). $p < 0.03$ (Wilcoxon, 2-tailed).

Fieve (1974) published a selection of 55 bipolar patients of whom 27 did not respond to lithium. The rapid cyclers were disproportionally highly repesented amongst the nonresponders: of 11 rapid cyclers only two responded to lithium. An intraindividual comparison of lithium and placebo in three of these rapid cyclers revealed, however, some improvement on the phase chart with lithium therapy. Analogous findings have been published by Prien et al. (1974) using another method. Recently, Goodnick et al. (1987) demonstrated that rapid cyclers receiving lithium have higher numbers of depressive symptoms per visit, more lithium side effects, more mood shifts, and more manic relapses. Misra and Burns (1977) also observed only partial response to lithium in nine patients with

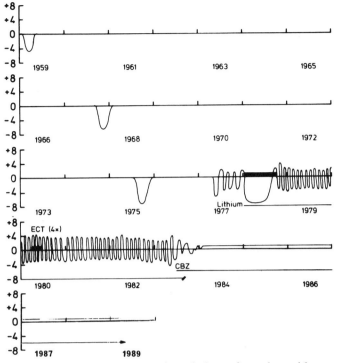

Fig. 5. Time course of the psychopathology of a patient with a rapid cycling bipolar affective disorder (ICD-9 296.2) receiving prophylactic long-term medication with carbamazepine (*CBZ*). *Symbols* as in Fig. 1; *ECT*, electroconvulsive therapy

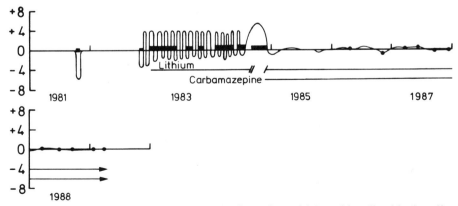

Fig. 6. Time course of the psychopathology of a patient with a rapid cycling bipolar affective disorder (ICD-9 296.3) receiving prophylactic long-term medication with carbamazepine combined with a low dose of lithium. *Symbols* as in Fig. 1

rapid cycling. The question then arises of whether lithium is indicated at all in rapid cycling patients, and what possible alternative therapies there are. This is also underlined by the fact that Baastrup and Schou (1967), in their classical work, described a single nonresponder, who was a rapid cycler, in their first series of lithium patients.

An important factor predisposing to rapid cycling is, apparently, continuous medication with tricyclic antidepressants. Kukopulos et al. (1980) and Wehr and Goodwin (1979) have provided examples in this regard. Wehr and Goodwin, for example, found a reduction of cycle length from about 100 days to about 30 days with tricyclics, which is of great therapeutic importance. Interestingly, however, in a patient with the extremely short regular cycle length of 48 h, Zerssen et al. (1983) observed the opposite, namely an increase of cycle length, using amitryptiline. An explanation of this discrepancy may be that this patient suffered from a unipolar disorder, so there was no chance for the induction of frequent manic episodes.

Anticonvulsants appear to be alternatives to lithium in rapid cycling. In the series of 12 patients treated with valproate, only one patient with a schizoaffective bipolar disorder was a rapid cycler. He has now been stable with valproate therapy (in combination with a low dosage of lithium) for more than 9 years. Similar findings have been reported by McElroy et al. (1988). The greatest experience regarding therapy of rapid cycling has been with carbamazepine. As early as 1973, Okuma et al. published a study of 32 patients of whom 15 were rapid cyclers. Ten of them showed a good or partial response to carbamazepine. Post et al. (1983) described seven rapid cycling patients all of whom responded well to carbamazepine treatment and Strömgren and Boller (1985) described five rapid cyclers, three of whom responded to carbamazepine. Müller-Oerlinghausen (personal communication) treated three rapid cyclers, two of whom responded to carbamazepine. Additionally, my group observed a good carbamazepine response in one rapid cycler (see Fig. 5). Taking these data together, of 31 rapid cycling cases treated with carbamazepine, 23 (i.e., 75%) responded to carbamazepine. Similar data have been accumulated regarding the combination of carbamazepine with lithium. Here, my group observed a response in 1 of 1 case, (see Fig. 6), Shukla et al. (1985) in 4 of 4 cases, Inoue et al. (1981) in 3 of 3 cases, and Nolen (1983) in 4 of 7 cases. In sum, 12 of 16 cases responded to the combination of carbamazepine with lithium, which again amounts to a 75% positive responses.

From this it may be deduced that carbamazepine (in some cases in combination with lithium) apparently has an about 75% success rate in rapid cycling, and valproate also appears to be promising.

Conclusions

The introduction of valproate and carbamazepine as alternatives and/or adjuncts to lithium prophylaxis has broadened the possible therapeutic strategies for prophylactic treatment of affective and schizoaffective disorders. At present, there is no clear indication which types of patient might respond best to which type of medication. Recently, however, Emrich et al. (1988) developed a visual dark-adaptation test which might, in the near future, be useful in predicting the clinical response to lithium. Also, regarding clinical indicators, the present data give some hints that carbamazepine may have a greater therapeutic potential in patients with schizoaffective psychoses than valproate, which is probably devoid of antipsychotic properties.

References

Baastrup PC, Schou M (1967) Lithium as a prophylactic agent. Arch Gen Psychiatry 16: 162–172

Ballenger JC, Post RM (1980) Carbamazepine in manic-depressive illness: a new treatment. Am J Psychiatry 137:782–790

Dose M, Apelt S, Emrich HM (1987) Carbamazepine as adjunct of antipsychotic therapy. Psychiatry Res 22:303–310

Dunner DL, Fieve RR (1974) Clinical factors in lithium carbonate prophylaxis failure. Arch Gen Psychiatry 30:229–233

Emrich HM, Cording C, Pirée S, Kölling A, von Zerssen D, Herz A (1977) Indication of an antipsychotic action of the opiate antagonist naloxone. Pharmacopsychiatry 10:265–270

Emrich HM, von Zerssen D, Kissling W, Möller H-J, Windorfer A (1980) Effect of sodium valproate on mania – The GABA hypothesis of affective disorders. Arch Psychiatr Nervenkr 229:1–16

Emrich HM, Dose M, von Zerssen D (1985) The use of sodium valproate, carbamazepine and oxcarbazepine in patients with affective disorders. J Affective Disord 8:243–250

Emrich HM, Wendl A, Zihl J (1988) Die Wirkung von Lithium auf die Dunkeladaptation. In: Beckmann H, Laux G (eds) Biologische Psychiatrie. Synopsis 1986/87. Springer, Berlin Heidelberg New York, pp 382–384

Goodnick PJ, Fieve RR, Schlegel A, Baxter N (1987) Predictors of interepisode symptoms and relapse in affective disorder patients treatment with lithium carbonate. Am J Psychiatry 144:367–369

Inoue K, Arima S, Tanaka K, Fukui Y, Kato N (1981) A lithium and carbamazepine combination in the treatment of bipolar disorder – a preliminary report. Folia Psychiatr Neurol Jpn 35:465–475

Kukopulos A, Reginaldi D, Laddomada G, Floris G, Serra G, Tondo L (1980) Course of the manic-depressive cycle and changes caused by treatments. Pharmacopsychiatry 13: 156–167

Lambert PA, Carraz G, Borselli S, Carrel S (1966) Action neuropsychotrope d'un nouvel antiépileptique: le Dépamide. Ann Med Psychol (Paris) 1:707–710

McElroy S, Keck PE Jr, Pope HG, Hudson JI (1988) Valproate in the treatment of rapid-cycling bipolar disorder. J Clin Psychopharmacol 8:275–279

Misra PC, Burns BH (1977) "Lithium non-responders" in a lithium clinic. Acta Psychiat Scand 55:32–40

Nolen WA (1983) Carbamazepine, a possible adjunct or alternative to lithium in bipolar disorder. Acta Psychiatr Scand 67:218–225

Okuma T, Kishimoto A, Inoue K, Matsumoto H, Ogura A, Matsushita T, Nakao T, Ogura C (1973) Antimanic and prophylactic effects of carbamazepine (Tegretol) on manic depressive psychosis. A preliminary report. Folia Psychiat Neurol Jpn 27:283–297

Post RM, Uhde TW, Ballenger JC, Squillace KM (1983) Prophylactic efficacy of carbamazepine in manic-depressive illness. Am J Psychiatry 140:1602–1604

Post RM, Uhde TW, Wolff EA (1984) Profile of clinical efficacy and side effects of carbamazepine in psychiatric illness: relationship to blood and CSF levels of carbamazepine and its 10,11-epoxide metabolite. Acta Psychiat Scand 69 (Suppl 313):104–120

Prien RF, Caffey EM Jr, Klett CJ (1974) Factors associated with treatment success in lithium carbonate prophylaxis. Arch Gen Psychiatry 31:189–192

Shukla S, Cook BL, Miller MG (1985) Lithium-carbamazepine versus lithium-neuroleptic prophylaxis in bipolar illness. J Affective Disord 9:219–222

Strömgren LS, Boller S (1985) Carbamazepine in treatment and prophylaxis of manic-depressive disorder. Psychiat Dev 4:349–367

Takezaki H, Hanaoka M (1971) The use of carbamazepine (Tegretol) in the control of manic-depressive psychoses and other manic-depressive states. Clin Psychiatry 13:173–183

Wehr TA, Goodwin FK (1979) Rapid cycling in manic-depressives induced by tricyclic antidepressants. Arch Gen Psychiatry 36:555–559

Zerssen D von, Dirlich G, Fischler M (1983) Influence of an abnormal time routine and therapeutic measures on 48-hour cycles of affective disorders: chronobiological considerations. In: Wehr TA, Goodwin FK (eds) Circadian rhythms in psychiatry. Boxwood, Pacific Grove CA, pp 109–127

The Heterogeneity of Schizoaffective Disorders

M.T. Tsuang[1]

The general assumption has been that schizoaffective disorders are a heterogeneous grouping mainly consisting of affective disorders or schizophrenia.

This assumption has been tested previously by using the sibling pairs method. Out of 71 pairs of siblings who were both hospitalized for psychiatric disorders, 35 pairs were selected after each sibling had been given a blind diagnosis of either schizophrenia or affective disorder by the late Eliot Slater, formerly Director of the MRC Psychiatric Genetics Research Unit at Maudsley Hospital, University of London. Case histories of each of these siblings were subsequently given to George Winokur, Professor and Head, Department of Psychiatry, University of Iowa. He made the diagnosis (schizophrenia, affective disorder, or schizoaffective disorder) of each sibling blindly, without knowing the sibling relationship or the original diagnosis (Tsuang 1979).

The diagnosis of schizoaffective disorder was based on (a) admixtures of schizophrenic and affective features or (b) an affective episode preceded or followed by an episode of concurrent schizophrenic and affective features or an episode with only schizophrenic symptoms. After this blind diagnostic exercise, the siblings were classified into the six possible pair combinations: schizophrenic (ScSc), schizoaffective (SaSa), affective (AdAd), schizophrenic-schizoaffective (ScSa), affective-schizoaffective (AdSa), and schizophrenic-affective (ScAd) disorder. Using these diagnostic pairs, the following two hypotheses were tested: (a) Is schizoaffective disorder genetically independent from schizophrenia and affective disorder? (b) If it is not independent, is schizoaffective disorder a variant of schizophrenia or a variant of affective disorder?

Table 1 shows the number of siblings given the diagnosis of schizophrenia, schizoaffective disorder, and affective disorder. If the assumption is made that each of the three diagnostic categories are independent from one another, the expected number of concordant pairs for each diagnosis can be calculated by dividing the number of siblings in each diagnostic category by half. It can be seen that there are not statistically significant differences between the expected and observed numbers of schizophrenic and affective disorder pairs. However, there is a statistically significant deficit of observed schizoaffective pairs in comparison with the expected number of pairs. This finding suggests that schizoaffective

---

[1] Harvard Schools of Medicine and Public Health, Brockton/West Roxbury, VA Medical Center, 940 Belmont Street, Brockton, MA 02401, USA

Affective and Schizoaffective Disorders
Edited by A. Marneros and M.T. Tsuang
© Springer-Verlag Berlin Heidelberg 1990

disorder may not be a genetically distinct condition, whereas schizophrenia and affective disorder may be genetically independent groups.

The second hypothesis can be tested by using the discordant pairs to see if schizoaffective disorder is a variant of schizophrenia or affective disorder. Table 2 shows the observed number and expected number of ScSa and AdSa discordant pairs. (Since ScAd pairs are not relevant to test this specific hypothesis, they are not used.)

The expected number of discordant pairs can be estimated by calculating the probability of ScSa (p_1) and AdSa (p_2) as shown on the bottom of Table 2. The expected numbers of pairs thus calculated for ScSa and AdSa are very similar to those which were observed. This indicates that all schizoaffective disorders, at least from the familial point of view, should not be considered merely variants of schizophrenia or variants of affective disorder, but that some schizoaffective disorders actually belong to schizophrenia and some belong to affective disorder.

The assumption that schizoaffective disorder is a heterogeneous condition consisting of both a variant of schizophrenia and a variant of affective disorder is supported by the familial data from this sibling pairs study. We should not waste our time arguing whether schizoaffective disorder is affective in nature or schizophrenic in nature but rather spend more time discovering and defining the characteristics which can help both clinicians and researchers further subtype the schizoaffective disorders into the categories of schizophrenia or affective disorder.

Table 1. Overall diagnoses of 70 siblings along with the observed and expected numbers of sibling pairs with like diagnoses

Diagnosis	No. of siblings	Concordant pairs		
		Expected[a]	Observed	
Schizophrenia	17	8.5	5	NS
Schizoaffective disorder	21	10.5	4	($p < 0.05$)
Affective disorder	32	16	11	NS

[a] Assuming genetically distinct disorders.
NS, not significant.

Table 2. Observed and expected numbers of discordant sibling pairs

Discordant sibling pairs[a]	Observed	Expected	
ScSa	5	4.33	NS
AdSa	8	8.67	NS

[a] ScAd not relevant for this analysis.
NS, not significant; ScSa, schizophrenic-schizoaffective disorder; AdSa, affective-schizoaffective disorder; ScAd, schizophrenic-affective disorder; P_1 – probability of ScSa = $(17/70 \times 21/70) \times 2$; P_2 – probability of AdSa = $(32/70 \times 21/70) \times 2$; expected value of ScSa = $[P1/(P_1 + P_2)] \times 13 = 4.33$; expected value of AdSa = $[P_2/(P_1 + P_2)] \times 13 = 8.67$.

Reviewing the available literature, we see some schizoaffective disorders that are similar to affective disorder and some that are similar to schizophrenia from the point of view of premorbid personality traits, precipitants, age of onset, symptomatology, course, response to treatment, outcome, and family data. This may be the result of the different study samples from which the schizoaffective disorder patients were selected. In addition, there are no universally agreed upon diagnostic criteria for schizoaffective disorder, hence, comparison of the results across studies is extremely difficult.

If one uses rather broad criteria for schizoaffective disorder, considering any case of endogenous psychosis with some schizophrenic and some affective features to be a case of schizoaffective disorder, this would result in a very few cases of typical schizophrenia, which have no affective features or in a very few cases of typical affective disorder, which have no schizophrenic features. The distribution of endogenous psychoses could be viewed as continuous, with schizophrenia at one end of the continuum, affective disorder at the other end of the continuum, and the majority of the psychoses in the middle, now classified as schizoaffective disorder. Essentially this would narrow the boundaries of schizophrenia and affective disorder and widen the boundaries of schizoaffective disorder. Consequently the term "schizoaffective disorder" becomes synonymous with "endogenous psychoses" and loses its meaning.

Although the continuous model is a plausible one, the current status of our understanding of major psychoses, from all the available literature, supports the view that they are probably heterogeneous. Unless we can narrowly define the diagnostic criteria of schizoaffective disorder, the boundaries between it and schizophrenia or affective disorder, become hazy and unclear.

Therefore, at this stage in our research on major psychoses, we should first make the effort to classify and schizoaffective disorder as either schizophrenic or affective in nature and only leave those cases which are undifferentiated or mixed to be called schizoaffective disorder. Then, rigorous research on this undifferentiated group should be pursued from biological, clinical, epidemiological and psychosocial points of views.

It is hoped that, out of this research, specific indicators and research criteria for this subgroup can be identified. In this way, further study can be done to validate or refute this nosological entity.

References

Tsuang MT (1979) Schizoaffective disorder: dead or alive? Arch Gen Psychiatry 36:633–634

Schizoaffective Disorders: A Separate Disease?

H. Häfner[1]

In the following I would like to present an impromptu summary of some of the important issues discussed at this most stimulating meeting and to address a number of problems which have remained unresolved even after excellent contributions.

Schizoaffective Disorders as "Cases in Between"

I would like to start by saying that it was very wise of the organizers of our meeting to choose the title "Similarities and differences of affective and schizoaffective disorders". It is a realistic rather than an extremely ambitious issue. They avoided the challenge of venturing into unexplored territories, which would have been implied by a title such as "The nature of schizoaffective disorders". Nevertheless, during our meeting speakers and discussants have repeatedly gone beyond the limitations of comparing symptomatology, course, and genetics of schizoaffective and affective disorders by inquiring into the nature of differences and similarities. This encourages me to ask some further questions.

After two days of excellent papers on schizoaffective psychoses followed by extensive discussions, it seems to me that we have reached our objective. Explicitly or implicity, our considerations have been based on Kraepelin's early dichotomy (1896) of functional psychoses, his division into two clearly discernible disease entities, namely schizophrenia and manic-depressive psychosis. The contestation of this paradigm through Kasanin's "The acute schizoaffective psychoses" (1933) and Schneider's makeshift diagnosis of "mid-cases" or "cases in between" (Marneros 1983) underlay most contributions and discussions at this meeting.

We have come to a straightforward conclusion: no matter which clinical variables we use to identify the cases with clearly defined schizoaffective psychoses, the cases generally occupy an intermediate position between the two great functional psychoses. This is true for the demographic variable, e.g., the distribution of the morbid risk across the sexes, for the age of onset, and for the directly disease-related variables such as symptomatology, course, and outcome. Unexpectedly, it is also true for indirectly disease-related variables such as

Zentralinstitut für Seelische Gesundheit, J 5, Postfach 122120, 6800 Mannheim, FRG

Affective and Schizoaffective Disorders
Edited by A. Marneros and M.T. Tsuang
© Springer-Verlag Berlin Heidelberg 1990

suicide risk or therapy response. Finally, the controlled study of first-degree relatives by Maier and Krause (1989) provided evidence of an intermediate position also in the genetic correlation of schizoaffective psychoses with both the familial risk of schizophrenia and the risk of bipolar affective psychoses. The unipolar major depressive disorders, on the other hand, show no apparent genetic specificity. They rather represent a common familial risk of all functional psychoses. No matter whether by cross-sectional or by longitudinal approach, the schizoaffective psychoses occupy an intermediate position between schizophrenia and bipolar affective disorders. This seems to be a consistent result in all important studies, e.g., Angst (1986), Winokur (1984), Tsuang et al. (1986), Kendell (1986), and Marneros et al. (1986). I do not hesitate to conclude that the metaevaluation of publications, as suggested by Dr. Maier, would merely confirm this result.

What Are the Causes of Schizoaffective Disorders?

The identification of similarities and differences between the schizoaffective syndrome and affective or schizophrenic psychoses is of considerable importance for clinical purposes such as prognosis or therapeutic decisions. All the currently available therapeutic measures do indeed interfere at the level of symptomatology. Nevertheless, and this is my first naive question, what are schizoaffective psychoses really? What does the intermediate position of schizoaffective disorders mean for the etiology of this disease? There are in fact several models of explanation, most of which have been mentioned or discussed during our meeting. I would like to refer to five of these models.

Combination Model

Schizoaffective disorders are the combination of two inherited diseases, schizophrenia and bipolar affective disorders, leading to a phenotype with features of both diseases. If this assumption were true and the genetic combination of both dispositions were purely accidental, then the disease expectancy rate for schizoaffective psychoses should be close to the product of the cumulative lifetime risks for bipolar affective disorder and schizophrenia. If the calculation is based on rates of 0.6%–0.8% for schizophrenia and of only 0.8%–1.6% for bipolar affective psychosis, the result will be a disease expectancy rate for schizoaffective disorders of approximately 1 per 10000. However, the cumulative morbid risk seems to be about ten times higher.

This calculation starts from a possibly incorrect assumption of an almost 100% penetrance of the two genotypes, schizophrenia and bipolar affective disorders. The concordance of the phenotype in monozygotic twins, which is no more than 30%–50% for schizophrenia and 50%–80% for bipolar affective disorders, suggests that there are at least twice as many persons carrying the gene than manifest cases in the population. Consequently, a higher rate of crossbreeds should be expected, which may not necessarily mean that there will also be an increase in the number of phenotypes of schizoaffective disorder. Nevertheless, it should be investigated whether the combination of the two genes increases the penetrance, i.e., the manifestation risk for schizoaffective psychoses.

Another factor which may contribute towards increasing the risk of a genetic combination of bipolar affective disorders and schizophrenia is assortive mating. An increased morbid risk of functional psychoses can be observed not only among the relatives of schizophrenic and manic-depressive individuals, but also among their normal marital partners (Saugstad and Odegaard 1987). This implies that assortive mating may have an enhancing effect on the combination of phenotypic manifest and latent gene carriers for the two major functional psychoses and thus on the morbid risk for schizoaffective disorder.

This combination model is not disqualified by the results of twin, family, and segregation studies. These results show that schizophrenia and schizoaffective disorder – with the exception of unipolar or major depressive disorder – have a clear tendency towards to be passed on within families, thus exhibiting a moderate degree of specificity to the two major functional psychoses (Tsuang et al. 1980; Kringlen 1987). On the other hand, it seems to be established beyond all doubt that the offspring of patients with schizoaffective disorders face a slightly increased risk of schizophrenia and of affective psychoses; this was confirmed by a methodologically sound family study of a large sample of patients with functional psychoses and their first-degree relatives (Maier and Krause 1989).

Kendell (1986) presented an interesting argument, which may bring into question the idea of a combination of schizophrenia and bipolar affective psychoses in the origin of schizoaffective disorders, namely that if schizoaffective patients carry one gene for schizophrenia and an additional one for affective disorders, the outcome of the psychosis must be poorer than in those patients carrying only one gene for either schizophrenia or bipolar affective psychosis, since a second pathogenic gene has a negative effect on the prognosis. This hypothesis may, however, coincide with the possibility that the more favorable tendency for the course and outcome of affective disorders counteracts those of schizophrenia. Blunted affect and deficits in cognitive and social competence may be positively influenced if at the same time affective disorders with severe mood swings are present.

The combination of the two genotypes underlying the schizoaffective psychosis, provided our first hypothesis proves true, does not generally lead to the occurrence of two largely independent phenotypes in the form of schizophrenic and bipolar affective episodes. Rather, the schizoaffective psychosis occurs mainly as a mixed type and is maintained as such with over 60% stability, as demonstrated by Marneros et al. (1986, 1989) in their follow-up study covering an average period of 25 years. The bipolar affective dimorphism of most schizoaffective courses, i.e., the occurrence of episodes of both manic as well as depressive character, is presumably derived from a single genetic subfactor, namely the genotype of bipolar affective psychosis. Whether the mixed type or the combination of the phenotypes of the two major functional psychoses is predominant in the symptomatology of schizoaffective episodes may be determined by the fact that, given a disposition for either of the two disorders, each manifestation of a psychosis triggers the other vulnerability and thus leads to the emergence of episodes with mixed symptomatology.

Continuity Model

The second model is a continuity concept, here called the "green disease" model, with schizophrenia being defined as the blue disease, and bipolar affective disorders as the yellow disease. The schizoaffective symptomatology would then be defined the rich green color obtained by mixing the two primary colors representing the major functional psychoses. This suggests that there is a continuum between unipolar, bipolar, schizoaffective, and schizophrenic psychoses. This model would cover all the gradations of color ranging from yellow through yellow-green and from blue through blue-green to green. There are in fact several such continuity models in opposition to the early Kraepelinian concept of "disease entities" within the group of functional psychoses. Gershon et al. (1982) and Crow (1986), for example, resumed, in slightly different form, Neumann's concept (1859) of a disease entity of the psychosis ("Einheitspsychose").

This leads to my second naive question, namely continuity of what? Should we assume a continuity of the functional psychoses confined to the symptomatology and thus phenotypic and of possibly polygenetic origin, or even a genotypic continuity of whatever definition? These maximum assumptions of continuity are partly contradictory to the above-mentioned moderate genetic specificity of the phenotype schizophrenia and bipolar affective disorder. The assumptions would be well in accordance with the mentioned position in between of the schizoaffective syndromes. The question would still remain open as to where the borderline should be drawn between the continuity model of functional psychoses and the nonpsychotic states on the fringe such as schizophrenia spectrum disorders or mild bipolar and unipolar affective disorders. In order to validate or disprove the phenotypic continuity model, an extensive first-degree relative study or an epidemiological population study is required in which the relevant data of the entire symptomatology and the course of functional psychoses are collected and can then be analyzed according to patterns of dimensional distribution and clustering.

Two-Level Model

The third model discriminate between the genetic level as the cause of the disease and a pathogenetic level which only explains the relatively stable typology of manifestations of the functional psychoses. This two-level model is based on the assumption that there are only a limited number of reaction patterns triggered by heterogeneous causes available to the brain. For the schizophrenic diseases, this hypothesis is to some extent plausible, as the reaction pattern of the schizophrenic psychosis can be triggered on the basis of a genetically mediated vulnerability, e.g., through chronic abuse of certain psychoactive substances such as amphetamines and through a limited number of brain lesions (Häfner 1988). This is also true to a certain extent for the bipolar affective diseases. If this assumption were applicable to all functional psychoses, then the kind of symptomatology or phenotype would be largely determined by the reaction patterns of the brain and would only be precipitated by the direct causes of the disease, including the genotypes. It would then be of secondary importance whether the schizoaffective psychosis is understood from the simultaneous triggering of the two reaction patterns schizophrenia and bipolar affective disorder, or as a reaction pattern of its own kind. Insofar as the two-level model does not attribute any specificity to the etiological level in producing the psychosis, but only in this respect, its plausibility in regard to the relative genetic stability of bipolar affective disorders and schizophrenia is not very great.

Giving some further consideration to the assumption of a continuously distributed morbidity dimension, one usually thinks of a continuous scale of severity or range of symptomatology or impairment. The best known continuity model in psychiatry is that of mental retardation; it is classified according to certain low IQ values, defined as low following the gaussian normal distribution in populations which reaches up to extremely high IQ values. This model can only partly be applied to the functional psychoses. Degree of severity of the disease or of an impairment are not suitable measures for the discrimination of the major functional psychoses. As a consequence, specific continuity models are presently preferred. Moreover, according to the findings of twin and family studies published so far, continuous dimensions of manifest psychopathology, as proposed by Kretschmer (1921) or Meehl (1962), seem to be rather unlikely. Vulnerability models such as latent trait models are, therefore, better suited to epidemiological and related data than are dimensions of manifest symptomatology (Häfner 1990). However, they have not yet been sufficiently validated.

In this context Propping's paper should be recalled, in which he demonstrated that between gene expression on the one hand and psychopathological processes on the other hand, there is a whole series of largely unknown neurochemical and pathophysiological processes. These can produce a varying but never infinite number of phenotypes. One example studied by Propping himself is metachromatic leukodystrophy, which is due to a hereditary deficiency of arylsulfatase A. It can lead to a comparatively wide range of mental disturbances, from mild personality disorders to the relatively rare clearly schizophrenic episode. But if we start out from the phenotypes and inquire into the nature or the causes of a disease, the basis is again ambiguous. Before any biological links in the chain of connections between psychopathological symptomatology and gene which indicate specific processes or reaction patterns have been identified we have to resort exclusively to epidemiological and familial data.

The three models discussed above taking the schizoaffective disorder as the combination of two genotypes, as part of a continuum of functional psychoses, or as the precipitation of two different preformed answers of the brain are at present only more or less plausible models, which have to be further tested.

Schizoaffective Psychosis as a Separate Disorder

A fourth model is based on the assumption that the schizoaffective psychosis is a third, extra disease largely independent of the two major psychoses. The cycloid psychosis theory of Leonhard (1954) and Perris (1986) could be mentioned as an example. In the light of the results of family studies, however, the plausibility of this model is questionable. The respective findings leave no doubt about a genetic overlap, especially in the occurrence of bipolar affective psychoses on the one hand and of schizophrenia on the other hand in the second generation, which cannot be purely accidental.

Moderator Model

The fifth model of explanation assumes that the majority of schizoaffective disorders are derived from a schizophrenic genotype, whereas their symptomatology and course are modified by the more intense affective reactions or mood anomalies. This is based on the observation that course and outcome of schizophrenic disorders are dependent upon several extrinsic or intrinsic moderating factors. In the normal psychological environment, a strong emotive or dynamic component of behavior is a positive predictor for similar behavior in the future.

Hence, it may be inferred that a very weak premorbid emotive and activity component in a person can, in the case of a schizophrenic disease, increase the risk of emotional, cognitive, and social deficits. A high intrinsic level of activity and affectivity, however, could reduce the risk of affective blunting and other negative symptoms. This would imply that types of schizophrenia with a strong affective component, such as the schizoaffective psychoses at the extreme end, would have a more favorable prognosis than nonaffective types of schizophrenia.

There are indeed arguments supporting this assumption, for example the correlation between a high measure of affective symptomatology and a favorable prognosis in schizophrenia. In their dimensional concept of functional psychoses, Berner and Lenz (1986) therefore hold that if at the same time a "bipolar axial syndrome" is present, or, in quantitative terms, high values on the bipolar affective axis, this will significantly improve the prognosis of a schizophrenia with respect to the development of deficits.

Nonetheless, I do have some doubts concerning the plausibility of this moderator model. It is one-sided as it classifies the schizoaffective psychoses mainly under schizophrenia from a genetic point of view and thus runs contrary to the repeatedly mentioned findings of genetic family and kinship studies. The polar position and the assumption of negative influences of schizophrenic or of mood incongruent traits (Winokur 1986; Tsuang 1986) on the course of bipolar affective psychoses is at present mainly speculative. In this context it should be remembered that in their longitudinal course study, Marneros et al. (1986) found simple affective symptoms to have no significant influence on outcome measures in schizoaffective psychoses. However, the issue of a moderating influence of affectivity on the course of functional psychoses, especially schizophrenia, has not yet been finally settled. It is merely inadequate in demonstrating why the schizoaffective psychoses clearly occupy a position in between the two major functional psychoses and thus probably also in explaining their true nature.

Genetic Factors

Finally, I would like to draw some preliminary conclusions. In Propping's contribution, the author pointed out that we have to differentiate between various levels of etiology; the level of direct gene expression in the form of transcription and translation processes is connected with the final reaction pattern of psychosis only through numerous intermediate links comprising a still unknwon number of variations of the same etiology. The correlation of the two levels does not seem to be purely accidental in the two major psychoses. The dimension of genetic specificity is reflected by the 30%–50% concordance of monozygotic twins in schizophrenia and 50%–80% concordance in bipolar affective disorders. In addition, there is a spectrum of unspecific patterns of disturbances, obviously expressions of the same genotype, which have yet to be studied more extensively by epidemiologists.

Only part of these disturbance patterns show features resembling the two psychoses and can thus be classified under the so-called spectrum disorders. The complex interaction of neurochemical and pathophysiological processes linking gene expression and psychopathology is still largely unknown. For our under-standing of the nature of functional psychoses and for the development of causal therapies, it is essential to learn more about it.

Leaving aside this issue for the time being, I would like to focus once again on the findings of twin and family studies and point out that part of the geno-types of both functional psychoses develop patterns of disturbances reaching from relatively specific, non-psychotic to apprently totally unspecific patterns. This suggests that the psychosis itself is presumably the extreme "negative" phenotypic end of this genotypic dimension of morbidity. The more restrictive the definition of the psychosis, the smaller the part cut off from the morbidity dimensions of schizophrenia, bipolar affective psychoses, and schizoaffective psychoses. Therefore, we must be aware that restrictive diagnostic definitions will lead not only to the exclusion of disturbance patterns from the disease concept, but also of an unknown number of cases with the same genotype. If, on the other hand, schizophrenia and bipolar affective disorders represent the ex-treme ends of two morbidity dimensions extending to milder patterns with less specific disturbances, this will again support the plausibility of the combination model in explaining the position "in-between" the schizoaffective psychoses.

However, schizophrenia is presumably not only the characteristic phenotype of an underlying genotype, but a comparatively stable uniform pattern of reactions (Häfner 1987), a "final common pathway" (Lewis et al. 1987) of the brain, possibly in response to specific genetic causes but also to less specific exogenous causes.

This leads to my last naive question. I am astonished it has not been asked and answered more often in the history of our discipline, namely how many such stable reaction patterns or final common pathways are available in our brain? These patterns include among others mental retardation, which has already been mentioned as an example of dimensional psychopathology, which is defined as a pattern of cognitive deficits, graded according to severity and represents a fairly uniform pattern of reactions to a multitude of heterogeneous causes. Epileptic phenomena are also included among these stable reaction patterns of the brain as are the exogenous reaction types described by Karl Bonhoeffer (1917). The latter and the symptomatic psychoses are preformed reaction patterns triggered by different kinds of exogenous functional impairments of the brain. Surprisingly, various genetic causes can prodcue the same patterns of functional impairment of the brain and of the psychopathology associated with them. There must be an answer to the question why not only a specific genotype but also both genetic and several exogenous causes can initiate or trigger schizophrenia, schizoaffective disorders, and affective disorders.

The question of how many such reaction patterns are available in our brain and which genetic or exogenous causes can trigger them is also directed expressly at genetic research. The functional structure of the brain is most likely to be as genetically determined as the genetic keys themselves, which may trigger such preformed dysfunctions or reaction patterns in the brain.

Concluding my remarks, I would like to ask one last question. Almost all our speakers point out that "further research is needed" and we all agreed. However, what kind of research is particularly needed now for elucidating the nature of schizoaffective disorders?

References

Angst J (1980) Verlauf unipolar depressiver, bipolar manisch-depressiver und schizoaffektiver Erkrankungen und Psychosen. Ergebnisse einer prospektiven Studie. Fortschr Neurol Psychiatr 48:3–30

Angst J (1986) The course of schizoaffective disorders. In: Marneros A, Tsuang MT (eds) Schizoaffective psychoses. Springer, Berlin Heidelberg New York Tokyo

Berner P and Lenz G (1986) Definitions of schizoaffective psychosis: Mutual concordance and relationship to schizophrenia and affective disorder. In: Marneros A, Tsuang MT (eds) Schizoaffective psychoses. Springer, Berlin Heidelberg New York Tokyo

Bonhoeffer K (1917) Die exogenen Reaktionstypen. Arch Psychiatr Nervenkr 58:58–70

Crow TJ (1986) The continuum of psychosis and its implications for the structure of the gene. Br J Psychiatry 149:419–429

Gershon ES, Hamovit J, Guroff JJ, et al. (1982) A family study of schizoaffective, bipolar I, bipolar II, unipolar, and normal control probands. Arch Gen Psychiatry 39:1157–1167

Häfner H (1987) Epidemiology of schizophrenia. In: Häfner H. Gattaz WF, Janzarik W (eds) Search for the causes of schizophrenia. Springer, Berlin Heidelberg New York Tokyo, pp 47–74

Häfner H (1988) What is schizophrenia? Changing perspectives in epidemiology. Eur Arch Psychiatry Neurol Sci 238:63–72

Häfner H (1990) New perspectives in the epidemiology of schizophrenia. In: Häfner H, Gattaz WF (eds) Search for the causes of schizophrenia II. Springer, Berlin Heidelberg New York Tokyo

Jablensky A (1986) Epidemiology of schizophrenia: A european perspective. Schiz Bull 12: 52–73

Kasanin J (1933) The acute schizoaffective psychoses. Am J Psychiatry 13:97–126

Kendell RE (1986) The relationship of schizoaffective illnesses to schizophrenic and affective disorders. In: Marneros A, Tsuang MT (eds) Schizoaffective psychoses. Springer, Berlin Heidelberg New York Tokyo

Kendler KS, Hays P (1983) Schizophrenia subdivided by the family history of affective disorder. A comparison of symptomatology and course of illness. Arch Gen Psychiatry 40:951–955

Kraepelin E (1896) Psychiatrie, 5th edn. Barth, Leipzig

Kretschmer E (1921) Körperbau und Charakter. Springer, Berlin

Kringlen E (1987) Contribution of genetic studies on schizophrenia In: Häfner H, Gattaz WF, Janzarik W (eds) Search for the causes of schizophrenia. Springer, Berlin Heidelberg New York Tokyo

Leonhard K (1954) Die zykloiden, meist als Schizophrenien verkannten Psychosen. Psychol Neurol Med Psychol 9:359–373

Lewis SW, Reveley AM, Reveley MA, Chitkara B, Murray RM (1987) The familial/sporadic distinction as a strategy in schizophrenia research. Br. J Psychiatry 151:306–313

Maier W, Krause K (1989) Ergebnisse einer Familienstudie bei affektiven, schizoaffektiven und schizophrenen Erkrankungen. Paper presented at the Seminar on Biological Psychiatry, Oberlech, Austria, 2–8 April 1989

Marneros A (1983) Kurt Schneider's "Zwischen-Fälle", "Mid-cases" or "Cases in between". Psychiatr Clin 16:87–102

Marneros A, Rohde A, Deister A, Risse A (1986) Schizoaffective disorders; The "cases-in-between". In: Marneros A, Tsuang MT (eds) Schizoaffective psychoses. Springer, Berlin Heidelberg New York Tokyo

Marneros A, Deister A, Rohde A, Steinmeyer EM, Jünemann H (1989) Long-term outcome of schizoaffective and schizophrenic disorders: a comparative study. Eur Arch Psychiatr Neurol Sci 238:118–125

Meehl PE (1962) Schizotaxia, schizotypy, schizophrenia. Am Psychol 17:827–838

Neumann H (1859) Lehrbuch der Psychiatrie. Enke, Erlangen

Saugstad LF, Odegaard O (1987) Inbreeding and the epidemiology of schizophrenia. In: Vogel F, Sperling K (eds) Human genetics. Proceedings of the 7th international congress, Berlin, September 1986. Springer, Berlin Heidelberg New York Tokyo, pp 466–473

Schneider K (1973) Klinische Psychopathologie. 10th edn. Thieme, Stuttgart

Tsuang MT, Winokur G, Crowe R (1980) Morbidity risks of schizophrenia and affective disorders among first degree relatives of patients with schizophrenia, mania, depression and surgical conditions. Br J Psychiat 137:497–504

Tsuang MT, Simpson JC, Fleming JA (1986) Diagnostic criteria for subtyping schizoaffective disorder. In: Marneros A, Tsuang MT (eds) Schizoaffective psychoses. Springer, Berlin Heidelberg New York Tokyo

Winokur G (1984) Psychosis in bipolar and unipolar affective illness with special reference to schizoaffective disorder. Br J Psychiatry 145:236–242

Subject Index